Angelina's Shake-a-Stick!
A Grandfather's Immersion into
Autism in America

By John Bryan

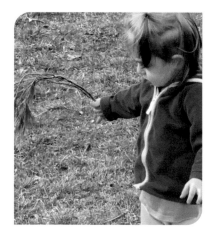

When Angelina started walking I would take her to the park where she always enjoyed finding a stick that she could pick up and shake – back and forth continually. She'd shake her stick happily in spite of her many challenges that began well before birth – more challenges than you can shake a stick at. Angelina demonstrated that her challenges were NOT more than SHE could shake a stick at.

So one day I found my own stick, washed it, sanded it, and painted it with bright colors. And from that point on, whenever I encountered any sort of challenge or situation that appeared to be more than I could shake a stick at, I'd prove that notion wrong by shaking my custom-created stick. I called it, "Angelina's Shake-A-Stick!"

I've made several Angelina's Shake-A-Sticks and have given them to friends – all of whom report that they keep them handy for whenever they face more than they can shake a stick at.

I've learned that in the world of autism, almost everyone has more challenges than they can shake a stick at. That's one reason for the title of this book. The other reason is something that's confirmed to me continually regarding autism's history, its research, its therapies, its controversies, its organizations, its books, etc.: there's far more in autismland than you can shake a stick at. Unless, of course, you have your own Angelina's Shake-A-Stick!

See this book's "One Last Thing" section to learn how to get your own authentic Angelina's Shake-A-Stick!

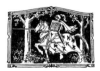

Charles Creek Publishing 2024
www.AngelinasShakeAStick.com

Book Design by ThinkFast LLC

ISBN: 978-0-9656314-2-6

Library of Congress Control Number: 2024908699

First Printing: Fall 2024. Printed in Canada.

Contents

2. YOUR AUTISM FAMILY (cont.)

3. AUTISM INTO AND THROUGH ADULTHOOD — 102

4. THE REAL WORLD — 127

* ANGELINA'S STORY SECTIONS

5. PROFILES BY AND ABOUT AUTISTICS — 147

6. BOOKS, MOVIES, TV SHOWS — 205

7. CONTROVERSIES AND VIEWPOINTS — 221

8. ONLINE RESEARCH AND DISCOVERY — 241

9. GRANDPARENTS — 253

CLOSING THOUGHTS — 277

INDEX — 303

* ANGELINA'S STORY SECTIONS

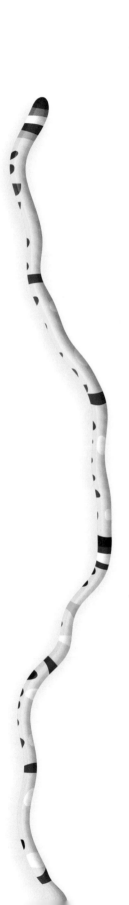

Preliminary Guidance

Dedication

THIS BOOK IS DEDICATED TO TWO AUTISM GRANDPARENTS who, sadly, are no longer with us: Virginia D. Robertson and Alan I. Kirshner. The legacies of Gin and Alan have each had an important and productive impact on my eight-year-old granddaughter, Angelina.

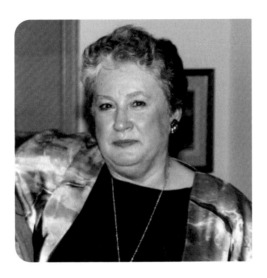
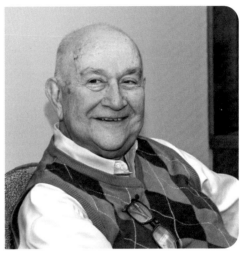

Gin, a loving and caring personal friend, provided my introduction to autism 30 years ago when she introduced me to her five-year-old grandson, Sam Hulcher. Gin was providing supportive and energetic involvement for our city's fledgling Autism Society of Central Virginia, including hosting meetings in her home. Thanks to the early involvement of Gin and others, the ASCV has grown to become a significant provider of services and events that today have a wonderfully productively impact throughout our region. Angelina's life is continually being made better by many of the ASCV's events and services.

I met Alan 23 years ago when he contacted me for assistance in establishing an annual "Art for Autism" event – a gala fundraiser for The Faison Center (named for his autistic granddaughter, Brittany Faison) which, at the time, was a start-up school for a few autistic children. And coincidentally, JC (my wife, artist JC Gilmore-Bryan) was at that time overseeing one of her VCU art classes in painting murals in what was the Center's small facility. Alan's generosity of time, energy, passion, persistence, and money enabled The Faison Center to grow to become a national leader in autism education and service, now providing direct engagement for hundreds of autistic children and adults. Angelina was wonderfully served during her early childhood years at The Faison Center.

It was just prior to Angelina's second birthday when we realized that she was autistic. I quickly called two persons for consultation: Bradford Hulcher (Gin's daughter, an autism trailblazer in Richmond) and Alan Kirshner. Both, although amid busy lives (Bradford an autism mother, and Alan a CEO of a Fortune 500 company) said yes to my requests for in-person meetings. Bradford provided a first-steps plan for Angelina, and Alan provided grandfather-to-grandfather consultation. I continue to be grateful for the benefits that came from those initial meetings.

AND this book is dedicated to autism grandparents everywhere.

It was a pair of wealthy and influential autism grandparents, Bob and Suzanne Wright, who, in 2005, provided the money, energy, relationships, and time that established the organization, Autism Speaks, that, right out of the gate, produced immediate and unimaginable advancement in three key areas: autism awareness, autism research, and autism advocacy. Suddenly, thanks to these grandparents, millions more persons, via the info-rich website and marketing efforts of Autism Speaks, knew about 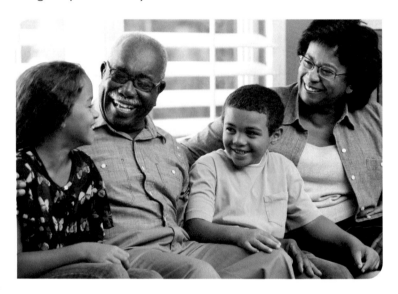 autism. And suddenly, tens of millions more dollars were available for research. And suddenly, via the influence and relationships of the Wrights and Autism Speaks, lawmakers began establishing legislation to fund a significant range of services for autism families, including requiring their insurance companies to pay for many of them.

Since becoming an autism grandparent myself, I have discovered hundreds of autism grandparents who, although not rich and powerful like the Wrights, have loving, helpful, productive, and even heroic roles in the lives of their autistic grandchildren. Autism grandparents throughout America are devoting priority components of their lives making the lives of their grandchildren ever better.

A few years ago, with assistance from key persons from throughout the nation, I conducted a national survey of autism grandparents. It confirmed that they (we) play vital and important roles in the lives of our grandchildren. You'll find the survey's Executive Summary in this book's Appendix.

Special Thanks

NOTE: *This book is a philanthropic project. Neither I nor anyone else who has provided content is paid. All financial proceeds are given to the Autism Society of Central Virginia in its work providing information and services that make lives better in Central Virginia and, via its robust website and virtual services, throughout the nation.*

A lead grant from the E. Rhodes and Leona B. Carpenter Foundation helped launch this book project and meet its goal to provide free copies to each of several nonprofit autism service organizations throughout the nation to support their work making lives better. Appreciation also goes to the Autism Society of Central Virginia for donating its fiscal agency as well as generous consultation and expertise.

I also express appreciation to additional donors whose funding has helped with production costs and donations of free books to families throughout central Virginia: Pam Royall, Jayne and Bobby Ukrop, and Gail and John Jay Schwartz in honor of their grandchildren. Special thanks also to David B. Robinson, CPA, for a variety of assistance including financial support in honor of the 100th birthday of his late mother, Frances Alyn McCrary Robinson, who had heartfelt empathy for all marginalized persons.

I appreciate the Dominion Energy Charitable Foundation's support for the Autism Society of Central Virginia as well as the company's demonstrations of understanding, compassion and respect for autistic persons and their families.

Thanks also to this book's printer, Friesens, a huge, 117-year-old, employee-owned, community-serving printing company that surpassed my best expectations for my last book, and, as I write this, continues to surpass expectations – "based on the philosophy of serving others, fine craftsmanship, and community building."

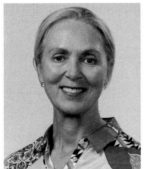
Pam
Royall

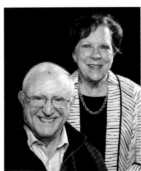
Gail and John
Jay Schwartz

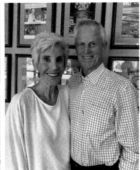
Jayne and
Bobby Ukrop

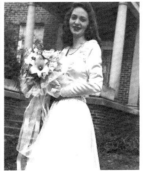
Frances Alyn
McCrary Robinson

My research for this book included a variety of books and other sources as well as informative websites of many respected experts and organizations. You'll see many of them referenced throughout the book. Special thanks goes to those who granted permission to reprint specific passages, and also to persons and organizations that provided writings, photos, and consultation.

<h2 style="text-align:center">They are, in alpha order:</h2>

Autism Society of Greater Akron	Kristin Carleton	Kathy Matthews	James Prosek
Autism Society of Greater Wisconsin	Jennifer Cook	Colleen McCluskey	Wendy Ross
Autism Society of Minnesota	Laurie Cramer	David Minot	Shelley Rotner
Autism Spectrum News	Jules Edwards	Anna Mooney	Andy Shih
	The Faison Center	The Peak	Jane Tobias
Chris Banks	Ann Flippin	Don Morse	Sabra Townsend
Ida Barksdale	Eron Friedlaender	Stuart Neilson	Judith Ursitti
Michael Bishop	Carol Hinch	Jason Nolan	Kellie Vanella
Elizabeth Bonker	Bradford Hulcher	Fred Orelove	Carol Vera Vincent
Virginia Breen	Anita Kelley	Ian Patrick	Olivia Visser
	Joan Babich Lipstock	Rachel Pretlow	Lori Waran
			Patricia Wright

Thanks also to those who provided consultation and services for the 2021 National Autism Grandparents Survey that composes this book's Epilogue.

The engaging visible appearance of this book, inside and out, is the work of designer Will Arnold (ThinkFast LLC), whose smiling professionalism, remarkable work ethic, and sincere enthusiasm have been invaluable to this project.

And finally and especially, I thank my family members: JC for letting me include writings and photos that include her, and for proofing various sections of the book; Thomas for letting me write a special article about him; Kelly and Justen for letting me include writings and images that include them, AND for allowing me to share so much about Angelina; and of course Angelina who brightens lives everywhere, and, as per one of her teachers "is a constant ray of sunshine!"

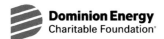 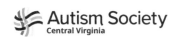 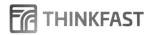

Introduction: My Observations on How to Improve Employment for People on the Autism Spectrum

By Temple Grandin, Ph.D., Professor of Animal Science, Colorado State University

EVERYBODY KNOWS THAT THE STATISTICS ON EMPLOYMENT for people on the autism spectrum are poor. There are two ways that this could be improved. The first is having jobs outside the home before the student graduates from high school and the other is availability of career-related classes such as skilled trades. In my own case, I had no speech until age four and I went onto a good career. I had excellent teachers, a mother who pushed me, and when I was a teenager, I learned how to work. When I was thirteen, my mother got me a job hand sewing for a seamstress. At fifteen I cleaned horse stalls and during college, I had two internships. In the first internship, I was a one-on-one aide for a child with autism. On the second summer internship, I worked in a research lab. For both internships, I lived outside my home in rented accommodations. It is essential for individuals on the spectrum to learn how to do a task on a schedule outside the home.

Successful old undiagnosed individuals on the spectrum in highly skilled jobs – For over 25 years, I worked with skilled metal workers and welders who built projects I had designed. These people are now in their 50's and 70's. Many of these individuals were the problem kid with awkward social skills. A welding class was their ticket to a good career. Today there is a huge shortage of electricians, plumbers, truck mechanics, and welders who can read drawings. These people are now retiring and they are not getting replaced. The young adult with autism who may be playing video games in the basement, might have had a path to a good career if he/she had been introduced to a skilled trade before they graduated from high school.

Today I am doing many speaking engagements. On one day I am doing a cattle industry talk and on another day, an autism talk. Grandparents of

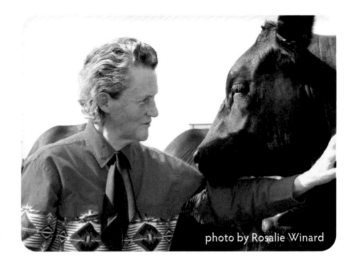

photo by Rosalie Winard

children with autism often come up to me and tell me that they discovered that they are on the autism spectrum after the grandchildren get diagnosed. The grandparents had paper routes when they were kids and they now have a good career in computer science, engineering or a skilled trade. In all these cases, the successful grandparent had learned both life skills such as shopping and they were working way before high school graduation.

What should we do today? There are simple ways that kids on the ASD spectrum can learn both work and social skills. When I was about eight years old, I had to put on good clothes and greet the guests that my parents invited over for dinner. All the kids in my neighborhood were taught to shake hands with the guests when they arrived.

At about age 11 or 12, it is easy to set up jobs outside the home that are on a schedule. Some examples are walking dogs for the neighbors and volunteer jobs at a house of worship or neighborhood center. Every week, the child has to put on their good clothes and pass out programs to the congregation. As soon as they are of legal age, they should get real paying summer jobs.

Some schools are already starting to put skilled trades, such as welding and mechanics, back into their programs. To really get kids interested, tools and making things need to be introduced in Middle School. Skilled trades are not for everybody. Another child may find a career interest by being in the school play or playing in the band.

I get asked all the time, how did you get interested in cattle? I was exposed to livestock when I was 14-15-years old. Students get interested in things they have been exposed to. After exposure, they can discover a career they may like or discover that they hate it.

When I go to autism meetings, I get two reports from parents of young adults. There appears to be two distinct paths. One mom will say I pushed my kid, gave him/her choices and now they are working and loving it. Another sad mom will admit that their kid is in the basement playing video games. There is still hope. Give the individual choices of work options and slowly wean them off video games. If they choose a skilled trade, such as electrician, welding, or mechanic they will have a high paying career, full health benefits, and a computer will not be able to replace their job.

Again, skilled trades are not a good option for everybody. For visual thinkers who are similar to me, a skilled trade is often a good choice. Algebra was impossible for me, but building things was easy. For another individual with a mathematical mind, computer science and programming may be the right choice. I have visited the tech companies in Silicon Valley. It is likely that half the computer programmers are on the autism spectrum. Many of their parents have avoided the labels and their kids are almost apprenticed into coding and programming.

In conclusion, students get interested in things they get exposed to. Interest in science or business can be fostered by having magazines such as *Nature, Science, Business Week, Fortune,* and other business periodicals in the high school library.

__Note from the author:__ I met Dr. Grandin a few years ago when she was a speaker at the Richmond Forum. At the time, Dr. Kathy Matthews and I had begun working on a book that we were calling, Autism in America. *The book was to contain brief profiles of 365 autistic persons – profiles provided by their families. Kathy and I told Dr. Grandin about the book and asked if she would consider writing the book's Introduction. She said yes and provided the Introduction seen here. The book that Kathy and I were attempting didn't progress. Most of the autism families that promised to write profiles for our book didn't follow through. The reason was obvious later, but we hadn't considered it: many autism families face continual 24/7 challenges and thus don't have a lot of "spare" time to write profiles. A year or so after Kathy and I abandoned that book, I began to envision this new version of* Autism in America. *Dr. Grandin's Introduction continues to be so relevant and so important that I am pleased to provide it here.*

Born in 1947, Temple Grandin is arguably the world's most famous and celebrated autistic person. Her career in animal husbandry included her singular innovations and designs that revolutionized cattle handling facilities for ranches, feedlots, and slaughter plants to reduce stress and improve animal welfare. She is a member of the faculty of Colorado State University's College of Agricultural Sciences and is also a frequent presenter and subject of media attention throughout the nation and beyond. She has written several books including, in 1986, Emergence: Labeled Autistic, *which was the first book about autism written by an autistic person. Dr. Grandin discusses her process of "thinking in pictures" in many of her talks and writings including in her 2022 book,* Visual Thinking *(discussed elsewhere in this book). The 2010 film, "Temple Grandin," starring Claire Danes, received seven Primetime Emmy Awards including for best film, best leading actress, and best director. I recommend a visit to Dr. Grandin's website, templegrandin.com, where you'll be fascinated by the six-minute video entitled "About Temple Grandin" in which she shares some of her thoughts about autism. Among the website's other contents is the "Ask Temple!" opportunity to submit a question. (She answers as many as she has time for.) In 2010* Time Magazine *included Temple Grandin in its list of the 100 most influential persons in the world.*

Preface

By Chris Banks

THIS BOOK PROVIDES A FRESH LOOK at the unique, challenging, and beautiful relationship between an autistic young lady and her grandparents. And it is filled with lessons for all in the autism community. We know well that the diagnosis of Autism Spectrum Disorder affects all involved in the life of the autistic individual. In today's American society, grandparents have more involvement than ever with their grandchildren out of both desire and necessity – sometimes not in equal proportions.

John Bryan was introduced to me by Ann Flippin, the Executive Director of the Autism Society of Central Virginia, which is one of the more than 70 affiliates of the Autism Society of America. At the time, John was involved with the affiliate and wanted to conduct a survey on grandparents in the autism community.

Through the survey John conducted in collaboration with Dr. Kathy Matthews, an autism parent with more than 20 years of professional experience, we learn of the need to involve grandparents in the approach to supporting the autistic individual. In the United States, there are approximately 4 million autism grandparents and nearly 80% of them have only a moderate amount of knowledge of autism.

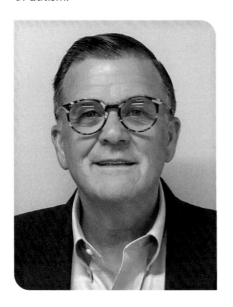

The survey finds that even though the majority of autism grandparents are involved in decision-making regarding therapies, education, etc. for their grandchildren, only 30% of grandparents receive information from the professionals who provide those therapies, education, and other services. The majority of grandparents receive their information about autism from the Internet and from their grandchildren's parents. Although 80% of autism grandparents say they have at least a moderate amount of knowledge about autism and about their own grandchildren's specific cases of autism, they desire to know even more about how to address their grandchildren's specific needs.

This is a glaring gap and yet a tremendous opportunity for the Autism Society and other autism organizations in our local communities. We need and can do more to provide opportunities for grandparents like John to help with more informed decision-making on behalf of their grandchildren as John is doing for his granddaughter.

There appears to be a gap between autism grandparents, who are ready and willing to help, and a clear pathway inviting them and guiding them to a closer connection with the professional service providers.

The Autism Society of America encourages the more robust involvement of grandparents when appropriate for meeting the needs of autistic individuals.

Christopher Banks is President and CEO of the Autism Society (aka Autism Society of America). He has a comprehensive background of serving the nonprofit community and has worked in a variety of organizations including medical centers, community hospitals, assisted living communities, secondary and higher education institutions, human service organizations and more.

Foreword: Autistic Existing

By Jules Edwards

Jules Edwards provided permission to reprint this article that I discovered on the website of the Minnesota Council on Disability, and it's so important, that I told Jules I wanted to position it as the book's Foreword. Jules, as stated on the website of the Autistic Women & Nonbinary Network (awnnetwork.org), "is a neurodivergent Anishinaabe writer, gardener, accountant, and disability justice advocate. She is the parent of neurodivergent Afro Indigenous people, and care provider to many neurodivergent children throughout the years." Jules is the co-author, with Meghan Ashburn, of a book that should be required reading everywhere: I Will Die On This Hill. *(The book is discussed elsewhere in this book.)*

F YOU HAVE NEVER FELT BUBBLES OF HAPPINESS from the depth of your belly, rippling through your entire body until it releases through flapping your hands or jumping in delight, you may not know that being Autistic can be joyful.

You may not know the satisfaction of clicking a fidget, the gentle comfort of pacing and rocking, the sense of fullness from lying under a weighted blanket, the feeling of flying that comes from listening to music panning from one ear to the other with your eyes closed.

The stories we hear about autism are often full of hardship. Stories about parents struggling with their Autistic children, bullied Autistic teens invited to prom by popular students, or adults who have endured a lifetime of barriers and someone shares a viral story about them "overcoming the odds." How would you feel if those stories were told about you from someone else's perspective?

Being Autistic is not all sunshine and rainbows, nor is it doom and gloom.

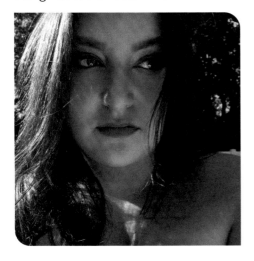

Autism is a social, communication, and sensory disability diagnosed based on observable behavior rather than a person's thoughts, feelings, or experiences.

Autism is a dynamic disability. Autistic people don't always experience the same strengths or support needs at any given time. An Autistic person's support needs fluctuate over time, and every autistic person is different. You may have heard people trying to classify autism with different severity levels or as high/low functioning. Neither of these are useful descriptors.

Often, when people say "severe" or "low functioning autism," they mean an Autistic person with co-occurring disabilities. Common co-occurring disabilities include apraxia of speech (nonspeaking), intellectual disability, learning disabilities, epilepsy, Attention Deficit/Hyperactivity Disorder (ADHD), sleep disorders, and gastrointestinal disorders. Saying someone is "low functioning" is inaccurate and hurtful. People with complex neurodevelopmental disabilities deserve to be accurately identified and supported with respect.

When people say "high functioning autism," they generally mean that a person has fewer visible co-occurring disabilities. In my experience, this view dismisses the perspectives of Autistic people and can invalidate the support needs of Autistic people and deny reasonable accommodations.

Autistic people experience barriers with social interactions, communication, and sensory experiences. All Autistic people should have access to the support we need to live full and self-directed lives.

The people struggling the most to access the support and services are Black Indigenous People of Color (BIPOC) Autistics. The lack of resources and the disparities we face is abhorrent. It begins with inaccurate diagnoses that misidentify Native Autistic children with Fetal Alcohol Spectrum Disorder and Black Autistic children with Emotional Behavioral Disorders. People point fingers at parents and children alike, rather than providing culturally responsive care that seeks to nurture our children and provide the support they need.

Poorly planned and inequitable special education leads our children down the preschool-to-prison pipeline. Fewer than half of disabled Black students graduate high school in my district, and more than half of all disabled Black people in the United States are arrested by age 28.

I am an Ojibwe woman identified as Autistic in adulthood. Statistically, I don't exist. Indigenous Autistic people are counted in such small numbers in data collection that no useful information can be extrapolated. There may be a footnote about the lack of data, but frequently, we're just erased.

Culturally, disability isn't a notable characteristic for Ojibwe people. Native cultures are built on connection, relationships, and caring for others. Disability is a natural part of life that we will all experience at one point or another.

I've met a few Indigenous Autistic women I've felt an instant connection with. One of the first things one said to me was, "I'm thrilled that you exist." And I am thrilled she exists. Being invisible is lonely, and I crave connection and community with other neurodivergent Native women.

I'm the parent of Afro-Indigenous Autistic children. Statistically, they don't exist either. But here they are, living full and authentic lives on their own terms. My children will succeed at exactly what they choose to – with my wholehearted encouragement and support.

Now is the part where I'm supposed to talk about how hard it is to parent disabled kids. But I won't because my kids are fantastic, and I am lucky to be their mother. Parenting my children is not the hard part. Surviving in oppressive systems is the hard part!

You can read more about my perspective on parenting in *I Will Die On This Hill*, a book I co-authored with Meghan Ashburn of Not An Autism Mom (notanautismmom.com).

Happy <u>Send an Autistic Person Crepe Cake</u> Month! (I made it up, tell the others.)

PS – Jules is a member of the Board of Directors of the Autism Women & Nonbinary Network. "The mission of Autistic Women & Nonbinary Network (AWN) is to provide community support, and resources for Autistic women, girls, transfeminine and transmasculine nonbinary people, trans people of all genders, Two Spirit people, and all people of marginalized genders or of no gender. AWN is committed to recognizing and celebrating diversity and the many intersectional experiences in our community."

How to Use and Make Sense of this Book

YOU'LL QUICKLY SEE THAT THIS BOOK IS A HODGEPODGE – just like my personal mission to continually learn as much as I can about autism. I suggest that you use one (or all) of the three following methods to benefit from this book. CONTENTS METHOD – Begin by reading every entry in the Contents section, and mark the parts that interest you. INDEX METHOD – If there are topics that you want to learn about, look for them in the book's Index. BROWSE MEDTHOD – Simply flip through the book and read sections that catch your attention.

What You'll Hate About this Book

NO MATTER WHO YOU ARE, YOU'LL FIND SOMETHING IN THIS BOOK THAT YOU STRONGLY DISAGREE WITH. Fighting words. Why? Because there is an ever-increasing amount of information and research and observations concerning autism, and each seems to be accompanied by strongly held opinions on at least two opposing sides.

Like what? Well, let's start with ABA (Applied Behavior Analysis) therapy – the long-time gold standard of therapies. Years ago, as autism was starting to become more widely recognized and diagnosed, a highly touted research study determined that 40 hours per week of ABA therapy, starting as early as possible (Angelina started at age 2), enables the child to act and behave much more "normally." But now those first ABA-treated children are maturing as adults and a lot of them are saying that ABA caused severe trauma, forced them to act and behave in extremely uncomfortable ways, and robbed them of their true selves. As I write this, the ABA controversy, already hot, is getting hotter. (More about ABA elsewhere in this book. And, by the way, Angelina had a very good experience with ABA.)

Equally heated are the opinions about the nation's biggest and most visible autism organization: Autism Speaks. Critics site Autism Speaks' history of funding research to find a cure for autism. (We of course now know that autism is an innate wiring of the brain; it can't be "cured.") They criticize Autism Speaks' record of research to "fix" children diagnosed with autism – as opposed to celebrating the good things about neurodiversity. But as you'll see, throughout this book I reference excellent resources and guidance that can be found on the website of Autism Speaks. And Andy Shih, the organization's Chief Science Officer, has written an excellent Afterword for this book. I'll leave it to you to determine your own opinion about today's Autism Speaks.

Are you someone who doesn't yet know much about autism? Who doesn't have autism in your family? Or in the families of any of your close friends? Even you will find something to hate in this book. Perhaps it will be my very strong opinion that most of those popular books and movies and television shows that focus on autistic persons are doing a disservice. Why? Because the movie, "Rain Man," is still what the majority of the American public thinks autism is like. Others think that Sheldon ("The Big Bang Theory") is what autism is like. Ditto with "Love on the Spectrum," *The Curious Incident of the Dog in the Night-Time,* and all the others. Here's the fact that everyone should embrace: IF YOU'VE MET ONE PERSON WITH AUTISM YOU'VE MET ONE PERSON WITH AUTISM. And autism's not a linear "spectrum;" it's an every-whichaway starburst!

This book discusses plenty of other fighting-words controversies: vaccinations, facilitated communication, even "Sesame Street's" Julia, and more. Hopefully the stuff you'll like and learn in this book will far outweigh the stuff you'll hate. Just saying.

What's this Book About?

'M AN AUTISM GRANDFATHER WHO HAS BEEN LEARNING AS MUCH AS I CAN since my granddaughter's diagnosis in early 2018. The more I learn about autism, the more I discover there is to learn, and the more I realize that I don't yet know what I don't know. (Read *In A Different Key – The Story of Autism* by John Donvan and Caren Zucker and you'll feel the same.)

Angelina's eight now. She and her mother, Kelly (my and JC's daughter), lived with us for Angelina's first four years. They now live in their own home with Kelly's husband, Justen. JC and I continue to enjoy spending time with Angelina.

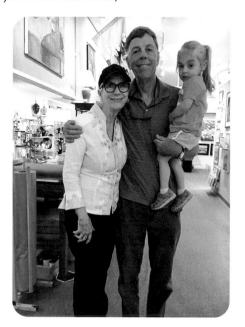

This book is two things. First is its throughline: Angelina's story. And second it's a hodgepodge of my discoveries in autismland – discoveries that are meant to be helpful for autistic persons and their families, for autistic adults, for autism service providers, and for the general public.

The book is an information smorgasbord that's meant to have at least some content that's helpful and interesting for every person: the basics of autism; advice regarding all sorts of challenges such as meltdowns, sleep disorders, eating issues, aggression, etc.; profiles by and about autistic persons; brief reviews of books, movies and television shows; descriptions of a few autism organizations; and even discussion about some of autism's major controversies. You'll see that the book is sprinkled with special content for grandparents; hopefully others will benefit from this special content too. My hope is that this book will give everyone, whether an autism newbie or expert, a bountiful look at autism's joys and challenges.

A Very Brief Message to Autism Families

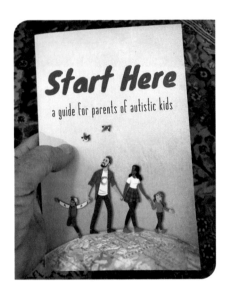

REALIZE THAT YOU'RE LIKELY BUSY WITH 24/7 CHALLENGES, but if you can find the time, and if you haven't yet read it, buy and read the booklet, *Start Here – a guide for parents of autistic kids* (48 pages, $6.99 on Amazon). And, since you're holding this book, read its Contents section; you are almost certain to find topics that can be both helpful and informative for your specific involvements with autism. I, like you, am a member of an autism family. My 39-year-old son is autistic, and my 8-year-old granddaughter who lived with JC and me for her first 4 years is autistic. I of course can't imagine what it's like to walk in YOUR shoes, but I, like you, am walking in the shoes of an autism family. And finally, if your community has a nonprofit autism services organization, join it. There you'll benefit from meeting and knowing other autism families.

A Message to Autistic Adults

YES, I KNOW WHAT YOU MAY BE THINKING: "NOTHING ABOUT US WITHOUT US." I'm not autistic but I've done my best to get a lot of guidance and consultation from autistics. And the book contains articles by and about autistic adults.

While preparing this book I interacted with a variety of autistic adults: verbal and nonverbal, high-support and minimal support, strong advocates and non-advocates. They expressed differing opinions regarding many things concerning autism.

I of course realize that I've spent only a few years thus far learning about autism – and you've lived with autism your entire life. You have my apology for any content in this book that you believe is misguided, ignorant, unkind, or just plain wrong.

But know that I mean well. I will of course never know what it's like to walk in your shoes or live in your brain, but I continue to learn as much as I can from autistics. All of us neurotypicals (or, as per John Elder Robison, "nypicals") need and welcome your patience and understanding.

"Neurotypicals are rubbish at understanding anything that's not neurotypical." – Dialog from the film, "The Reason I Jump"

A Message to Autism Service Providers: Healthcare Workers, Therapists, Teachers, Social Workers, Etc.

JUST ONE WORD: GRANDPARENTS. Many of us grandparents can be helpful. Please be proactive in asking autism parents if the grandparents are willing and able to help. JC and I have been involved with almost all of Angelina's providers since birth, and all have welcomed our involvement and have observed that it has been very helpful. BUT, even though they've been thrilled to have our involvement – zero of them were proactive in asking Kelly and Justen if Angelina has grandparents who can help. Zero. And grandparents from throughout America have told me the same: their involvement is welcomed and helpful, but was not proactively suggested.

In most cases, we grandparents have much more "free" time available than our grandchildren's parents. So put us to work in productive ways.

What can we do? Lots of things. I'll mention five of them. First, we can attend physical and occupational therapy sessions and learn how to do those exercises when our grandchildren are in our care. Second, we can establish a rapport with school teachers so that when our grandchildren are in our care we will know how to be most helpful with homework and how to work with our grandchildren on their weak areas. Third, we can be members of, and have a rapport with, our local nonprofit autism organization so that, when our grandchildren are in our care, we can involve our grandchildren in the organization's events. Fourth, if there are dietary concerns, we can do some of the grocery shopping. And fifth, since parents' schedules are often busier than ours, and since healthcare appointments are so difficult to schedule, let US take our grandchildren to those appointments when the parents' schedules won't allow.

Bottom line: ask parents if there are grandparents who are willing and able to be involved, and then put us to work!

Also, take a look at the National Autism Grandparents Survey in the Appendix of this book.

A Message to Persons Who Don't Know Much About Autism

FIRST OF ALL, YOU <u>SHOULD</u> LEARN A FEW THINGS ABOUT AUTISM. Why? Because it's everywhere: in your neighborhood, in your workplace, in your children's schools, in your friends' families, and on and on. The CDC's most recent ratio for autism prevalence is 1 in 36.

An easy way to start your autism education is to watch the 10-minute, 2009 film, "Autism Reality," by Alex Plank who is an autistic adult. Find it by searching YouTube: "Autism Reality Plank." Next, read two brief sections in this book: "I'm Still Not Good at Explaining What Autism Is," and "Autism 101." After that, just poke around in the book randomly. But DON'T make the mistake of thinking that "Rain Man" or Sheldon or any other autistic persons depicted in popular film and print singularly represent autism. As everyone who knows about autism can attest, "If you've met one person with autism you've met one person with autism."

If you don't have personal involvements with autism, you're likely to say things that are well-meaning but are off-putting to autism families. And you're often at a loss regarding what is good to say. Following are some examples.

Don't ask about or mention vaccinations. This is an extremely contentious issue. Some persons are certain that vaccinations can cause autism. Other persons believe the scientific studies that have shown that there is no relationship between vaccinations and autism.

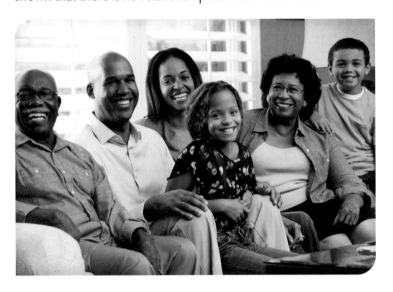

Don't mention Temple Grandin or Rain Man or Sheldon Cooper. Almost everyone who is involved with autism knows who these folks are and they resent those three stereotypes being heralded as any sort of norm for the autism spectrum. (Sort of like expressing your admiration for Louis Armstrong or Joe Louis to a Black person in the 1950s.)

Don't question the diagnosis: "Perhaps it was a misdiagnosis," "He seems so normal; I bet next time he won't receive that diagnosis," "Are you sure he really is autistic?" etc. The diagnosis is personal and is something that the family is already dealing with in their own way in consultation with specialists.

Don't ask the parents "How is [child with autism]?" without also asking about the other siblings. DO ask about all siblings at the same time.

Don't offer autism expertise: "I've heard that . . ." But do offer this: "If you need any research done on resources or anything, I'd be glad to help. I'm really interested in learning more."

Don't mention the family's genetics: "Did either side of the family have autism in it?" This implies blame.

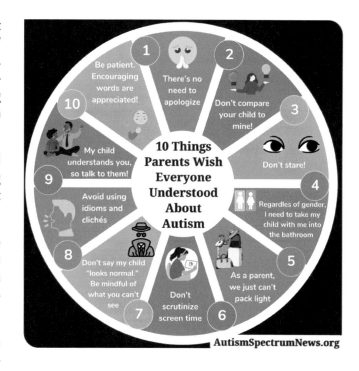

Don't say, "I think I'm a little autistic at times," or "I have sensory issues too," or "I also feel like I don't fit in." This confirms your ignorance of autism and also signals your insensitivity to the autism family.

Don't ask whether the autistic person takes medication. This implies that you think there are negative things for which he <u>should</u> take medication.

When you learn that someone is autistic, DO say things like, "Well that explains a lot about [actions or characteristics of the person with autism]. Thanks so much for sharing this with me."

It's much better to say, "Tell me about autism," rather than pretending to know.

DO say things like, "Would you like to come play with us?" or "Let's schedule a time for us to get together." or "Come join us!"

Don't say, "He's not at all like [another person you know who is autistic]." Autism is complex spectrum; each person is different from all the others.

Don't say things like, "I don't know how you do it," or **"Life doesn't give us anything we can't handle."** The person/family likely already feels the load without you confirming it. They would rather hear things like, "Pick a day next week for me to babysit."

Don't say, "Be sure to take care of YOURSELF." The parent will likely think, "Yeah, right." Or, "Where do you expect me to get the time or energy to take care of myself?"

Don't say things like, "I wish he would calm down," "I wish he would just look me in the eyes," "I wish she would stop that [repetitive motion]" etc. Autistic persons are compelled to display a variety of behaviors that are not "normal" and that often bother or concern other persons. But often such behaviors have beneficial functions for the autistic person.

Don't say, "He must have high-functioning autism." Terms such as "high-functioning" are broad labels and are dismissive of the fact that everyone is different.

Do say, "He's lucky to have you as a parent!" [Or grandparent, or brother, or family member.]

David Minot, founder of the online publication *Autism Spectrum News* (autismspectrumnews.org) provided permission to reprint the chart shown above. *Autism Spectrum News*, written by leading professionals, is a source of evidence-based information including current research, treatments, advocacy, and more – while not promoting unproven and/or unsafe treatments and procedures. "Autism Spectrum News exemplifies leadership in journalism that is vital to advancing acceptance for the Autism community." – Chris Banks, CEO, Autism Society of America.

A Message to Autism Grandparents

I F YOU'RE LIKE ME, YOUR GRANDCHILD WAS YOUR INTRODUCTION TO AUTISM. And, like me, you're continuing to learn as much as you can. This is the book that I wish I'd had when Angelina was diagnosed, and it contains lots of stuff meant specifically for us grandparents. The Contents section will introduce you to the book's wide range of topics, and if you're looking for something specific, you're likely to find its listing in the Index.

If you haven't yet done so, join my favorite Facebook group: Grandparents of Children on the Autism Spectrum. It's hosted by Carol Vera Vincent (2 autistic grandchildren). You'll like her. And every week or so she convenes us for a Zoom meeting: never any agenda, we just talk about whatever's on our minds, grandparent to grandparent to grandparent. (It's so nice to be able to talk with, and get to know, others who have similar joys and challenges.)

And of course, feel free to contact me at any time. (Contact info in the "About the Author" section.)

This Book's *"Grandparent Confidential"* Boxes

SPRINKLED THROUGHOUT THE BOOK YOU'LL SEE LITTLE BOXES containing quotes from real autism grandparents from throughout America. Each quote is a first comment from a grandparent who has just joined the Facebook group, Grandparents of Children on the Autism Spectrum, and/or the Autism Grandparents Club (www.autismgrandparentsclub.com). Hopefully their words will broaden your awareness of the issues, opportunities, and needs that involve autism grandparents. (I've slightly modified the quotations to disguise their identities.)

> ## GRANDPARENT CONFIDENTIAL
>
> *"My 6-year-old granddaughter is autistic, and my 8-year-old granddaughter has ADHD and Sensory Processing Disorder. I've been helping to care for them since birth. Their mother (my daughter) is neurodivergent. What can I do to be most supportive?"*

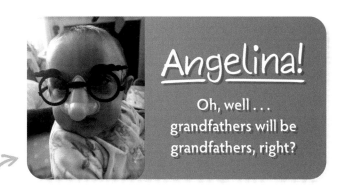

Angelina!
Oh, well . . . grandfathers will be grandfathers, right?

This Book's *"Angelina!"* Boxes

SPRINKLED THROUGHOUT THE BOOK ARE LITTLE BOXES with random photos and info about Angelina. They provide a variety of glimpses into the workings of her remarkable brain.

Angelina's Story: Hard to Predict

KELLY CALLED YESTERDAY AND ASKED IF ANGELINA CAN STAY WITH JC AND ME all day tomorrow. Kelly and Justen both have to work tomorrow from 7am until 7pm. Kelly's a nurse and Justen's a respiratory therapist, both at the same huge urban hospital. I'll get up at 4:30, and later drive to their home to arrive at 6am as they depart for work. I'll awaken Angelina, get her dressed, feed her some breakfast, and then take her to school which starts at 7:20 and is walking distance from their home. JC and I will pick her up when school lets out at 2:10 and then take her to our house. Kelly and Justen will arrive around 7:45pm to take her home.

"Hard to predict" is my and JC's watch-phrase. Kelly and Justen's schedules are continually subject to change and we can't predict when we'll be called on to watch Angelina. Kelly and Justen are always nice and appreciative and even apologetic for late-notice requests. Angelina is always thrilled to be with us – and vice versa!

It's common for autism grandparents to be willing and able to provide both planned and unplanned caretaking for their grandchildren. And I suspect that "hard to predict" is a watch-phrase that's embraced by most members of most autism families – all of whom can likely make use of their own Angelina's Shake-A-Stick!

The Importance of Richmond – The Author's Hometown

THESE DAYS THERE ARE OF COURSE LOTS OF "AUTISM FRIENDLY" COMMUNITIES. JC and I lived in Manhattan for four years. Such mega-populated cities obviously have many more resources than a "middle-market" city like Richmond, Virginia (metropolitan statistical area of 1.4 Million), but mega-populated cities can have mega-populated waitlists for services. We also lived for four years in tiny Ailey, Georgia (population 519, 100 miles from the nearest airport) where the lines weren't long for services, but where services were meager. Richmond's size is perfect in that it is large enough to have great services and small enough to be able to access them. Plus, I can list nine nation's-best superlatives why my city – Richmond – is one of the nation's best cities for autism.

1:   Richmond is the headquarters of the **Autism Society of Central Virginia (ASCV)** which was named the 2022 Affiliate of the Year from among the 70+ local affiliates of the Autism Society of America. Just take a look at the website (ascv.org) and/or become a member and you'll see the wide variety of in-person and virtual ways (many each week) that ASCV serves autistic persons, family members, and the general public. Plus, the website contains a wealth of information that can be helpful for autism families, autism providers, and the general public. And you don't have to live in central Virginia to be an ASCV member! There are plenty of online opportunities – for neurotypicals and autistics – that anyone anywhere can benefit from. For example, last week 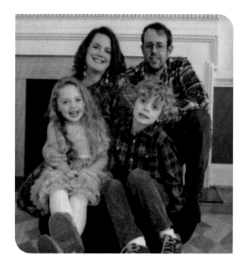 JC and I attended ASCV's Zoom support group for grandparents. We also attended ASCV's online/Zoom presentation of the widely-lauded film, "Life Animated," that included a post-film Zoom discussion with the film's star, Owen Suskind. (Ann Flippin, ASCV's Executive Director, is a friend of Owen and his family.) And of course Angelina LOVES the ASCV's events and activities!

One indicator of a strong nonprofit organization is its Board of Directors. I recently met one of the newest board members when I was one of dozens of volunteers doing autism advocacy with elected officials at the Virginia General Assembly. Her name is Ida Barksdale, and here is the photo and article that ASCV posted on its website to announce her membership on the Board. The Barksdales: Ida and Will, daughter Dylan, and son Nathan.

Ida Barksdale is an autistic advocate who enjoys life with her husband and two kids in Hanover, Virginia. Ida's son Nathan is also autistic and is a regular participant in ASCV programs, especially summer camp, RCIG gymnastics, and bowling. Ida and her family also enjoy attending our member events, and she's a strong champion of the ASCV and our growing programs. Ida is thrilled to join the ASCV in this leadership role, as well as being a liaison and mentor to ASCV's Self-Advocate Council.

Ida is currently a Consulting Engineer at Dominion Energy where she supports their nuclear fleet. She is on the leadership team of the DiverseAbility ERG at Dominion Energy where she is working to build up their self-advocate presence. When Ida is not advocating for neuro-affirming environments for her autistic kiddos or tending to her profession, she can be found knitting, sewing, or at least organizing her craft supplies.

2: **The Faison Center** provides nation-leading educational opportunities for autistic children. A few years ago I had lunch with Dr. Louis Hagopian, Director of the Neurobehavioral Unit at the Kennedy Krieger Institute (affiliate of Johns Hopkins Medicine where Dr. Leo Kanner was the nation's first and leading pioneer in recognizing, naming, and researching autism). I asked Dr. Hagopian

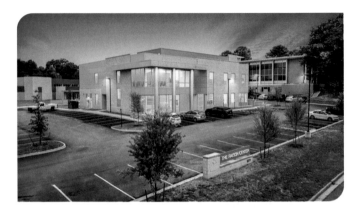

how The Faison Center compares nationally with other educational autism facilities. His response: "There is none better." He went on to punctuate the fact that The Faison Center accepts clients that other facilities probably wouldn't accept. I am of course aware that there are bigger, more prestigious, better-funded, larger-staffed centers elsewhere, and that Dr. Hagopian may say even better things about other centers that he visits, but he DID say that to me about The Faison Center. And as you'll see elsewhere in this book, Angelina's early education included The Faison Center. "At The Faison Center, our mission is to give children and adults with autism and related challenges the best opportunity to improve their life's journey through evidence-based practice. We provide world-class services and programs through our unique lifespan model, which offers enriching opportunities from early diagnosis to adulthood. No matter when our services are needed, we are committed to improving the lives of the individuals we serve."

3: **Virginia Commonwealth University's School of the Arts** is not only the nation's largest art school (nearly 3,000 full-time students), but is also one of the very best (#4 among the 226 art schools ranked by *U.S. News & World Report*), and VCU's School of the Arts was also the school that Qatar enlisted to initiate its "Education City" that now includes Cornell Medical School, Carnegie Mellon University, and six other universities. I was a faculty member and administrator for VCU's School of the Arts for more than 20 years, and I saw first-hand the extraordinary creations of diverse brains that were anything but "typical." A third of the School's graduates stay in Richmond to make their careers – thus the city's bounty of neurodiversity and its multitude of visual, performing, and design arts creators and organizations, all of which not only embrace neurodiversity but also embody it.

4: Search YouTube for "**LIVE ART** Short Film" and you'll see another evidence of Richmond's superlative attention to autism. The six-minute film, First Place Winner of the national PBS Short Film Festival, documents a grand performance in one of Richmond's premiere concert venues, by a multi-dozen cast of neurotypical and neurodivergent high-school-age performers. "Live Art," produced by SPARC (sparcrichmond.org), went on to be an annual performance event that included guest stars such as k.d. lang and Jason Mraz. To repeat: First Place in the whole nation!

(Have tissues handy when you watch the film.)

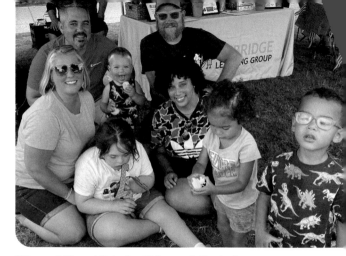

5: Richmond's annual **Festival of Inclusion** (full name: RVA Duck Race and Festival of Inclusion), hosted by the Autism Society of Central Virginia, is a free, sensory-friendly festival designed to include individuals with autism and other developmental disabilities. It includes music, family activities, and thousands of plastic ducks racing down the river. And it takes place downtown on Brown's Island in the James River – named the nation's best urban river by *Outside Magazine.*

(Pictured Above) Enjoying Richmond's Festival of Inclusion on Brown's Island: John Nemetz (red shirt), Neville Morrison (black), Priscilla Nemetz (pink), Chrystal Hall (camo), Kaysen Nemitz (dino), Tonia Nemetz (white), Stella Payne (lavender), and Lincoln Payne (dino, blue glasses).

6: Richmond Raceway is the only one of the 26 **NASCAR** Cup Series tracks whose President is not only an autism parent but who has also made the raceway autism-friendly. (See the article about Lori Waran elsewhere in this book.)

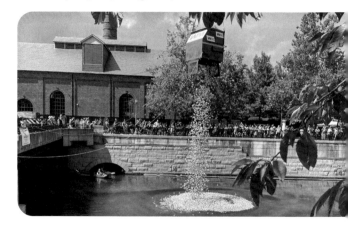

7: Certainly neurodiversity has a lot to do with Richmond's **Martin Agency** more than once being named the nation's best ad agency. It's the creator of those Geico commercials as well as the long-lived "Virginia Is For Lovers" slogan and campaign that is enshrined along the Madison Avenue Advertising Walk of Fame.

8: **GWAR!** Ten years ago I was at a gathering of marketing professionals from throughout the nation, and at one of our informal events we started talking about rock and roll bands: favorite concerts, favorite musicians, etc. At one point someone asked, "Who would get your vote as the most outrageous band of all time?" The unanimous vote: GWAR. (If you're unfamiliar, go to YouTube – but caution, parental guidance is required.) This home-grown band, founded in 1984 and still touring, is a direct product of Richmond's fertile atmosphere for even the most extreme diversity of mind, culture, and even body. You can find GWAR leader Michael Bishop's article elsewhere in this book. (And when

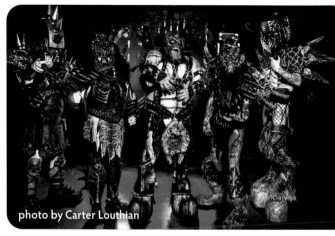

photo by Carter Louthian

you're in Richmond, be sure to eat at the GWARBar – disgusting menu names, but really good food!)

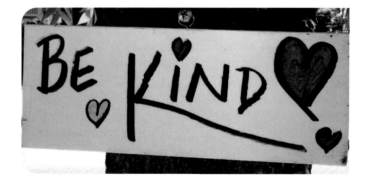

9: Have you seen this **Be Kind sign**? The one with the honest, unsophisticated lettering? The one that appears to be homemade and heartfelt? Well, it is. In 2017 Richmonder Gini Bonnell painted the first sign on a simple, scrap piece of wood and displayed it outside of her house. It was her way of dealing with the increasing onslaught of news about shootings and wars and other toxic things. Her neighbors liked the sign and asked her to make signs for them. And then word and visibility spread, and spread, and spread. To date Gini, along with helpers, has given away more than 100,000 signs. Others, in schools and companies and clubs, have made their own signs similar to the original. As of this writing Gini's "Be Kind" signs are displayed in every state and in dozens of countries, even as far away as Australia. She's been interviewed many times, and one publication quotes her as saying, "It's divine inspiration. I just believe I'm the messenger and this is a message that needs to go out right now." [Note: The Internet has lots of information about Gini Bonnell and her Be Kind sign, and, unlike a bunch of the other Be Kind initiatives that have now sprung up, there is no website and nothing to purchase.]

BONUS: (I'm sure lots of other cities have things like the following.) Angelina's fortunate to live here in Richmond – not only because of the wonderful services of the Autism Society of Central Virginia, but also because of the abundance of autism service companies and organizations – many of which I encountered last weekend at the annual "Disability Expo" presented by the Friendship Circle of Virginia.

"The expo will feature non-profit organizations and businesses that provide services and resources for individuals across the lifespan from infants through senior citizens and their families." The ASCV was there as well as other entities that serve the autism community. I learned about additional services that can be helpful for Angelina.

For example, I talked with an instructor at Humble Haven Yoga – a company that provides yoga for persons with disabilities, and, thanks to JC teaching her, Angelina loves yoga. And the instructor whom I met looked like Wednesday Addams – black outfit, black hair, etc., which is especially appealing given that Angelina dressed up as Wednesday Addams for Halloween.

I talked with lots of other organizations: Children's Assistive Technology Service that provides refurbished assistive devices at no charge; the YMCA's "Miracle League," a baseball league for children "with diverse abilities;" Virginia Career Works that helps ". . . 18-24-year-olds begin their career . . ." and several others.

The Friendship Circle of Virginia was founded in 2012, and "is a 501c3 (81-5132419) non-profit organization that aims to create an inclusive community by facilitating friendships and social opportunities for people with and without disabilities to connect through meaningful social experiences at home and throughout the community. We celebrate the differences and similarities of every person, valuing each of us as an integral part of the community. Friendship Circle was founded on the Jewish principle that every person has a unique purpose in this world that only they can achieve with their specific abilities and challenges. Our role is to create an inclusive community where each soul can shine and truly belongs."

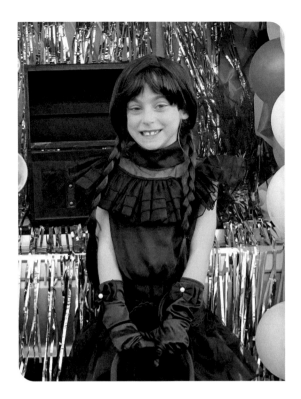

1

The Basics
of Autism

Anna Mooney and the Starburst

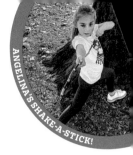
ANGELINA'S SHAKE-A-STICK!

ONE OF THE MOST INSIGHTFUL TAKEAWAYS from Autism Advocacy Day at Virginia's General Assembly was from Anna Mooney, one of the volunteers in my group. Anna had just left a 15-year white-collar position with a major organization. I asked if she was willing to tell me about her departure: basically, the company experienced a deficiency in tailored leadership strategies aimed at optimizing employee performance. Anna stated: "The treatment I received could be characterized by a lack of understanding and support regarding my needs as an autistic individual. Regrettably, leadership frequently deflected responsibility and attributed team challenges solely to my deficits rather than recognizing the need for accommodations and education regarding neurodiversity. This failure to acknowledge and address the unique requirements of autistic individuals was ableist and created an environment of frustration and marginalization, hindering my professional growth. Recognizing the imperative of prioritizing my mental well-being, I made the decision to depart from the organization."

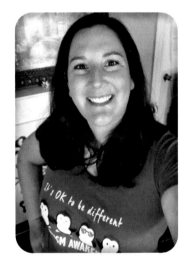

Anna's education includes an MBA, and she describes herself as a *"self-proclaimed autistic data-savant and strong data* systemizer. Experienced in incorporating data analytics with innovation by intuitively figuring out how things work, extracting underlying rules that govern databases, and discovering patterns in unorganized data."

As our group was attempting to provide insight regarding autism to one of our state's legislators, Anna showed him a quickly hand-drawn starburst-looking diagram and explained that autism isn't best described as a linear spectrum but as a starburst – with each of the "bursts" – some small, some large – representing a specific characteristic.

I'd never seen such a diagram and later I had no success with Google. So I e-mailed Anna.

Here is her reply:

"Understanding the history of autism is crucial for comprehending the development of how we perceive the spectrum. Initially misunderstood in the early 1900s when the term was first coined, it took over four decades of research for autism to be officially acknowledged as a distinct condition. The concept of the 'autism spectrum' emerged in the 1970s, introduced by Lorna Wing to encompass the condition's diverse manifestations. By the 2010s, Asperger's Syndrome, an outdated term indicating someone with mild autism, was integrated into the broader autism diagnosis, which came to be portrayed as a linear continuum, delineating varying degrees of severity from mild to severe.

"The linear representation is depicted as a one-dimensional bar, indicating the severity of autism within an individual (ranging from low to high functioning or level 1 to 3 indicating level of support needed or severe to mild). However, this simplistic portrayal fails to encompass all the diverse experiences that define the individual, thereby providing an inaccurate reflection of the autistic person. In recent years, both autistic self-advocates and allies have begun to challenge the linear spectrum model. They advocate for a shift towards a holistic look that better represents the wide range of characteristics observed in autism, which emphasizes the unique strengths and challenges of each individual on the spectrum. The diagrams below are commonly encountered examples.

"The best way I like to describe the diagram is to think of it as a column chart, where each column symbolizes a distinct characteristic arranged around a central point. Below is how I see the transformation.

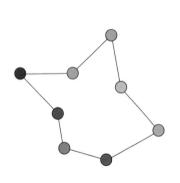

Looks like a Constellation, Polar Chart, or Spider Chart

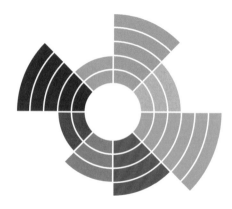

Looks like a Wheel or Starburst

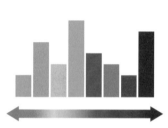

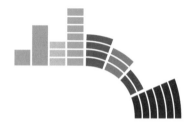

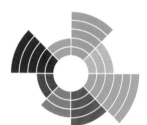

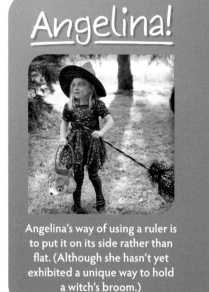
ANGELINA'S SHAKE-A-STICK!

"While some may label the diagram as a pie or starburst chart, observe how each color segment is formed from an equal angle (slice) indicating no segment holds greater weight over another. The outward extending length illustrates the individual's position within each category. Another way to view this is through the constellation, polar, or spider diagram, which serves as an excellent visualization for plotting an individual's placement across the traits. In contrast to the linear spectrum, which emphasizes external factors such as assimilation into the neurotypical world, the newer autism diagrams empower autistic individuals to articulate their own experiences. As a result, no two diagrams will appear identical, nor will they encompass identical categories of characteristics or traits.

"Anyway, these types of images better represent a spectrum, showing the multifaceted complexity that is ASD."

Thanks to Anna Mooney, a "data-savant," Starburst is now my new single-word descriptor for the characteristics of each member of the universe of autistic persons.

I'm Still Not Good at Explaining Autism. Is Anyone?

YESTERDAY ELMER'S SON JOHN CALLED to tell me that Elmer had died in his sleep. He was my 101-year-old friend. Brilliant, thoughtful, clicking on all cylinders mentally, worn out physically. "I don't recommend it," is what he told me last month about being 101. I visited him for a couple of hours every month. We discussed deep issues and solved the world's problems. He was one of those rare friends with whom no topic is off limits and with whom you can be honest.

Although Elmer's career included business involvements all over the world with all sorts of persons, and although he was a voracious reader of important nonfiction books, he apparently never had much opportunity to become acquainted with or knowledgeable about persons with developmental disabilities. He regularly asked about Angelina and I would tell him and he would remain confused about just what autism is. One of his nurses had a Down syndrome son and more than once Elmer would sort of conflate Down syndrome with autism. And no matter how much I told him about autism, he never did get it.

Last week a smart, 70-year-old white-collar professional friend of mine

Angelina!

Angelina's way of using a ruler is to put it on its side rather than flat. (Although she hasn't yet exhibited a unique way to hold a witch's broom.)

asked me about my granddaughter and I told him that she's autistic. His reply: "Isn't that like Down syndrome?" Also last week, a friend told me that her 3-year-old son had just been diagnosed with autism, but her husband, who is a physician, discounted the diagnosis because he thinks that autistic children do things like beating their heads against the wall and their son doesn't.

It continues to amaze me that so many smart, experienced, educated persons – even doctors – know very little about autism. In each case, I try to explain, but I'm still apparently not good at it.

My late friend Phil Meggs, former head of VCU's Department of Communication Arts and Design, continually stressed to me that when communication is not understood, it is always, ALWAYS, the fault of the communicator, not of the person being communicated to. Which confirms that I am still – even now with several years of knowledge and research – unable to explain autism in a way that's understandable. I wonder if this is the nature of autism – that it's simply too jumbled to relegate to a straightforward explanation?

Angelina's Story: Kelly Moves Back Home and is Admitted to the Hospital

A COUPLE OF WEEKS AGO I finally cleaned out all of the stuff in the downstairs bedroom that belonged to Kelly and Angelina and that has been in there ever since they moved to their own place 4 years ago. Their residency here began during Kelly's pregnancy in late 2016 when she moved back home with us – a pregnancy that gradually had more and more warning signs.

The big turning point came on February 12, 2016. I was smack in the middle of hosting and coordinating an important symposium with a couple of hundred attendees, several presenters, and a special out-of-town guest presenter from the Bill and Melinda Gates Foundation. (A result of months' worth of more moving parts than I could shake a stick at – and this was of course prior to me having my own Angelina's Shake-a-Stick.) My mobile phone rang: Kelly had been admitted to the hospital – significant bleeding. Serious. I left someone else in charge of the symposium and drove to the hospital.

Kelly had gotten married a few months prior, and her husband (psychological challenges) had left her shortly after her pregnancy got underway. (She hasn't seen him since; he moved to parts unknown. They divorced and Kelly eventually found Justen, her wonderful new husband and father to Angelina.) Then on February 12 she was admitted to the hospital

Angelina!

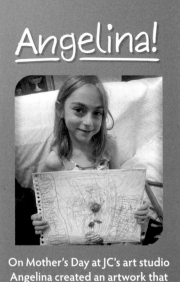

On Mother's Day at JC's art studio Angelina created an artwork that she entitled, "Magic Flowers," and about which she said, "Magical flowers spreading happiness all around, making happiness grow on the planet Earth."

for the duration of her pregnancy, and she was put under the care of a doctor who specializes in high-risk pregnancies. Translation: fingers tightly crossed. JC and I took turns being with Kelly at the hospital each day. We befriended the nurses. We learned where to find the free sandwiches and snacks that our local Ronald McDonald House delivered for family visitors of labor and delivery and pediatric patients. And we discovered all the tricks for finding the best parking spaces – including those adjacent to the helicopter pad. The hospital was Kelly's new home; it was my and JC's second home.

We quickly learned the meaning of 24 weeks: babies born before 24 weeks have almost zero chance of surviving; full-term is 40 weeks. The first goal: make it to 24 weeks. Kelly's bleeding lessened, but the doctor continued to use the term "high risk," with emphasis on "high." They monitored everything constantly: bleeding, amniotic fluid, heartbeat (yes, the machines allowed us to hear the tiny heart.) Even though things continued to look bleak, the doctor never gave up hope. The best she could muster, and with raised eyebrows and a bit of a smile, was, "I've seen worse."

Then one day the nurses came in with a fancy cupcake. It was a celebratory cupcake; the pregnancy had reached 24 weeks. The baby now at least had a chance for survival.

Autism 101

A FEW WEEKS AGO I WATCHED A VIDEO OF A PRESENTATION by Rachel Pretlow (autistic young adult) entitled "Autism 101." You can find lots of information on the Internet entitled "Autism 101," and Rachel's is the best I've experienced thus far. Following are 25 nuggets (in no particular order) from the presentation.

1: Autism is a lifelong developmental disability, a brain difference that affects communication, bodily movements, and senses of the world.

2: Autism is a spectrum disorder. Each person is unique regarding communication, motor skills, executive function, and senses.

3: Autism is found in every ethnicity, every culture, and every socioeconomic demographic.

4: Four times as many boys than girls are autistic.

5: It is very common for Black women to be undiagnosed until later in life.

6: Self-diagnosis is valid; not everyone has money or access for formal diagnosis.

7: Identity-first language (autistic person) is preferred to person-first language (person with autism). (An analogy is that we say Black person rather than person with Blackness.)

8: The sentence, "Everyone is a little autistic," is false. Persons think saying this is empathetic, but it shows ignorance about autism.

9: The sentence, "You don't look autistic," isn't valid. There are no shared physical traits among autistic persons. (Down syndrome, for example, has common physical traits.)

10: Autism traits usually appear before age three.

11: The cause of autism is unknown, but there is a strong correlation with heredity in many cases.

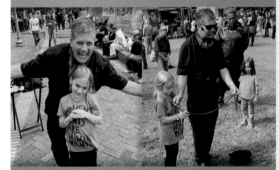

Angelina!

Angelina loves magicians, and her favorite is Jonathan Austin! (But her unconventional brain usually solves MY magic tricks that fool everyone else.)

12: Don't use the term "treatment." It implies a disease or affliction that can be cured. Do use the term, "support services."

13: Many autistic persons crave attention and camaraderie, but when seen playing by themselves, others often assume that they want to be alone. Often this is not the case.

14: A common belief among neurotypical persons is that autistic persons don't have empathy. It is dangerous and unfair to assume that autistics are heartless and don't care about others.

15: It is common for autistic persons to be unable to understand gestures and facial expressions.

16: It is common for autistic persons to have either exaggerated or minimal facial expressions.

17: Eye-to-eye contact is often difficult (sensory overload) for autistic persons.

18: It is common for autistic persons to have difficulty understanding what is not explicit: jokes, sarcasm, small talk, implication, etc.

19: Many autistic persons have a unique tone and rhythm of speaking.

20: One third of autistic persons are either non-verbal or minimally verbal. But many of them can benefit from AAC (augmentative and alternative communication: pointing at letterboards, or using iPads and other high-tech mechanisms).

21: Even among autistic persons who speak well, there are times when they can't speak, and AAC can be very helpful.

CHAPTER I: The Basics of Autism

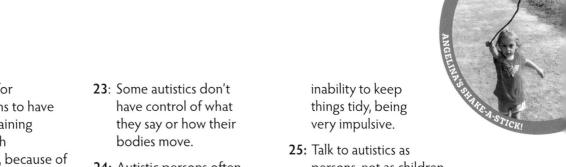

22: It is common for autistic persons to have trouble maintaining back-and-forth conversations, because of unpredictability.

23: Some autistics don't have control of what they say or how their bodies move.

24: Autistic persons often have challenges with executive function: planning and completing tasks, concepts of time, inability to keep things tidy, being very impulsive.

25: Talk to autistics as persons, not as children.

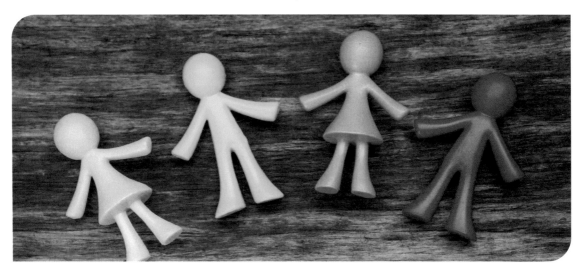

Categories of Autism

T HOSE OF US IN THE AUTISM COMMUNITY OFTEN HEAR THIS QUESTION: "What type of autism?" Formerly used terms such as "high-functioning," "disintegrative disorder," and "pervasive development disorder" are no longer recommended – the reason being that autism is so unique with each individual that it's simply not possible to come up with a descriptive list of three or five or even five hundred specific categories.

Here's an accurate statement: "Autism Spectrum Disorder is an umbrella term for complex neurodevelopmental disorders that affect communication and behavior." Each person with autism is affected differently. Even the often-used adjectives "mild" and "severe" are too loaded with assumptions to be effective.

Each autistic person is probably best "typed" with a couple of sentences that are custom-developed. Here's an attempt at typing Angelina: "Angelina is in regular school, is an active and happy child, and doesn't exhibit any of the more noticeable autism traits such as odd communication, flapping hands, and meltdowns. Her challenges include staying on task, following multi-step instructions, and fine motor skills such as writing. And she approaches a variety of things atypically such as eating bananas from the side and using a white crayon to color on white paper."

When you research autism you find continual references to the American Pediatric Association's 2013 Diagnostic Statistical Manual of Mental Disorders (DSM-5 – meaning this is the fifth and most recent such manual they've issued). The DSM-5 is the most recognized and accepted reference, and it has lumped everyone on the autism spectrum into three categories according to how much support is required.

LEVEL 1	LEVEL 2	LEVEL 3
"Requires Support"	"Requires Substantial Support"	"Requires Very Substantial Support"
These persons may have noticeable differences with verbal and non-verbal communication skills, difficulty changing focus or action, etc.	These persons may exhibit things such as inflexible behaviors, interactions that are limited to narrow special interests, etc.	These persons may be non-verbal, may exhibit great distress when changing focus or action, etc.

Although DSM-5 groups autistics into three giant categories, there are of course millions of "categories," and it's misleading (at best) to relegate any autistic person simply to one of the three.

Profound Autism – 24/7

THE TERM "PROFOUND AUTISM" WAS INTRODUCED BY DR. CATHERINE LORD (UC-LA's Center for Autism Research and Treatment) in September, 2021 at the Autism Science Foundation's "Day of Learning."

The term is offered as a substitute for other terms such as Severe Autism and Level Three Autism. Simply put, profound autism is a condition that usually requires 24/7 care, support, and supervision.

One learning tool is the 2020 book, *WE WALK: Life With Severe Autism*, by Amy S.F. Lutz – mother of a profoundly autistic son. Embraced by glowing reviews, the book's *New York Times* review by Judith Newman, concludes with this: "*WE WALK* clears a path for us toward kindness and understanding."

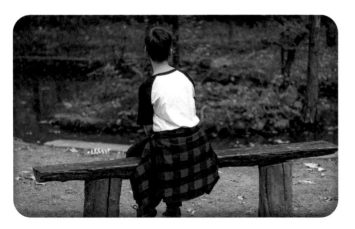

Profound autism often manifests in infancy and becomes more and more noticeable through pre-school. Symptoms can include absence of verbal communication, extreme sensitivity (crowds, lights, noises), low IQ, repetitive behaviors such as violent rocking and door slamming, moaning, sleeplessness, self-injury, hitting, biting, kicking, fecal smearing, wandering, running away, inability to self-soothe or form bonds, inappropriate responses (laughing when someone is hurt), limited eye contact, no acknowledgment of others, blank facial expression, inability to communicate hunger or pain, intense fixations, and on and on . . .

Usually several professionals are needed: pediatrician, occupational therapist, speech therapist, psychologist, psychiatrist (to prescribe medications), behavioral therapist, and perhaps a music or art therapist. All of this is expensive, and often there are intense negotiations with insurance companies regarding who pays how much for what.

Unfortunately, the long-term future for profoundly autistic children isn't usually bright – thus the need for as much therapy and love as possible as early as possible. Hospitals and jails are being used more and more as "residences" for profoundly autistic persons when their behaviors are too severe or dangerous for family members or other caregivers. When social services and other programs fall short, profoundly autistic teens and adults are routinely spending weeks and months restrained, sedated, and/or confined to mesh-tented beds in hospitals nationwide.

"There is no safe place for the client to go," is a recurring lament among public agencies. There are waiting lists everywhere for programs, services, and residences – waiting lists that are growing.

While there is no silver bullet for profound autism, intense therapies sometimes help, and usually the earlier the better.

Masking – Being Someone You're Not

N THE WORLD OF AUTISM, "masking" means making exhausting efforts to act and communicate in ways that appear neurotypical in order to blend into society and meet social norms. Common examples include interactions at social gatherings, discussions at medical or legal appointments, job interviews, and even telephone conversations. Masking is usually difficult and exhausting for autistics and it commonly results in the need for extensive rest or even depression and/or long-term therapy.

All neurotypicals mask. And the reason we've never thought much about masking or even known that there is a name for it is that it's second nature for us. It's easy. It's just something that we do. And there are lots of well-known examples. Take that old Motown song by the Miracles, "The Tracks of my Tears": "Outside I'm masquerading, inside my hope is fading . . ." Or Lou Christie's "Two Faces Have I": " . . . one to laugh and one to cry." Or the famous 1964 "Twilight Zone" episode entitled, "The Masks." Four folks seem likeable, but they are masking their true personalities which are revealed in the episode's climactic ending in which their faces are contorted grotesquely into their true personalities: a sniveling coward, a miser, a brutish buffoon, and a narcissist.

And regarding the daily lives of us neurotypicals, we mask when we have job interviews, when we're dating, when we join groups, when we interact with almost everyone. We wear different masks for different situations: an empathetic mask when we're doing volunteer work, an intelligent mask when we're in a strategic planning session, a "love-the-food" mask when we're at a dinner party, an "I'm-perfect-in-every-way" mask when we're meeting our girlfriends' parents, and a mask of reverence and sadness at funerals.

All of these examples, while second-nature to us neurotypicals, are usually frighteningly and anxiously difficult for autistics.

2

Your Autism Family

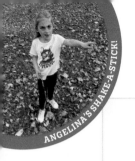

ANGELINA'S SHAKE-A-STICK!

Angelina's Story: Diagnosis

I GUESS IT WAS AT TEN OR ELEVEN MONTHS that I began to notice some "different" things about Angelina, most notable of which were not smiling and not making eye contact. And she didn't babble, much less say a first word. Her developmental pediatrician wasn't concerned. After all, Angelina was born over 3 months early and so at 12 months old, her "real" age was only 9 months.

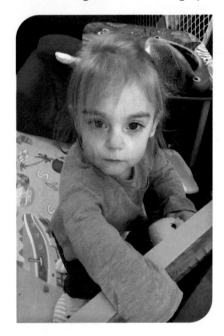

Speaking of developmental pediatricians, I've learned that not only in my community, but almost everywhere, there is a long line to get an appointment. Even though we live in a 1.4-million metropolitan area, we had to drive to a smaller city an hour away for the quickest appointment – thankfully with a physician who was wonderful. (And for her GI doctor, we had to drive 2 hours in the opposite direction.)

Angelina's home-visit therapists worked with her on various things, but the absence of smiles and eye contact caused me to begin to suspect autism. And finally one of the therapists said the word – not regarding Angelina, but regarding another child with whom she was working. That child was autistic, and perhaps one of the communication methods that were helping that child might help Angelina. (This was when Angelina was around 17 months old.)

I called my friend Bradford Hulcher, an autism pioneer in our city. She said that we should have Angelina evaluated by a specific professional organization in town. We did. It was an ADOS (Autism Diagnostic Observation Schedule) session that took an hour or so and consisted of them watching Angelina play in various ways. Their on-site diagnosis was autism. We weren't surprised. She still wasn't walking or speaking.

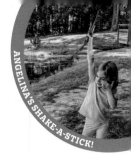

After Angelina's diagnosis, her developmental pediatrician labeled her "high functioning." Ever heard of Tiffany Joseph? Her Facebook site is called Nigh.Functioning.Autism. It's her humorous play on words – on the label "high functioning." That label continues to be used widely, and, as I now know, ignorantly. Such labels unfairly and inaccurately imply a whole set of traits and characteristics, but of course every autistic person is different from every other autistic person. It's simply misleading to assign group labels.

Early on, Tiffany Joseph was thought to be <u>unable</u> to function – the opposite of "high functioning." But now that she communicates mostly via AAC and can function quite well in certain areas, she has, with tongue in cheek, labeled herself "Nigh Functioning." I recommend a podcast interview with her, presented by Two Sides of the Spectrum (learnplaythrive.com), and entitled, "Nigh Functioning Autism: From Shame to Empowerment." About Learn Play Thrive: "Our mission is to provide resources and continuing education trainings that promote the use of strengths-based, ethical, neurodiversity-affirming practices for professionals (including OTs, SLPs, social workers, and psychologists) working with Autistic people."

The American Academy of Pediatrics recommends that all children should be screened for autism at their 18- and 24-month checkups. Parents usually have their hands full tending to all of the daily tasks associated with babies and toddlers, and they may not notice possible traits of autism. Grandparents are often the first persons to notice.

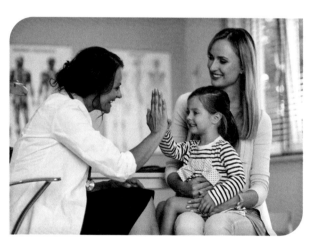

The American Psychiatric Association's most recent Diagnostic and Statistical Manual of Mental Disorders (DSM-5) presents the following criteria for an "official" autism diagnosis.

There must be "persistent deficits" in all three of the following:

✓ Social-emotional reciprocity (e.g. relating appropriately to others with back and forth communication and sharing of emotions).

✓ Non-verbal communication behaviors (e.g. eye contact, facial expressions, gestures).

✓ Understanding and maintaining relationships (e.g. making friends, sharing play, interest in others).

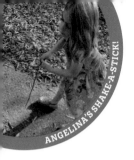
ANGELINA'S SHAKE-A-STICK!

AND there must be persistent deficits in at least two of the following four:

✓ Repetitive motor movements (e.g. lining up objects, idiosyncratic phrases).

✓ Insistence on sameness (e.g. same food, same routines).

✓ Abnormally intense fixations (e.g. excessive preoccupations with specific things or topics, strong attachments to unusual objects).

✓ Hypo- or hypersensitivities (e.g. indifference to pain or temperature, fascination with lights.)

The pediatrician is usually the frontline professional who monitors and evaluates a child's health. But there is no lab test, no x-ray, no blood test, etc. that can diagnose autism, and autism includes a very wide range of traits. Autism can range from severe mental disabilities to very high intellect. Three typical milestones that a pediatrician looks for are smiling by six months, mimicking sounds and facial expressions by nine months, and babbling by twelve months. (Angelina was delayed on all.)

The pediatrician may ask questions such as whether there is sensitivity to light or noise or temperature, whether there is a tendency towards anger, whether there are problems with eating or sleeping, and whether there is appropriate response when you attempt to get the child's attention.

Other professionals who may be involved to help with a diagnosis include child psychologists, speech-language pathologists, occupational therapists, developmental pediatricians, and neurologists. If a child is suspected for autism, this team of professionals may do periodic evaluations up until the age of 5 or longer.

One caution is that it is still common for pediatricians not to be well-educated about autism and to be unconcerned about behaviors and traits that should cause suspicion of autism. Specialists – "developmental pediatricians" – are equipped to recognize these concerns, but in many communities there are long waiting lists for appointments with developmental pediatricians. Parents should be proactive and if they suspect autism they should have their child evaluated at an autism diagnostic center.

The sooner an autism diagnosis is made, the sooner appropriate therapies and supports can begin. And research has shown that the earlier the better.

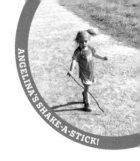

What's in YOUR Notebook?

B ACK WHEN ANGELINA AND KELLY LIVED WITH US it took me a few months to conceive and put together a special notebook and get it fully operational. My "Angelina Notebook" was a mainstay in our household. Simply put, it was a reference and guide for JC and my interactions with Angelina – almost all of which were times when Kelly was at work: nursing shifts at a big urban hospital. Angelina's long stay in the NICU had influenced Kelly to embark on a new career: nursing. So during the immediate years after Angelina's birth, even though she already had a B.S. degree, she got another one, this time in nursing, while also being a new mother. Since she and Angelina were living with us, JC and I were able to do a lot of caretaking for Angelina. Kelly stayed busy with classes, clinicals, and studying – then spending an hour or more each night putting Angelina to sleep by reading and singing to her, then doing homework until well past midnight.

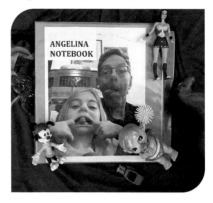

Following is the list of tabs and contents of the Angelina Notebook.

CONTACTS – This was the list of persons whom I might need to contact, and their cell/home/office contact information: Kelly's several telephone numbers at work as well as the exact location (building/floor) of her work/school, as well as the numbers of a couple of others if I couldn't reach her direct; ditto for Angelina's primary care physician and her other healthcare providers.

EMERGENCY MEDICAL INFO – Here I listed the top priority things that healthcare workers needed to know (including insurance information) if ever I had to take Angelina for emergency medical attention.

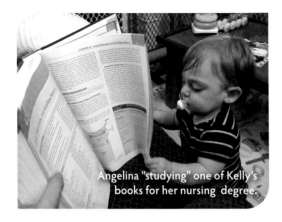

Angelina "studying" one of Kelly's books for her nursing degree.

FOOD – This was a continually-added-to list of food/drink that Angelina liked. (She had significant eating issues during her first couple of years – so it was wonderful to discover new things that she liked to eat.) Simply having this list to refer to was great when it was time to prepare meals and snacks.

ROUTINE MAINTENANCE – This was an ever-decreasing list of things that JC and I were required to do when Kelly was away. It started as a very long list when Angelina was finally released from the

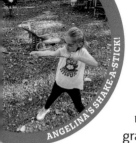

ANGELINA'S SHAKE-A-STICK!

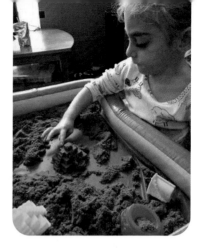

hospital: feeding tube, pulse/ox wire, nasal cannula, various medicines and of course the g-tube. Those responsibilities gradually disappeared.

FUN STUFF – This was a continually changing list of things that Angelina enjoyed doing. I remember adding Flying a Kite to the list. An indoor activity that got removed from the list was playing with kinetic sand. (I recommend that you never have this on your list; try it, you'll see.) The Fun Stuff section also included photos. It was so nice to be able to show Angelina the photos when we were deciding what to do next.

GOALS – This was a short but continually changing list of a very few goals/accomplishments – each small enough to be attainable – that we tried to work on with Angelina. When she accomplished a goal, we would add a new goal. I remember when one goal was for her to enunciate the "f" sound. She was saying it like "b." She eventually let me fold her lower lip up under her upper front teeth to make the "f" sound. Each time we worked on a specific goal, I put a mark next to that goal in the notebook.

VIDEOS (TV shows, movies, YouTube stuff – anything that can be seen on a television) – This was a continually changing list of things that Angelina really enjoyed watching on television. This section included photos.

My Angelina Notebook was a continual work in progress, and it was worth it.

Angelina's Story: The 24-Week Talk

WHEN KELLY'S PREGNANCY REACHED 24 WEEKS they told her that she was required to have a difficult and emotional meeting with members of the healthcare team. The meeting was to determine Kelly's wishes regarding using extreme measures to save the life of an early-term baby that may well have all sorts of lifelong disabilities (cerebral palsy, blindness . . .) and may well have a severely shortened lifespan. For example, if the baby can't breathe (extremely probable), does Kelly want them to attempt to insert a tiny breathing tube? (The lungs won't be adequately functional for weeks.) They told Kelly about a variety of other survival challenges that were likely; to what extent does Kelly want them to attempt to keep a baby alive that may not live long and that may well have severe lifelong disabilities? Kelly's final decision was straightforward: do everything to keep her baby alive.

Money and Services for Early Intervention

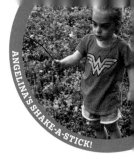

THIS MORNING'S NEWSPAPER has an Associated Press article written by Claire Savage: "Early Intervention crisis hits families hard." The article is about the fact that even though nearly 30 years ago the national Individuals with Disabilities Education Act required that Early Intervention would be provided for children with developmental delays, adequate resources just aren't available. The CDC says that one in six U.S. children has at least one developmental disability or delay, and "Since all U.S. states and territories accept federal funding for Early Intervention, they are obligated to provide services . . . But providers are scarce in almost all states. Some children wait months or years for the care they need, and many age out of the program before they access any services at all."

The article goes on to point out that families with private insurance and families with financial means are able to get Early Intervention therapies much more quickly than others, and that families of color, especially Blacks, are at the end of the line.

"When children turn 3, the responsibility for providing special education services shifts from Early Intervention to school districts. But those systems are understaffed and booked up . . . "

> ## GRANDPARENT CONFIDENTIAL
>
> *"My grandson will soon be 2, and he does not respond to his name, is toe-walking, and doesn't yet speak. I think he's going to be diagnosed with autism and will be starting early intervention. His father is in denial."*

So bottom line, something I hear from autism families not only in my community but throughout the nation, is that even though these services are required by the government, they're way short of being adequately provided. And, as with everything, the families who have the time and ability to be very squeaky wheels are getting served first.

ABLE Savings Plans

A COUPLE OF YEARS AGO I MET ANITA KELLEY, *Savings Director for the Alabama State Treasurer's office which oversees the Alabama ABLE Savings Plan, and she wrote the following article for me to share nationally. Even though she is the Alabama expert, ABLE plans are similar everywhere.*

Gene Perret once said, "What a bargain grandchildren are! I give them my loose change, and they give me a million dollars' worth of pleasure."

I'm sure you understand exactly where he is coming from. But perhaps you are looking for a way to provide your grandchild with some of your loose change. An ABLE (Achieving a Better Life Experience) account is a great vehicle for persons to save for their loved ones with a disability.

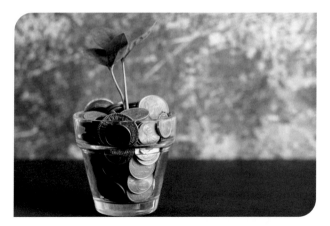

The ABLE ACT was signed into law in 2014. Since its passage, 44 states and D.C. have established programs that provide tax-free savings accounts for individuals with disabilities. These programs allow for individuals with a disability to save without impacting resource-based benefits such as SSI, SSDI, or Medicaid.

Nationwide,101,000 ABLE accounts have been opened, with an average savings in each account of $8,600 and a total amount of $874 million dollars.

ABLE accounts are limited to $15,000 in annual contributions unless the individual is working and not contributing to a retirement plan. Accounts can have up to $100,000 in balances without impacting SSI or SSDI and these funds will not affect Medicaid. If the individual is not receiving SSI or SSDI, they can save more than the $100,000 (amount depends on what state plan you open).

ABLE participants may use the savings for a wide range of qualified disability expenses – from medical costs to education, assistive technology, service animals, housing, transportation, basic living expenses and more.

The Alabama ABLE Savings Plan has a low annual fee of $35.00 and is administered by the State of Alabama Treasurer's Office. Contributions into the account can be deposited into an FDIC savings account or one of three Vanguard portfolios. Contributions may also be deductible for Alabama residents up to $5,000.00 per filer on their state income tax. Remember to check with your own state for any tax benefits or fee expenses.

With greater savings comes increased financial security and flexibility for the disability community.

When and How Children Should be Told They are Autistic

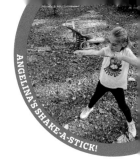

YOU DON'T EVEN NEED TO READ THIS SECTION if you'll just watch this 5-minute video on YouTube: "6 Things You Should Do When Telling Your Child He/She Has Autism" (But watch it even if you do read this section.)

Hopefully you've now watched the video. Following are nine things that may be helpful.

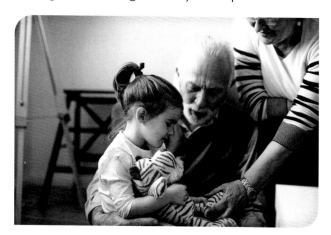

1: Determine **WHO** is the best person to initiate and continue this conversation with the autistic child. It should be a person whom the child feels comfortable with and trusts and respects. In some families this person might be a grandparent.

2: Start the conversation as **SOON** as possible – hopefully very soon after the diagnosis. The content of the initial conversations will depend on the child's age and cognitive abilities. For example, if the child has been diagnosed at two years old and isn't yet verbal and isn't likely to understand words and sentences, you can still begin. Just as you say things such as "I love you," you can also say things like, "I love you, and one of the reasons you are so special to me is that you are autistic, and that means that you see the world differently from typical children. I am so excited to watch you grow and to learn things from you." Again, even though a two-year-old isn't likely to comprehend any of this, if you say it on a continual basis and gradually expand over the weeks and months and years, it won't be a sudden surprise as his cognitive abilities get stronger. Always talk about autism in an upbeat way, and regardless of the child's age, the conversation should be ongoing rather than a single, major session.

3: Start these conversations only after you are **COMFORTABLE** with his autism diagnosis and have worked through your own fears and doubts and anxieties.

4: You don't want the child to **FIND OUT BY ACCIDENT** that she is autistic: overhearing a teacher, being told by a playmate, seeing a television show about someone like her, etc. Your child's healthcare workers, therapists, teachers, playmates' parents, and many others will need to know that she

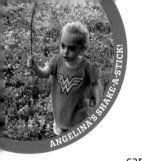

is autistic – and it's not helpful for that knowledge to be hidden from her. If she starts asking questions such as, "Why do people say I'm weird?" or "Is there something wrong with me?" or "What is autism?" then you're overdue in telling her that she is autistic. But it's great that you can now begin.

5: Initiate the autism conversation and have ongoing conversations only when your child is **CALM AND IN A GOOD MENTAL AND EMOTIONAL STATE** – not, for example, after a meltdown.

6: A good way to start is by discussing the fact that all persons are the **SAME IN SOME WAYS AND DIFFERENT IN OTHER WAYS**. For example, "Grandmother wears glasses but Grandfather doesn't. But Grandmother and Grandfather both like pancakes." Then, for example, "You and [playmate] are the same because you both like Peppa Pig. But you and [playmate] are different because purple is your favorite color and yellow is her favorite color." Then let her know that all people are the same in some ways: everyone has times when they are happy and also times when they are sad, etc. Then move on to the fact that everyone is good at some things but struggle with other things. Then, for example, "You are very good at dancing, but you sometimes need help walking down a flight of stairs."

> **GRANDPARENT CONFIDENTIAL**
>
> *"My grandson is really smart and does well in kindergarten, but he has outbursts, isn't potty trained (afraid of the toilet and of water) and needs structure. His parents are exhausted."*

7: Then proceed to talk about the child's **STRENGTHS AND CHALLENGES**. Be specific and emphasize the strengths: "You are so good at smiling at people. It makes people feel good when you smile at them." Be less emphatic about challenges: "Have you noticed that you sometimes try to run away from us?" Let the child know that you will help with challenges: "Running away can be dangerous, but I will always be here to help you with this. Everyone has challenges and things that they are not good at, and it is wonderful when there are people who can help."

8: **WHEN CHILDREN FIRST LEARN ABOUT THEIR AUTISM WHEN THEY ARE OLDER**, it is often a relief. They now know why they feel different, why they are treated differently, and why they may have difficulty making friends. Learning that they are autistic can help eliminate their feelings of failure, of inadequacy and guilt, and of low self-esteem. And it can eliminate their wrong ideas such as having a terminal disease or being from another planet. The knowledge allows them to become more self-aware and able to understand their identity.

9: Let the child know that **EVERY AUTISTIC PERSON IS DIFFERENT** from all the others, and that the autism community is big. You may be able to name other persons whom she knows or knows of who are autistic.

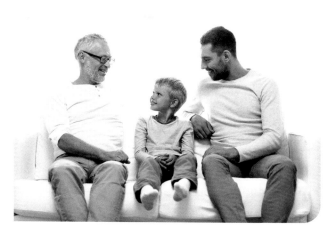

BOTTOM LINE: The **SOONER AND CALMER AND MORE UPBEAT** you can start talking to the child about her autism, the better. Sometimes grandparents – because parents often have more hectic and time-consuming challenges – are the ideal persons to lead these conversations, but even if not, grandparents can be empowered by their grandchildren's parents to participate in meaningful ways.

P.S.: A helpful project for many children is creating an ongoing artwork/poster entitled "All About Me." There may be a photo or drawing of the child surrounded by appropriate words and images.

When to Say the A-Word

A FEW YEARS AGO Angelina was playing with another little girl at a public playground and the girl's mother and I started talking. She asked me where Angelina goes to school. I told her and she said she wasn't familiar with The Faison Center. I told her that it's for autistic persons and that Angelina was on the autism spectrum. The mother's response was, "I bet Angelina is really good in math." I told her no, but that she has lots of good qualities.

When is it appropriate for us to tell another person that our child, or grandchild in my case, is autistic?

When JC was a university faculty member, occasionally a new student would bring her a letter from the school administration that described the student's learning disability and asked for special accommodations from JC – for example, the student's need to sometimes have an assignment explained in writing rather than verbally. JC never saw the word "autism" in any of those documents. It's the same with the classes that JC teaches at the Visual Arts Center of Richmond: a descriptive note, but never a label.

Who needs to know that Angelina is autistic? When is it helpful? When can it be counterproductive?

It was in 2013 that the American Psychiatric Association established "Autism Spectrum Disorder" as an umbrella term to encompass a vast range of characteristics. And today, even though almost everyone has heard of autism, it is common for the general public to associate autism with a single stereotype that is based on the latest movie or book or television show that features an autistic person. The general public doesn't yet have an adequate appreciation for the sentence, "Meet one person with autism and you've met one person with autism."

Thus, when I tell someone that Angelina is autistic, there is no way to know how that person will process the information.

Following are ten things that can help us determine whom to tell and when.

1: Dr. Temple Grandin says that throughout her life she has, when necessary, told others about the **challenges rather than the diagnosis**: "I can accomplish that task better if it is written down in precise steps." Or, if a child were to have a meltdown at a store, "She sometimes has overwhelming sensory issues when there are a lot of people . . ."

2: Terms that are meant to describe **levels of autism, such as "high-functioning," can create inaccurate assumptions**. Even if an autistic child has an exceptionally high IQ, she often still has significant challenges with certain social constructs.

3: Challenging behaviors of autistic children are often blamed on poor discipline. If there is a need to respond, **it's best to be positive**: "He can sometimes become intensely fixated on things, and we're proud that he's working hard to lessen episodes like this."

4: Even though disclosure of a child's diagnosis should help others to be understanding, **disclosure can sometimes be counterproductive**. For example, there are some persons who are uncomfortable around persons with disabilities. I take Angelina for swimming lessons, and if the swim teacher were to have this level of discomfort, I wouldn't mention autism. But, assuming a comfort level, I might mention it to the overall director of swimming. And that way she would be in position to be a champion for Angelina.

5: Should JC and I tell our friends and neighbors and colleagues, etc. that Angelina is autistic? **If it can be helpful to tell, yes. If not, probably not.**

6: **Disclosure profoundly changes the relationship.** Hopefully the change is for the better, but sometimes it's not. Families need to give careful consideration to this and not treat disclosure in a cavalier manner.

7: **Disclosure is absolutely necessary in certain situations**. Doctors, teachers, therapists, public service officials, and immediate family members are among those who need to be aware of the autism diagnosis.

8: As autistic children get older, they sometimes find it helpful to carry **small cards** that provide a brief explanation of their diagnosis of autism. They sometimes also feel good about wearing t-shirts with statements about being autistic.

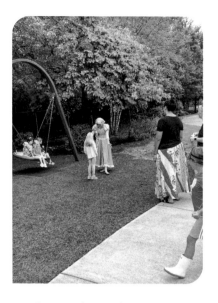

9: The child's legal guardians are the persons to determine when and how to **tell the child that she is autistic**. In most cases it's better if she learns it at home before hearing it from others. It can be wonderfully helpful for a child to have an understanding of himself – why some things are hard and other things fun and easy. It is also empowering for him to know that he is among a large community of others who are on this diverse spectrum.

10: **Playground education usually doesn't work.** Next time I'm talking with a stranger at a playground I probably won't – unless there is a situation that requires it – mention that Angelina is autistic. The moment I do that, I automatically prejudice the other person. And the playground usually is not the place at which an education session about autism can be very effective.

The bottom line is that we autism families should do three things regarding disclosing a child's autism diagnosis: first, continue to learn as much as possible about autism and the child's specific characteristics and challenges; second, know what we're talking about when we do disclose the diagnosis; and third, disclose the diagnosis only when it can be helpful.

Angelina's Story: Birth

AS KELLY'S PREGNANCY BECAME INCREASINGLY HIGH-RISK, meaning that an emergency C-section delivery might be necessary at any time, JC and I took turns staying with her at the hospital 24/7. It was on my watch – the morning of March 23, 2016 (25 ½ weeks into a normal 40-week term) – that the medical team rushed in and then ran as they rolled Kelly down the hall to the delivery room. Someone then came for me and after I put on sterile hospital garb they ushered me into the delivery room where Kelly was being attended to by a 12-person (I counted) team. There was already a lot of blood when I entered, and they seated me next to Kelly's head – an area that was draped from the blood. Between her continual screams of pain, Kelly would calmly say, "Dad, are you okay?" (I'd had a history of not doing so well at the sight of bloody surgery.)

Angelina weighed 1 ½ pounds, and the first thing they did was hand her to a neonatologist

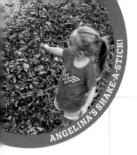

ANGELINA'S SHAKE-A-STICK!

(doctor who specializes in a baby's care immediately before, during, and after delivery) whose job it was to attempt to insert a breathing tube into Angelina's miniscule airway and then hope for the best. It was perhaps an hour later – Kelly and I were back in her hospital room – that a nurse entered with a smile and with the news that the breathing tube had been successfully inserted and that Angelina was alive. Although Kelly would be able to view Angelina, her skin was so thin and delicate that it would be a few days before she could actually touch her and even longer before she could hold her.

IEPs

EP STANDS FOR INDIVIDUALIZED EDUCATION PROGRAM. Every child who is eligible for special education is required to have an IEP. The school convenes an annual meeting to determine the IEP. Grandparents are allowed to be extremely involved in the process – that is, of course, if that's what the parents want and if the grandparents are available.

I am involved in Angelina's education, and when we thought she would enter a specific public school for kindergarten, I attended my first IEP meeting and I made lots of mistakes. My biggest mistake was thinking that all I needed to do was show up and allow the school's experts to develop an appropriate program for her.

I now have a much better handle on how to have the best involvement. The following information and suggestions cover the basics.

The U.S. government requires that every child receive "free appropriate public education . . . in the least restrictive environment." And, thanks to a 2017 Supreme Court determination that centered on a student with autism, IEP goals for special education students must be "appropriately ambitious." That is, schools are not allowed to aim for simply <u>minimal</u> progress. "Every child must have the chance to meet <u>challenging</u> objectives."

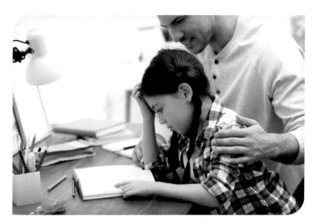

Angelina's school has the responsibility of

ANGELINA'S SHAKE-A-STICK!

determining whether she is eligible for special education and associated services. The school does this via an evaluation process that is initiated by parent request. The evaluation covers a lot of ground, and if the evaluation determines that the child is not eligible for special education, the parents can request that the school district conduct an IEE (Independent Education Evaluation).

After the student is determined to be eligible for special education, the school will arrange for a meeting to determine an IEP. The meeting attendees typically include the child's case manager, the school's special education teacher, a general education teacher, a school administrator, perhaps a school psychologist or social worker, and perhaps other teachers and/or therapists who know the child. Parents attend the meeting and can bring others with them who know the child: therapists, doctors, close friends, attorneys, grandparents, etc.

The parents (and grandparents if involved) can prepare for the IEP meeting by knowing (and listing) the child's strengths and weaknesses both in and out of school, by doing research on the various types of programs and supplemental aids (e.g. speech therapy, assistive technology, special seating, etc.) that might be appropriate for the child, and listing their own goals for the child's school year.

Parents (and grandparents) should always be aware that THEY know the child best, and should be advocates for what THEY believe are the best components for an appropriate IEP. And parents should come to the IEP meeting with a positive attitude and very high expectations.

The IEP goals should be measurable, and there should be a clear understanding of how and when progress will be measured for each goal. Goals should be measured at least quarterly. And any recommended supports and services should be clearly defined.

When children enter middle school, the IEPs should begin addressing plans for transitioning into adulthood.

I knew none of this in advance of my first IEP meeting for Angelina. I thought it was simply an education meeting that her parents asked me to attend. It was both intimidating and unnerving to sit there and hear a half-dozen "experts" talk about Angelina's strengths and challenges, and watching them determine a best-case education program for her. They were all nice and well-meaning, but their in-person involvement with Angelina had been far less than mine. As was their knowledge of her abilities. Had I come prepared I would have been able to provide valuable input.

One interesting thing is that if there is not a public school that can accommodate the child's IEP, the child can attend an appropriate private school at public expense.

How involved should parents/grandparents be in the child's education and IEP development? VERY! And what is the best way to be very involved? Basically, be involved in the school and have good relationships with the appropriate teachers and administrators. Take part in school activities and volunteer for school events. Ask the teachers what sort of communication (and how often) they want from you: e-mails, meetings, telephone, etc. – and comply accordingly.

I've learned that although schools welcome the involvement of grandparents at IEP meetings and in other aspects of the child's school life, they are rarely proactive in asking about or recommending the possibility of grandparent involvement – even though lots of us grandparents have the time and energy.

There is of course a lot of information about IEPs on the Internet. Autism Speaks' website is a great place to start: www.autism-speaks.org.

Postscript: When Angelina entered public school, she wound up not needing an IEP, but rather a 504 Plan (sort of like an IEP but less extensive and requiring fewer supports).

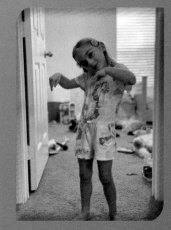

Angelina!

Once when Angelina and I were talking about geography I told her about the North Pole. She responded, "Where is the West Pole?" And she followed with, "Where is the East Pole?" (I had to find out from Google why those two poles don't exist.)

Sleep Disorders

IT'S COMMON FOR PERSONS ON THE AUTISM SPECTRUM – children and adults – to have chronic sleep disorders: difficulty falling asleep and difficulty staying asleep. For months and months after Angelina came home from her long stay in the NICU she had terrible challenges falling asleep – tossing and turning and kicking for what seemed like hours, her eyes wide open the whole time. A 2019 research study found that 80% of autistic preschoolers experience abnormally disruptive sleep. Another study showed that autistic children spend only 15% of their sleep time in the REM (rapid eye movement) stage, while neurotypical children average 23%. REM sleep is critical for learning. And too little sleep exacerbates a variety of other autism challenges.

There are things that can sometimes be helpful. The first thing to do is to get a medical analysis. For example, is the child taking a medication (such as for ADHD) that contributes to sleep problems? Are there gastro-intestinal problems (common with autism)? You can even get a professional sleep assessment, but it takes place in a laboratory and includes a variety of wires and sensors – an environ-

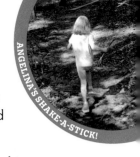
ANGELINA'S SHAKE-A-STICK!

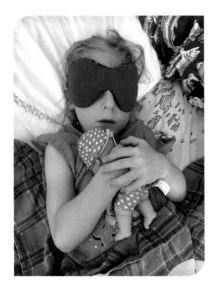

ment that doesn't appear to be sleep-friendly and thus may not be appropriate for many persons. (We never did this with Angelina.)

Once a medical analysis has been completed, the next thing to consider is the sleeping environment. Is the lighting too dark or too light? (Angelina tossed and turned regardless.) Some autistic children respond well to wearing a sleep mask. (A sleep mask does wonders for Angelina, and she loves wearing it!) What about sound? Some persons sleep better with zero sound, others with a soft "white" noise such the sound of a gentle rain. (With Angelina we tried various white noise machines with mixed results.) Headphones or earplugs can be tried. What about the temperature in the room? For most persons colder is better than warmer. What about dolls or stuffed animals? Many children sleep better when holding a favorite "friend." (Angelina needs to hold a stuffed animal; she has a big variety that she selects from each night.) Constant experimentation with the sleeping environment may eventually result in a condition that greatly approves sleep.

Many professionals recommend that an established bedtime "routine" is helpful for sleep – a routine that begins from 15 to 30 minutes prior to sleep time. They also recommend that the routine be written, or demonstrated by pictures or objects, in a way that the child can comprehend. The pre-sleep routine should not include television or any sort of tablet or computer screen. It should include normal pre-bedtime things such as brushing teeth, putting on pajamas, going to the bathroom, etc., and should also include calming things such as reading or listening to music. And once a routine is established, the recommendation is to stick to it until it becomes ingrained. (Of course routines sound good in theory, but the schedules of many families are simply too haphazard and unpredictable to adhere to routines on a regular basis.)

Regarding food, it is almost unanimously recommended that there be no meals within at least a couple of hours prior to bedtime.

There are other unanimous recommendations that may seem obvious: don't allow late afternoon naps; get lots of physical exercise during the day; and no caffeine (including that found in chocolate and some sodas) within 5 hours of bedtime.

Autistic adults may be able to take sleep aids such as Ambien for improved sleep, but children shouldn't take it. Melatonin supplements can often be helpful for children. (Angelina loves eating a melatonin gummy before bedtime, but she seems to sleep just as well when she doesn't.)

If your autistic child has developed a need for a parent to sleep in the bed with him, it is usually beneficial if he can be weaned of this need. You can begin by telling him that you'll sleep with him for most of the night, but not all of it – and that he'll be fine by himself after you leave. You may want this initial stage of weaning to include only a 10% reduction in the time you stay in the bed. Then gradually increase the amount – with appropriate praise each morning – until you stay in the bed only until he falls asleep.

The next stage is to begin bedtime with you sitting on the bed, perhaps with your arm around the child. Then after a few nights of this, begin bedtime with you sitting in a chair next to the bed. Then over the coming days move the chair farther and farther away while giving the child less and less attention. You get the idea. The duration of this weaning process varies from child to child – sometimes taking as long as several months. But successful weaning will have long-term benefits. (We went through a weaning process with Angelina.)

Autism Speaks (www.autismspeaks.org) has website information on sleep problems, and one idea that is suggested is a "Bedtime Pass" – a coupon that the child can use just one time during the night in exchange for a kiss or hug or drink of water or whatever. And if the child goes the entire night without using the Bedtime Pass, he might be rewarded with a sticker in the morning. And a certain number of stickers might result in a store-bought prize.

Fortunately Angelina now goes to sleep readily and sleeps through the night.

Diet and Eating and Meals

CHILDREN ON THE AUTISM SPECTRUM are at risk for all sorts of gastrointestinal and nutritional challenges: gastroesophageal reflux disease (GERD), chronic diarrhea or constipation, food regurgitation, food allergies and intolerances, feeding problems, etc.

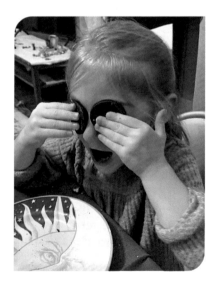

The GFCF diet (gluten-free/casein-free – no wheat, barley, rye, milk or dairy) is currently being claimed as something that is therapeutic for autism: they say that it can lessen problem behaviors, it can enhance speech development, it can even "cure" autism. The Ketogenic diet (high fat, low carbs) is another diet that many autism parents are embracing; they say it relieves seizure disorders. There's the yeast-free diet (no yeast or sugar), the Feingold diet (no additives or chemicals), and a wide variety of custom-concocted diets that all claim to do positive

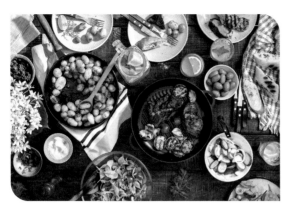

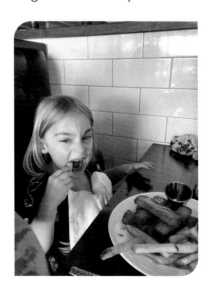

things for autistic children. Each of these special diets is accompanied by heartfelt praise from parents who claim to have seen its success in their own children. The same is true for all sorts of dietary supplements.

Sadly, in spite of claims to the contrary, no diet has yet been scientifically (evidence-based) proven to be effective at diminishing or eliminating any of autism's challenging characteristics or behaviors. You can find them discussed on the websites of the nation's leading medical centers, and you'll see the results of research. The GFCF diet, for example, has scientific merit to its reasoning, but its effectiveness is not supported by medical research. Perhaps a beneficial autism-specific diet will one day be discovered and proven, but thus far it doesn't exist.

Every special diet – whether for autism or not – is accompanied by challenges. The GFCF diet, for example, comes with a need to make up for lost fiber, nutrients, calcium and Vitamin D – all of which are vital for healthy growth and development. The Keto diet leads to poor growth, poor weight gain, and increased cholesterol. Dietary supplements – vitamins, minerals, probiotics, etc. – come with the risk of taking too much and/or significant contraindications with other supplements and medicines.

Many families aren't aware that dietary supplements receive very little oversight by the Food and Drug Administration. For example, the FDA does NOT review them for safety and effectiveness; manufacturers of dietary supplements oversee themselves. The FDA gets involved only after there are significant complaints. Thus the information we receive regarding a specific bottle of Vitamin C or Calcium pills is provided totally by the manufacturer and without review or confirmation by the FDA or by any other regulatory agency.

Every autistic person is different, and each person's diet and therapy should be tailored to that person's specific medical challenges. For example, constipation requires one type of diet, diarrhea another. Someone who has difficulty swallowing requires one type of diet, someone who overeats requires another.

Dieticians and nutritionists agree on one fundamental thing: diets that include fewer processed foods are best. They are not only easier to digest and absorb, but they also contain fewer toxins.

During Angelina's first few years she had a lot of eating issues. She received treatment from developmental pediatricians, gastro-intestinal specialists, nutritionists, OT therapists, etc. Thankfully, today Angelina's eating issues are mostly gone. There has been no magic bullet or wonder-cure or miracle therapy – just lots of worry, lots of trying all sorts of food, lots of professional care, lots of praise for each small improvement, and lots of love.

Even when the healthcare team has determined what sort of diet is best, there are often challenges with the act of eating. **There are a several things for autism families to consider:**

GRANDPARENT CONFIDENTIAL

"The only way to get my grandson to poop is to put him in a bath – of course NOT where we want him to go. How should I deal with this?"

1: Medical and/or dental problems can be causes of eating issues. One research study (Buie & Krigsman) suggests that at least 50% of children with ASD have significant gastrointestinal symptoms such as GERD, chronic constipation, abdominal pain, etc.

2: It is common for parents to be blamed for their children's eating issues, but such blame is not warranted when it concerns children on the autism spectrum.

3: Autism professionals recommend a variety of feeding therapies and protocols – some that may be productive, and others that may be counterproductive. But whichever is selected, it should result from careful research of information provided by reputable professional sources, and not simply from information provided by the practitioner.

4: It is common for autistic children to have sensory aversions. This means that they respond negatively to specific smells or tastes or colors or textures (for example, they may like crunchy foods, but not smooth), or food temperatures (it is common for autistic children to prefer foods at room temperature and be intolerant of foods that are either hot or cold), or noise level (e.g. lots of ambient noise during meals), or bodily sensations (e.g. chair too high or too hard, etc.), etc.

5: It is common for autistic children to be extremely selective with foods. Some children eat mostly foods that are either sweet, sour, bitter, or salty. Some learn that all foods are better with certain condiments (such as catsup).

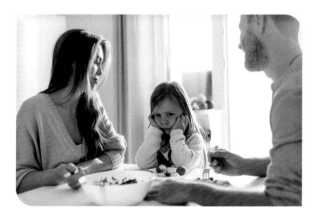

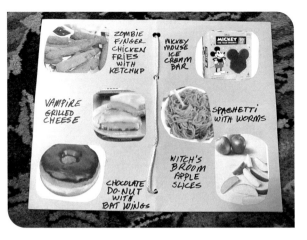
6: Other things can be issues, such as visual appearance (specific plates or napkins, location of food), socialization (whether or not other persons are there), transitioning from finger food to utensil food, etc.

7: Often autistic children don't feel hunger pangs or exhibit signs of hunger or answer "yes" when asked if they are hungry. Therefore it is usually a good idea to serve food at regular intervals whether or not there are signs of hunger.

8: As with most issues and challenges with autism, the focus should be on achieving and celebrating a series of <u>tiny</u> steps of progress. (For example, rather than an initial goal of eating a full helping of a newly introduced food, have an initial goal of simply tolerating the existence of that food on a separate plate during the meal.)

9: Parents of autistic children often hear, even from some medical professionals, words such as, "Don't worry; she'll eat when she gets hungry enough." Or, "All children go through phases with food issues." Such comments are not founded in a knowledge of eating issues among autistic children.

There are several things that families can do to be helpful with eating issues.

1: We can refrain from scolding or being negative regarding feeding issues. We can be positive during meals (rather than viewing them as battles) and be liberal with praise for every bit of success.

2: We can see that the child is involved with physical activity or exercise prior to meals. (Often such activity stimulates the appetite.)

3: We can try to make food and meals fun. (Making up songs or stories about food items, pretending with toy food items and dishes prior to the meal, allowing the child to "play" with the food, etc.)

4: We can accept the possibility of meltdowns, and put emphasis on praise when warranted.

5: We can eat together (unless socialization is off-putting) so the child can observe and possibly mirror our actions.

6: We can refrain from food "tricks" such as hiding vegetables in spaghetti sauce etc. (Once the child recognizes a trick, he may decide not to trust any foods.)

7: We can keep a feeding journal. Such documentation can often lead to a recognition of patterns of behavior that will enhance an understanding of the child's issues and thus result in strategies for progress.

There are many different strategies and therapies that are recommended by a variety of autism experts regarding eating issues. What works for one child may not work for another. But learning about current expert advice can help families better understand and empathize with the significance of this challenge for autistic children.

Stephen Mark Shore is a 58-year-old autistic professor at Adelphi University. He says this about how he processed food as a child:

"Brown or black food wouldn't be eaten, as I insisted that they were poisonous. Canned asparagus was intolerable due to its slimy texture, and I didn't eat tomatoes for a year after a cherry tomato had burst in my mouth while I was eating it. The sensory stimulation of having that small piece of fruit explode in my mouth was too much to bear and I was not going to take any chances of that happening again. Carrots in a green salad and celery in tuna fish salad are still intolerable to me because the contrast in texture between carrots or celery and salad or tuna fish is too great. However, I enjoy eating celery and baby carrots by themselves. Often as a child, and less now, I would eat things serially, finishing one item on the plate before going on to the next." [From his book: *Beyond the Wall – Personal Experiences with Autism and Asperger Syndrome*]

Parents often have trouble understanding why their autistic children won't eat this, won't try that, and won't even taste the other. Even when they demonstrate how much THEY like it. Even when they do time-proven tricks like flying the airplane into the hangar. And even when they offer rewards.

When Angelina was younger it was a major accomplishment to get her to open her mouth for a tiny spoonful of food. We didn't understand, we didn't have solutions, we consulted specialists, and we tried all sorts of things. We don't know whether it was any one thing or any certain therapy that "cured" her, but my guess is that in her case it was mostly a combination of persistence and time.

> ## GRANDPARENT CONFIDENTIAL
>
> *"Pizza is the only thing my 5-year-old granddaughter will eat. But she has GERD and the sauce aggravates it. I've tried recipes for non-acidic sauce but she won't eat it. Any suggestions?"*

The term "eating disorder" can refer to many different things ranging from simple aversions to, and preferences for, certain foods, to extremely harmful things like anorexia nervosa, pica (eating non-foods such as cigarettes, paper, dirt, etc.), rumination (regurgitating food and re-chewing it), rapid eating (including binging, and accompanied by the danger of aspiration or choking), and on and on.

Autism can be accompanied by a whole range of things that can have a negative effect on eating, including "abnormal" sensory experiences that relate to sight, taste, smell, and texture – any or all of which can cause an aversion to certain foods, and even a perception that certain foods are harmful or dangerous. I found one research site that says that 69% of children with autism are unwilling to

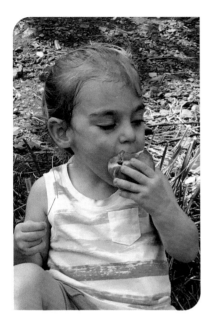

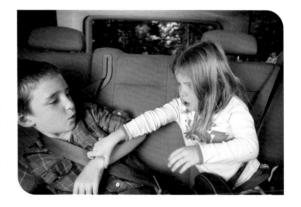
try new foods, and that 46% have rituals regarding eating.

While there may be no obvious therapy for, or easy solution to, or simple understanding of any eating disorder, families can be helpful in three fundamental ways:

1: We can realize that it's probably not our cooking or our menu or our presentation that has resulted in a negative eating reaction. We can understand that it's likely a manifestation of the child's unique type of autism. And we can act in a loving and understanding manner rather than the opposite.

2: We can make "eating" a priority topic for ongoing discussion with all family members, including grandparents, who host meals for the child, keeping everyone informed and welcoming their advice.

3: We can happily cheer and congratulate the child each time there is even the slightest bit of "progress."

I remember when Angelina first ate a peach by herself – not sliced, not peeled, not being held by us between bites. She did the whole thing by herself. And a week later she ate another one! One thing about autism families is that we receive so much joy from so many things that other families often take for granted.

Aggressive Behavior

A 2010 SURVEY OF 1,380 CHILDREN with autism, conducted by Stephen M. Kanne and Micah O. Mazurek, found that 68% displayed aggressive behavior with their caregivers and 49% with non-caregivers. Other studies have shown lower percentages. But the bottom line is that aggressive behavior is common among autistic children, and it can be bad: biting, kicking, breaking things, head banging, and on and on.

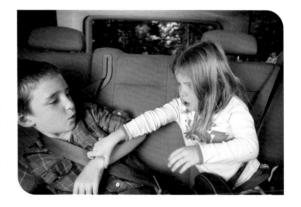

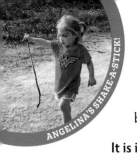

Are there things that can lessen aggressive behaviors? Following is some information that can be helpful.

It is important to know that aggressive behavior is very often an attempt to communicate. The child is trying to tell us something, trying to get us to understand something. She is either nonverbal and thus unable to talk, or if verbal, she doesn't know how to explain it in words.

It can be helpful to conduct an assessment of the aggressive behavior. Assessment is most helpful when it is accomplished in careful detail. This means documenting each aggressive behavior: when each episode begins and ends, what was happening just before and just after (location, persons present, environmental happenings, etc.), and what may have caused it to stop. Assessment also includes documenting what the caregiver's actions were before, during, and after. The assessment should be recorded in a multi-week or multi-month diary. And the aggressive behaviors should be videoed as often as possible. Assessment also includes determining times/locations/happenings when aggressive behavior almost never happens.

Such assessment can often help identify things that trigger aggressive behaviors. Did aggressive behavior usually occur when there was a change from one activity to another? When there was an attempt to touch or hug the child? When the television was turned on or off? Any of a zillion things can trigger aggressive behavior. It can be as seemingly simple as irritation from a scratchy label in an article of clothing, or as vague as a weather condition. Again, a careful assessment can often help determine the triggers.

There are five main things that are most important during aggressive behaviors: stay calm (don't rush around, don't raise voices, etc.), say as few words as possible ("Sit." rather than, "Thomas, come over here right now and sit yourself down!"), move to a safer and quieter place if possible (no shelves to knock over, no crowds of people), perform physical restraint only if absolutely necessary (physical restraint can be harmful to the child and can increase anxiety and make everything worse), and give praise or positive reinforcement when the behavior ends.

> ## GRANDPARENT CONFIDENTIAL
>
> *"My 8-year-old grandson says bad words and calls me bad names and has meltdowns and hits and bites. There are never punishments, only rewards. He has a virtual therapist. I don't want him to visit me anymore unless he can behave better. Any suggestions?"*

Be careful about providing rewards (candy, tablet time, etc.) when the aggressive behavior ends. Obviously if the aggressive behavior results in something the child wants, he will do it again.

Caregivers can help the child <u>prepare</u> for things that normally trigger aggressive behavior. For example, if turning off the television is a trigger, we can give him an advance heads-up: "In 5 minutes we will turn off the television. In 4 more minutes. Only 3 minutes left . . ." A visible timer – such

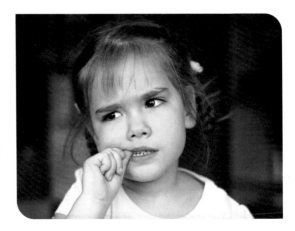

as many cell phones offer – can be a visible notice of the time limit and countdown. And/or caregivers can show him advance photos or picture boards that demonstrate a "trigger" that is forthcoming: a photo of him brushing his teeth, a photo of food being served, etc. Caregivers can understand that sudden and/or unexpected events and people and changes in schedule, etc. can trigger aggressive behavior. And caregivers can provide choices. For example, rather than saying that the child must eat broccoli, a choice can be offered to select from among three vegetables. Or telling him he must prepare for bedtime in a certain order – use the toilet, wash hands, wash face, brush teeth – he can be allowed to choose his own order.

It is important to know that aggressive behaviors can be caused by medical conditions: as straightforward as a toothache, and as complex as epilepsy. Medication is indeed effective for some persons who exhibit aggressive behavior. Medical assessment should be ongoing; it shouldn't stop after one physician gives a clean bill of health.

Regarding aggressive behavior, praise and positivity rule! One autism professional recommends a ratio of at least 8 praises for every 1 negative comment. So for every time I tell Angelina, "Stop that!" I need to praise her 8 times for other things. Every time she exhibits good behavior, I need to smile and applaud and hug her. Every time she doesn't get upset when it's time to turn off her tablet, I can praise her for it. Every time she brushes her teeth all by herself I can praise her. Generally autistic children progress much better when being praised rather than scolded.

Stimming

STIMMING, OR "SELF-STIMULATORY BEHAVIOR": it's simply the word used to identify a lot of the repetitive behaviors that most of us do – and that are often more pronounced and prevalent among autistic persons. When an autistic person continually shakes a stick, it's referred to as stimming, as in stimulation. Stimming usually consists of repetitive body movements or behaviors. It's common for autistic persons to stim: flapping their hands and arms, fluttering their fingers, rocking back and forth, turning lights on and off, opening and closing doors, etc. Stimming can have a variety of purposes: calming anxiety, reducing pain, relieving stress, etc. And unless the stimming activity is causing some sort danger or harm, it's not a good thing to forcefully stop it – even if it seems publicly embarrassing.

Among those of us who are neurotypical, our stimming-type behaviors include things such as tapping our fingers, biting our nails, clicking pens, jiggling our feet, etc. Among autistic persons common stimming behaviors include, but are not limited to, rocking, flapping hands and fingers, bouncing, twirling, walking on tiptoes, jumping, repetitive blinking, continual rubbing of the skin, staring at rotating objects such as ceiling fans, turning lights on and off, etc.

It's helpful to be aware of three basic things about stimming among autistic persons:

1: Stimming is not something that should be stopped unless it's physically harmful (biting, kicking, head-banging, etc.). Stimming is often beneficial, and causing it to stop can be detrimental. A stimming session can last from a few minutes to a few hours. Of course if stimming is a major disruption for specific situation, it may be appropriate to remove the stimmer from the situation.

2: Occasionally stimming can be an indication of medical problems. For example, stimming may be a reaction to a toothache or stomach ache. Or it may relate to something more complex such as epilepsy.

3: It isn't possible to predict whether stimming will increase or decrease as the child gets older.

The current opinion of many autism professionals is that stimming usually provides a variety of benefits: it feels good, it calms anxiety, it helps focus attention, it helps alleviate sensory overload and emotional stress, it helps express frustration, etc.

In previous years various extreme "therapies" were used to try to cause stimming to cease – therapies such as shock treatments, corporal punishment, and drugs. But today it is generally agreed that there is no medicine or therapy that has the singular result (without significant side effects) of stopping stimming.

However . . . there are ways to sometimes lessen the intensity and frequency of stimming that is harmful and/or dangerous. It's a three-step process.

FIRST, keep a log of when/where the stimming happens, including its duration and intensity and whether there is some sort of situational shift that coincides with the stimming's cessation. The log may provide clues regarding what conditions enable stimming to thrive. For example, does it happen mostly when there is more than one source of noise, or when it is nearing time for the next meal, or when a specific television show is on, or when there are two or more persons in the room, etc., etc., etc.

SECOND, but only if we are able to gain some prospective theories from our log, we can try to determine what emotions or stimuli are prevalent when the stimming starts. For example, if it occurs mostly when there is an overload of sounds, we may want to assume that stimming is a way of dealing with auditory overload and thus put in place things to lessen the frequency and intensity of such overloads. Or if it occurs mostly when it's nearing time for a specific activity, we may want to offer a substitute for dangerous stimming – such as offering a squeeze-toy.

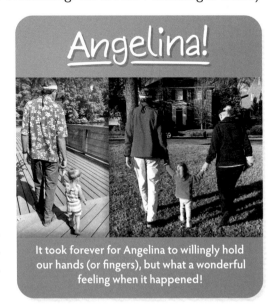
THIRD, if the previous two steps are successful, we can do a deeper evaluation of our log, consider additional theories, and offer a variety of things to substitute for harmful stimming.

The bottom line is that all of this takes a generous amount of time and thought. And stimming, unless it is harmful or dangerous, should be allowed and considered beneficial.

There is another thing about stimming that is especially worrisome to autism families: social isolation and bullying. Stimming can make it harder to attract friends and playmates, and can cause unfair and inaccurate judgments. Families can be proactive by explaining stimming to persons with whom their children socialize. The message is straightforward and has three parts. First, explain that the repetitive things are called stimming and that it's common among autistic persons. Second, observe that all of us stim; for example jiggling our feet while we're eating or tapping our fingers while we're waiting for something. And third, explain that stimming isn't an indication of intelligence or personality; it's just something that happens and is more noticeable among autistic persons.

As JC knows, whenever we take walks together, I like to find a long stick that I can use to poke at things, slap at bushes, punch the ground in cadence with my steps, make trails in the dirt or sand, etc. That's stimming. Ever find yourself tapping your fingers or humming? That's also stimming. Recent popular examples of stimming fidgets include those little spinners and push-pop toys: "fidget sensory toys" is the generic description.

There is an article in this morning's *Richmond Times-Dispatch* by Marcel Schwantes entitled, "BACK TO THE DRAWING BOARD?" The subtitle: "Research suggests doodling may spark creative juices at work." A lot of us doodle, not realizing that it's a type of stimming. The article: "According to a study by Drexel University . . . doodling can activate the reward pathways in the brain, which is known to boost mental health and creativity." And, "When you are facing a challenging project or problem at work and feel stuck, the solution may be to start doodling." And, certainly akin to stimming's effects for autistics, "Studies have shown that doodling can help reduce stress and create a focused mindset."

Years ago I attended a panel discussion that featured 4 famous American artists. Prior to the program a friend of mine placed a pencil and a pad of white paper on the table at each panelist's seat. After the event and the artists' departure he collected the left-behind pads, all of which contained stimming-doodles by the famous artists – albeit unsigned.

Angelina!

It took forever for Angelina to willingly hold our hands (or fingers), but what a wonderful feeling when it happened!

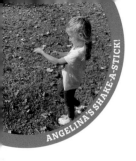

ANGELINA'S SHAKE-A-STICK!

Toilet Training

TOILET TRAINING IS OFTEN ONE OF THE MOST IMPACTFUL CHALLENGES for families of autistic children. Research has determined that children on the autism spectrum begin toilet training at an older age than do neurotypical children, and that it takes a lot longer. A 1992 study by Dalrymple and Ruble found that toilet training takes an average of 1.6 years, and longer for bowel training. I remember when Angelina was enrolled at The Faison Center and they told us they were going to initiate toilet training for her. I asked how long it would take (while thinking to myself six weeks or so) and they replied that they'd been working with one student on toilet training for nearly two years.

It is common for autistic children not to show "normal" signs of having to use the toilet, such as holding themselves, crossing their legs, nervous "dancing," etc. (Sometimes a child's "sign" is simply a certain way of looking at you.)

Frequency of bowel movements varies – from 2 or 3 per day to 2 or 3 per week. And it is common for children on the autism spectrum to "hold" the bowel movement until they are away from the toilet.

It is common for autistic children to have anxieties or fears associated with bathrooms: fear of a big hole with water in it, anxiety about being in a small enclosed room, sensitivity to the flushing sound, etc.

Medical problems should be ruled out prior to toilet training. (The child's developmental pediatrician can often do this.)

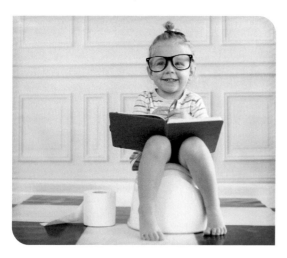

Praise and reward are often necessary for satisfactory long-term success and pride. Punishment and scolding usually negates self-pride and is counterproductive to long-term success.

Developing a toilet training plan requires extensive thought and research. The professionally developed and proven plans for toilet training for autistic children include details such as time schedules, visual aids, specific rewards, specific communication, types of praise and reward, necessary motor skills, hydration schedules, etc.

Praise can be very important, even for the small

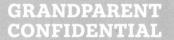

initial steps such as being able to sit on the toilet for five seconds. Sometimes rewards and special treats (favorite candy, use of the iPad, surprise toy, etc.) can be helpful. These were very helpful with Angelina's toilet training.

When there is an accident it's important to react and clean up in a matter-of-fact manner and without emotion. I remember once when I took Angelina to Story Time at a public library she had massive diarrhea in her pants. Fortunately, I was able to calmly take her to the family restroom, clean her, and change her clothes. (I always took along wipes and tissues and changes of clothes.) The key word is "calmly."

It can be helpful to document every aspect of toilet training (specific times each day, successes, accidents, circumstances that may have contributed to successes and accidents, etc.). I of course realize that such documentation isn't easily practical in most autism families.

The bottom line regarding toilet training is that it usually takes time, it requires loving patience, and sometimes it never happens.

There is a wealth of toilet training information on the Internet, including free online guides available from Autism Speaks, *Autism Parenting Magazine*, Marybarberra.com (private company that also sells things), and others.

Transitioning – A Common Big Challenge for Autistic Children

TRANSITIONING – CHANGING FROM ONE ACTIVITY OR SETTING TO ANOTHER – is a common challenge for autistic persons. They are often most comfortable with sameness and predictability; shifting attention from one thing to another in an environment that feels confusing and overwhelming can be not only a challenge but can cause a meltdown. Research has shown that approximately 25% of each day – whether at school, at home, at work, or wherever – is spent transitioning.

There are four things that can often help with transitioning.

1: **EXPLANATION** – Explain what the next thing (location, activity, project) will be. "Next we will go into the kitchen. The kitchen is the room where we prepare food for our meals. It has a refrig-

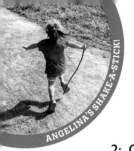
ANGELINA'S SHAKE-A-STICK!

erator and a stove . . . While there we will prepare our lunch."

2: **CUE** – A cue is a visual and/or verbal symbol for the next location or activity or project. For example, saying the word "kitchen," or showing a photo of the kitchen or the word "kitchen" written on a small card, are examples of cues. A cue can be a helpful part of a transition.

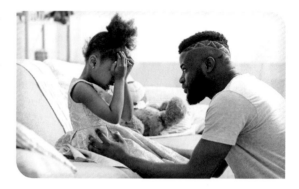

3: **COUNTDOWN** – A countdown is simply the allowance of a certain amount of time to pass between the cue and the actual transition. "In 3 minutes we will go to the kitchen . . . 2 minutes left . . . now only 1 minute . . . " The countdown can be long or short depending on the type of transition. For example, if you are at a playground getting ready to go home, you may use a 10-minute countdown: "In 10 minutes we will go home, so enjoy these remaining minutes here at the playground. . . Still 9 minutes left to play . . . etc." A clock can be an effective countdown device if the person understands clock movements. If not, there is a clock-like device called a Time-Timer that shows the remaining time in an ever-shrinking section of red. Another idea is to use color Post-It notes that are removed each minute. Regardless, a countdown of some sort can be helpful. But one warning. Phrases such as "Just a second," "In a minute," and "In a while" are often not easy for an autistic child to comprehend appropriately. It's best to stick to precise time intervals.

4: **POSITIVE REINFORCEMENT** – "Wonderful! You walked into the kitchen without any problems. I am so proud of you! Here is a special sticker." Positive reinforcement can consist of praise or a reward (candy, screen time, etc.) or both. "You did so well leaving the playground, and I'm proud of you. As a reward, you can now play with your Amazon Fire."

GRANDPARENT CONFIDENTIAL

"My daughter and her autistic child just moved in with me so I can help. I need to learn more."

Successful transitioning is often not as simple as those four steps, but they can provide an effective foundation.

Autistic persons often have trouble with sequencing and understanding relationships between steps, so when transitioning it's best to focus on as few steps as possible. Also, autistic persons often don't recognize "clues" to forthcoming transitions: other students packing their backpacks, putting purchased items into the bag at the store, etc. Thus the need for cues, etc.

A variety of factors can contribute to the difficulty level of a specific transition: length of time, enjoyability, loudness, crowdedness, etc.

In Nancy Mucklow's book, *Grandparent's Guide to Autism Spectrum Disorders,* she offers "The Ten-Second Room Zoom." When you take your child to a new place, stop at the entrance and narrate what you see and what you're thinking: "This room has a lot of people, some sitting and some standing and some walking around. We will have to decide which we will do. And we will want to move carefully so we don't bump into other people . . ." She notes that this raises awareness and helps them learn to transition to specific situations.

And finally, it's a good idea to always have a meltdown contingency plan – what you'll do in case of a meltdown.

The bottom line is that transitions are often problematical for autistic persons.

Education About Sexuality

THE WEBSITE OF THE AUTISM SOCIETY OF MINNESOTA contains information about the importance of educating autistic persons about sexuality. The Society gave me permission to share the information with the readers of this book. The title of the Society's information is, "7 Things to Know about ASD and Sexuality Education," and it includes the following:

Sexuality is a natural and healthy part of being human. All humans have the right to their sexuality and to express their sexuality in a safe and comfortable way. Sexuality is a multidimensional construct, of which sexual well-being is one component.

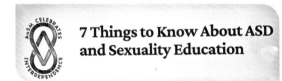

According to the World Health Organization, sexual well-being is defined as "not only the absence of sexual problems and inappropriate sexual behavior, but also a positive orientation to the emotional, psychological, and social aspects of sexuality."

1: Autistic individuals vary across the sexuality spectrum; they are not inherently asexual (an umbrella term referring to lack of sexual attraction).

2: Studies indicate that autistic individuals report higher rates of gender variance and non-heterosexuality than non-autistic individuals. Studies also indicate that autistic individuals who are non-heterosexual and/or gender non-conforming have increased health disparities.

3: Autistic children and adults experience disproportionately high rates of victimization, including sexual assault, in comparison to non-autistic peers.

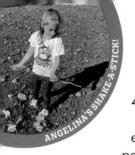

ANGELINA'S SHAKE-A-STICK!

4: Autistic individuals are less likely to receive information related to sexuality education from caregivers, school, and peers. This impedes access to sexuality education and restricts sexual well-being. A lack of sexual knowledge has been shown to be one factor related to increased risk of victimization. The most common perpetrators against individuals with developmental disabilities are service providers, acquaintances, neighbors, family members, and peers with disabilities.

5: Sexuality education is important regardless of a person's interest in gender expression, romantic relationships, or sexual activity.

6: Sexuality education promotes independence, safety, self-awareness, and self-determination for autistic individuals.

7: Sexuality curricula should be adapted to account for the challenges and strengths of autistic individuals, incorporate the use of evidence-based practices, and be delivered proactively.

Puberty

UBERTY IS OF COURSE WHEN EVERYTHING CHANGES – especially physically and emotionally. There are three fundamental rules for helping an autistic child navigate puberty. First, be explicit, literal, and graphic in providing very detailed information to the child. Second, be patient and understanding regarding the arrival of extreme and unpredictable emotions. And third, start preparing the child well before the onset of puberty – as early as 10 years old.

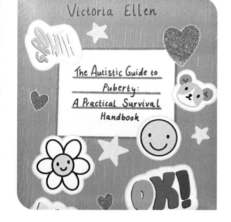

Puberty is of course filled with complexities, but they can be grouped into four categories.

Physical Changes

You will want to very carefully explain (repeatedly) – with photos and videos – each of the expected physical changes. For both sexes this includes the arrival of the enhanced need for cleanliness: daily bathing (including detailed washing instructions), use of daily deodorant (including electing a preferred scent), facial scrubbing (acne), etc. It also includes the arrival of hair in new places and precise, demonstrated instruction on shaving (electric razor for safety).

Educate girls about the arrival and growth of breasts, including details about bras. Educate girls about menstruation and their periods, and detailed information on how to use tampons and pads (including checking to see if they change them).

Educate boys about erections and wet dreams. And educate both boys and girls about masturbation: that it's okay to do it alone privately, but not in public or in the presence of anyone else. Also educate boys and girls about sexual arousal – that it's normal, and how to react and how not to react.

Again, it's important to be very specific, including the use of visual images, with explanations of physical changes.

Emotional and Social Changes

It's important to be aware that many autistic children experience high levels of stress and anxiety during puberty. Higher functioning children can be especially susceptible to thoughts and/or actions regarding suicide. And social acceptance is a commonly increasing challenge for autistic children as they enter puberty. Parents can often lessen or even prevent much of this stress and anxiety by doing the following, well in advance of puberty: enlisting the child in interest-based groups such as music ensembles, sports teams (player or manager), church organizations, game clubs, art classes, etc.; and/or getting professional social skills training regarding responses to social cues, what to discuss at the lunch table, etc. And of course sometimes medications can be helpful, but careful consideration should be given as to whether the benefits outweigh the often serious side effects.

Educational Changes

During puberty years educational expectations shift from memorization and repetition to more abstract thinking: discussion of "meanings," analyzing events, creative writing, etc. – all of which present significant challenges for many autistic children. This is often the time for shifting IEP accommodations (such as giving more time on tests), for individual tutoring, and even transferring to a school that can provide better services for autistic children. It can also be a time for consideration of a future educational path directed toward specific employment opportunities.

Thinking about Adulthood

It is during middle school that autism families should begin serious consideration of the eventual transition from school (accompanied by a variety of publicly-funded supports), to adulthood (when most publicly-funded supports vanish). Read Bradford Hulcher's article in this book: "Preparing for Life after High School – Avoiding the Cliff."

And Finally . . .

Google can lead you to a wealth of information regarding puberty. I recommend that you start with the Child Mind Institute's (childmind.org) section entitled, "Autism and Puberty," that's written by Caroline Miller with consultation from clinical expert Dr. Margaret Dyson. And Google will also lead you to a variety of books regarding puberty. For boys, you may want to consider, *What's Happening to Tom?*, by Kate E. Reynolds. For girls (and for Angelina), I've purchased *The Autistic Guide to Puberty*, by Victoria Ellen.

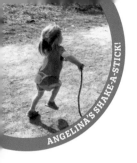

ANGELINA'S SHAKE-A-STICK!

Autistic Children in Public Places

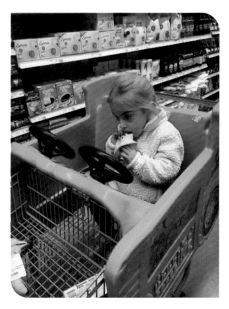

AKING AUTISTIC CHILDREN TO PUBLIC PLAC-ES – grocery stores, restaurants, playgrounds, medical offices, etc. – can offer unpredictable challenges.

Public places can present a smorgasbord of sensory information that can produce significant stress. This can result in difficult and even dangerous behaviors. The general public usually doesn't realize that "effective parenting techniques" often don't apply to autism, and thus autistic children can be the focus of judgment from strangers.

One of Angelina's regular outings is for healthcare appointments. She does great now, but there used to be significant problems. She usually screamed, always had to be forcibly held to be weighed and measured, fought blood pressure and temperature gauges, and on and on. And everything about dental appointments was just awful.

But the good thing about healthcare appointments is that many healthcare workers now have empathy and understanding – but that's usually not the case with other public settings. So how can we prepare and what can we do?

Here are some suggestions:

- **Role Play** – At home go through the motions of what the forthcoming public outing might be: entering the grocery store, getting the cart, selecting items for purchase, checking out, etc.

- **Start Small** – The initial grocery store outing might include simply parking and walking across the parking lot and entering – then immediately leaving and going home.

- **Involve** – For example, get the child to put the items in the cart. (Angelina loves doing this.)

- **Distract** – Have a favorite toy ready if needed.

- **Reward** – A favorite candy or use of the iPad.

- **What about significant negative behaviors such as a full-blown meltdown?** How can we prepare? What can we do? Following are some things to consider:

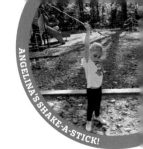

- **Teach and practice some basic things** such as walking together and standing in line.

- **Scout out the location in advance** – and/or call and ask questions.

- **If a bad situation does happen, s**top everything and make the child's safety your priority. And stay calm.

- **Ask bystanders to help:** "My child is autistic; it will help if you can give us some space." Or, "Can you please remove [dangerous object] from this area?" Or, "Please get the manager." Or, "Please call 911."

- **Some parents carry explanatory cards to give to nearby strangers:** "My child is autistic. She is not misbehaving." There are some excellent examples of cards on Pinterest.

- **The website of RWJBarnabus Health (rwjbh.org) Children's Specialized Hospital** has great information about public outings and also has links to other sites that provide helpful information regarding managing challenging behaviors in public places.

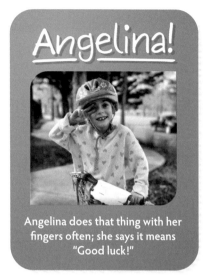

Angelina!

Angelina does that thing with her fingers often; she says it means "Good luck!"

If you're like me, you're anxious regarding public outings with autistic children. Will she "behave"? Will she do inappropriate things that involve other persons? What "rewards" should I have handy? And if you're like me, it's so much easier to just stay at home and forego any public outings – but of course public outings are helpful for the child's continued progress in being able to relate to "normal" society.

Helpful information can also be found on the website of Autism Speaks: https://www.autismspeaks. org/expert-opinion/parents-child-autism-seek-help-public-meltdowns

Meltdown at the Post Office

SPEAKING OF MELTDOWNS, yesterday while I was waiting in line at the post office a middle-aged couple came in with a girl – presumably their daughter – who looked to be around 13 or 14 years old. The couple looked tired. The girl, although dressed nicely, looked disheveled: messy hair, untied shoes, etc. She was wearing noise-cancelling headphones and she was struggling to loosen her hand from her mother's grip. I watched as she struggled harder, broke loose, and then started shouting and flapping her arms and stomping her feet. The father managed to grasp her and

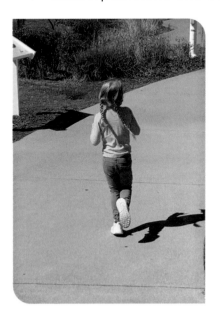

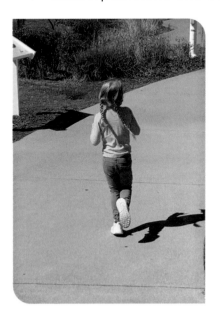ANGELINA'S SHAKE-A-STICK!

sort of carry her out of the post office while the mother stayed.

All of which caused me to regret not having said something to them. Maybe, "Let me know if I can be helpful." Or maybe to the stay-behind mother, "Please get in front of me in the line; I'm not in a hurry."

I've learned that often the worst thing I can do to "help" an autistic child who is a stranger and is having a meltdown is to give physical involvement without being asked: saying "calming" words to the child, providing a calming touch or hug, giving a small toy or sticker, etc. And often the best thing I can do is to help clear the area of sensory challenges: moving obstructions, opening doors, turning off background music, dimming lights, etc. Yesterday at the post office I could have even said to the line of waiting persons, "Let's all let her go in front of us." And I could have tried to catch the mother's eye to offer a smile.

Maybe next time.

Elopement

VARIOUS STUDIES HAVE FOUND THAT AROUND 50% OF AUTISTIC CHILDREN have eloped or have tried to. And of course many autistic children attempt elopement on a regular basis. Elopement means wandering or running – without permission – away from caregivers or secure locations. It's often difficult to determine the reason for a specific episode, but it's usually for one of four reasons: to get away from a stressful situation, to get to a desired thing or place, because the act of running relieves stress, or because of the sheer enjoyment of running or being chased. Elopement is of course always cause for concern: such as suddenly running into the street, leaving a school classroom to go outside, even exiting a vehicle.

Families who have concerns about elopement install locks and alarms on all exits of the home, including windows. And when outside of the home they employ harnesses, walking reins, and car harnesses. They dress their children in bright clothing so they can be seen better if they elope. And they attach tracking devices to their children. (Google can locate many brands and styles.)

Families tell their neighbors about the possibility of elope-

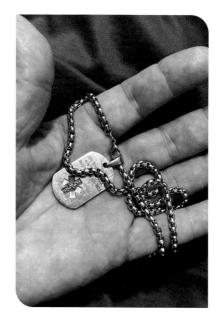

ment, and they give their neighbors info sheets with the child's name and photo, telephone numbers of caregivers, the child's communication abilities, advice for calming the child, and a list of places where the child has eloped to in the past. Families also have similar sheets available to give to police and other searchers if the child can't be quickly found.

There is no easy remedy for elopement. Sometimes psychologists and behavior analysts can provide therapies or exercises that can be helpful, such as "Stop" drills: sessions that encourage the child to stop when he hears the word said with a specific tone and loudness.

Elopement is a serious cause for concern, and each of a child's caretakers should be well educated regarding the safeguards and search procedures.

A Necessity for Emergencies

SEVERAL YEARS AGO I STARTED WEARING A MED-ICAL ID NECKLACE – you know, one of those tags with a caduceus along with contact and medical info. I was in good health, but I just wanted to make sure that info was available to anyone who might encounter me if I were incapacitated from some type of emergency.

I've become as attached to the necklace as my cell phone. I don't go anywhere without it. And I've become an advocate for everyone, regardless of age or health, wearing such identification. It would surely make things easier for EMTs and others – plus it would likely save lives.

Which makes me wonder why I haven't yet been proactive in seeing that Angelina has something similar. She goes to school, plays in parks, goes swimming, rides in cars, and does all sorts of normal things that might present an emergency for which that information could be helpful if not life-saving.

Autistic persons often lack danger awareness, are often prone to wandering, and often have health issues. Plus, autism is not easily identified by first responders. Some autistic persons are nonverbal and/or have intellectual disabilities. And anyone can be overwhelmed by emergency situations and unable to communicate clearly. And these days, since schools have to keep up with every student's allergies, a wristband or bracelet can be a great way to always have that information readily available.

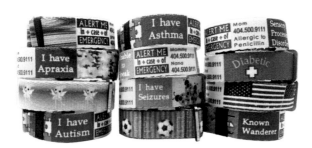

Autism Speaks is a good first stop for learning about the various options: https://www.autism-speaks.org/safety-products-and-services.

I've learned that there are many options for wristbands and bracelets, including a variety of colors and designs. I suspect that Angelina would pick something in her favorite color, pink. And they can be customized to match anyone's interests.

Do you know what ICE means? In Case of Emergency. The ICE telephone number is the most important piece of information for any wristband or bracelet. After that, there should be name, diagnosis, medications, and allergies. Some bracelets offer a QR code option: anyone who scans it will link to a site with all of the information. And there are all sorts of GPS tracking devices that can be attached to clothing, inserted in backpacks, etc. It would be great to know where your child is if the bus she is riding on doesn't show up on time.

There are also anklets, patches, pins, clips, ID cards, shoe tags, etc. But the most important thing is to use something that won't (can't) be removed and that is waterproof, convenient, and comfortable.

If your child is resistant to the whole idea, you can start by wearing something similar yourself and talking about it and being happily proud of it.

Then you can use the small-step-by-small-step method to attract the child's interest and enthusiasm. First, show the wristband and ask the child to simply TOUCH it. "Wonderful! You did it! I'm so proud of you!" Then, later or perhaps the next day, "Now let's put it around your wrist and leave it there while I count to three." Then more praise. You get the idea. And sometimes a visible timer can help. And of course rewards (special candy, special TV show, etc.) are often helpful.

You can make up stories to help introduce your child to the wristband. For example: "Can you say hello to this little wristband? His name is Charlie and he is very lonely and sad. He doesn't have any friends and nobody will play with him. Would you like to hold him?" And you can go from there . . . Eventually Charlie and your child may become inseparable.

Just two rules about getting your child to wear an identification device: make it fun and don't give up.

Is there any downside to wearing such identification? I've learned that some persons believe that it can be like placing an unfair "label" on someone. (Like my medical necklace perhaps labeling me as old or sick.) I prefer to view it as a statement rather than a label. And the statement is the same for everyone: In case I need help in an emergency, I want to make it easier for the helpers to help me.

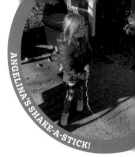

Children don't fully understand that all sorts of emergencies are possible each day, and that an identification band can be a lifesaver. And if you're like me, you'll first get your own bracelet or necklace.

Medication for Autism

MEDICINES HAVE BEEN EFFECTIVE WITH AUTISTIC PERSONS in reducing self-injury, aggression, irritability, repetitive behaviors, anxiety, tantrums, depression, obsessive-compulsive behaviors, hyperactivity, withdrawal, lack of focus, panic disorders, seizures, etc.

There are ten basic things that autism families need to know:

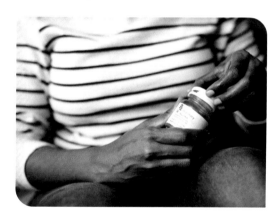

1: No medication cures autism. Even though some medications can help with challenging behaviors, no medicine has yet been found effective at <u>eliminating</u> any problem behavior.

2: All of the few dozen medicines that are prescribed for autism behaviors come with negative side effects, and some with very serious side effects.

3: All medicines for autism are most effective when combined with non-medicine therapies.

GRANDPARENT CONFIDENTIAL

"My 4-year-old autistic grandson gets speech therapy and OT and takes medicine for seizures. I'm looking for other grandparents who can commiserate and help me learn things."

4: Medicines for autism are always prescribed on a trial basis. It may take weeks or even months to determine whether a specific medicine is helpful and what dosage maximizes its effectiveness.

5: In many cases it's best to use only one medicine at a time.

6: Medicine should be tried only when non-medicine therapies have been ineffective.

7: Medicines for autism are expensive, so you should determine whether there is insurance coverage.

8: There are six major reasons for using medicine if other therapies have not helped sufficiently: aggression and/or

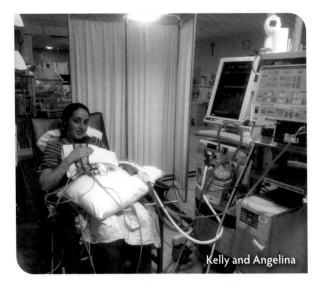

self-injury, too much stress at home and/or elsewhere, problems at school, problems with community activities, problems that affect learning, and problems that affect sleep.

9: The following four things are usually not helped by medicines: following directions, slow learning, communication skills including speaking, and social skills.

10: All members of the child's "team" should be informed about the child's medicines: teachers, therapists, caregivers, healthcare providers, etc.

AND FINALLY, autistic children with ADHD are often prescribed Ritalin and/or Adderall. Families should be aware of the potential problems with both. A good place to start is *Scientific American's* April 24, 2017 article, "Autism's Drug Problem." https://www.scientificamerican.com/article/autisms-drug-problem

Angelina's Story: 130 Days in the NICU

ANGELINA'S DELIVERY WAS FOLLOWED BY 130 DAYS IN THE NICU (Neonatal Intensive Care Unit, and actually the final few days in the Pediatric Intensive Care Unit because the NICU overflowed) and lots of scares and emergencies and procedures and surgeries and on and on. (Wish we'd had Angelina's Shake-A-Stick!) Kelly, JC, and I took turns spending lots of time in the NICU with Angelina. She was always attached to various wires and tubes and was usually bandaged in various places. We all came to know and love the NICU nurses. I still recall the day Angelina reached two pounds; it felt like a huge hurdle had been accomplished. Of course she didn't yet

Kelly and Angelina

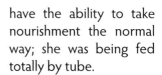

have the ability to take nourishment the normal way; she was being fed totally by tube.

We eventually learned to be sort of comfortable with the rhythms of the NICU: the continual sounds of warning buzzers and bells, the continual scurry of nurses and

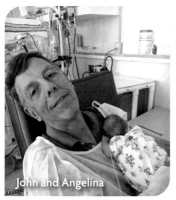

John and Angelina

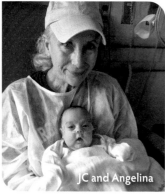

JC and Angelina

respiratory therapists and other healthcare professionals, the continual view of Angelina's machines and monitors – and being anxious about their meanings . . .

Marijuana and Autism

DID YOU SEE THE TELEVISED "CNN SPECIAL REPORT: WEED 6: MARIJUANA AND AUTISM"? This hour-long program featured CNN Chief Medical Correspondent Dr. Sanjay Gupta (a brain surgeon in Atlanta) visiting with and interviewing autism families that have been helped by marijuana, and medical researchers who are involved in a variety of clinical trial studies of the effects of marijuana on persons with autism. The findings thus far are stunningly encouraging.

The program featured specific autistic children who exhibited aggression, self-injurious behaviors, repetitive behaviors, and a lack of social communication and interaction. Their parents had – mostly illegally – experimented with exposing their children to marijuana, and in every case there were positive results. There was significant decrease in irritability, meltdowns, aggression, and self-injurious behaviors. And there was improvement in the ability to speak and communicate.

BUT . . . but. . . .

Even though marijuana is now legal in many states, it is largely unregulated. It's impossible to know much about its specific variety, its concentration of CBD and THC, whether it has been exposed to dangerous herbicides, and whether it has experienced sanitized handling and packaging.

The parents featured on the CNN program had no real guidelines regarding marijuana doses, fre-

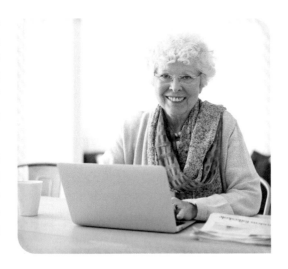

quencies, etc. They often relied on advice posted on the Internet by other parents.

The program pointed out that in most cases of profound autism, the commonly prescribed medicines are those used for psychotic patients and other similar cases, and that all of those medicines come with significant side effects. The program noted that marijuana is mostly absent of bad side effects.

The program advised that, because of so many unknowns, marijuana use is not yet advisable for autistic persons. But there is hope that there will one day be FDA-approved marijuana use for many of the challenges that come with autism.

FaceTime with Autistic Children

SOMETIMES I'LL DO FACETIME WITH ANGELINA, but since she lives in our city and since we see her all the time, FaceTiming certainly isn't a requirement for our relationship. But for folks who live at a distance and whose best option for face-to-face interaction is FaceTime (grandparents, relatives, friends), I've learned some useful tips.

But first it's important to realize that autistic children often have challenges interpreting cues such as tone of voice and facial expressions. And nonverbal children may use sign language and/or language devices that we don't know how to use. But it's is possible for us to have meaningful FaceTime interactions.

Just three rules:

1. **PLAN THE CALL IN ADVANCE.** The normal "How are you doing?" or "Tell me what you did today?" or "When are you coming to see me again?" types of random conversation often don't result in engaging interaction. It's best to plan something that is immediately engaging.

2. **HAVE LOW EXPECTATIONS (but high hopes).** The first FaceTime call may well result in zero interaction; it often takes time and persistence to develop a strategy for meaningful FaceTime calls.

3. **MAKE IT SHORT.** A one-minute happy and engaging interaction is cause for celebration; a five-minute, one-sided "conversation" isn't cause for celebration.

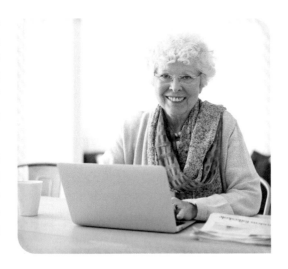

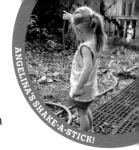

How do you plan for a FaceTime call? It's often best to base the call on something that the child likes: a favorite movie ("Frozen"?), a favorite topic (dinosaurs?), a favorite activity (bowling?), a favorite celebrity or group (the Wiggles?), a favorite relative (his mother?), etc.

Angelina loves Peppa Pig, so I gain her immediate attention and interaction when I begin a FaceTime session while holding a Peppa Pig figure and having it "talk" to her.

If the child likes cooking or helping to cook, perhaps the following would be a successful 3-minute FaceTime experience. "See this carton of eggs? I need your help. How many eggs should I crack so I can cook scrambled eggs? Ok, now watch carefully so you can give me advice on how to crack them . . . And I want to add some milk. I'll start pouring and you tell me when to stop . . . You tell me when it's time to scoop them out of the frying pan . . ."

Making silly faces can sometimes be a way to both entertain and engage autistic children. "Let's see who can make the happiest face." "Let's see who can make the angriest face." "Let's see who can make the silliest face." You get the idea.

You may also want to consider making your FaceTime interaction a part of the child's ongoing routine: "FaceTime with Nana" – Thursday afternoons at 4pm. Or "Silly Faces with Nana," or "Peppa Pig with Nana," or "Storytime with Nana," etc.

OR, perhaps the child likes to talk about his own special interests. This may well provide your opening for wonderful FaceTime interactions: "Hi Devon! I'm calling because I need you to give me an update on your dinosaur collection." Or, "I called to hear your latest song." Or, "I need to find out what your dog has been doing."

Once you find a successful strategy, you may be able to gradually increase the length of the call and make it more and more interactive. The important thing is to have endearing interactions.

Additional topics/strategies for FaceTime:

- **ARTS/CRAFTS** – "Cut a Snowflake With Nana"

- **FAVORITE TOYS**– "Toy Time With Nana"

- **PACKAGED GIFTS** – Fill a box with a toy or toys and wrap and address it on FaceTime. Then FaceTime again when he receives and unwraps it.

- **FUNNY NOISES** – See who can laugh the loudest or make sounds of farm animals or make clicks and gurgles, etc.

- **EXERCISE OR YOGA** – Angelina likes to copy JC's yoga ex-

GRANDPARENT CONFIDENTIAL

"My 6-year-old grandson lives in another state and won't do FaceTime or Zoom, and his mother doesn't relate to me and doesn't try to get him to either. When I visit, although he's very sweet, it takes a day or so for him to warm up to me. I wish I could be more involved with his life."

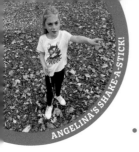

ercises (often engaged for as long as 15 minutes).

- • DANCING – You can copy each other's dance moves.

- TEA PARTY – Get out your cups and saucers at both ends of the line.

- MEAL – Eat together.

- I SPY – Move your camera around your residence to "spy" things.

- PUPPET SHOW – Use toy animals or figurines.

- STUFFED ANIMALS DANCE TO MUSIC – Favorite songs.

And finally, if you're not successful at first, keep trying. Don't give up after one or two or three tries. Often it takes several attempts before arriving at a successful strategy for meaningful FaceTime. But it will be worth it!

Social Media: Should We Display our Autistic Children?

ARE YOU LIKE ME IN PROUDLY POSTING IMAGES AND INFORMATION about your family, including autistic children, on social media? Do you agree with me that social media is a great way to keep folks updated about the amazing doings of autistic children (my granddaughter Angelina)? And are you like me in never (until now) having developed a social media policy or set of guidelines regarding posting that information? And finally, are you like me in never (until now) having done much research regarding the dangers of social media?

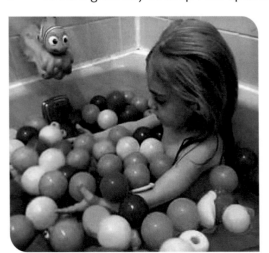

I've now investigated five categories of bad stuff – most of which JC and I had never really thought about. After all, JC and I raised our own children before there was social media.

BAD PEOPLE – There are dangerous folks out there. Photos of children are continually "borrowed" from social media and then used for awful purposes such

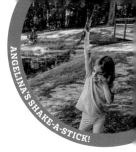

as on child porn sites and accompanied by awful captions and information. Other dangerous folks have involvements in custody battles and abuse situations, and they can determine where to find children by looking at location tags and landmarks in social media images.

DIGITAL KIDNAPPING – There are folks out there who "kidnap" photos and videos of children and give them whole new identities. Research has found that some of these folks are childless persons who use social media to give the impression that they have children.

POLITICS – I may think that posting a photo of Angelina holding a sign in favor of my favorite political candidate is important, but I haven't (until now) considered that when she gets older she may resent it. Or worse, it may cause others to assume incorrect things about her and her family. I now realize that it's not a good idea for me to post anything about Angelina that relates to politics.

BULLYING – Angelina is 8 years old now, but what if, when she is 24, one of her friends discovers that "cute" video that I posted of her trying to crack eggs for breakfast? And what if her friend shares it with her own friends and they share it with theirs and on and on? And what if Angelina is embarrassed by it? And what if everyone starts calling her a "cute" nickname that they came up with because of the eggs? You see where this is going . . . And much, much worse: the photo of her playing in the bubble bath, the video of her screaming, the story about her and the squirrel . . . What if a future potential employer discovers the old posts as she is being evaluated for possible employment?

OWNERSHIP – Who "owns" the rights to Angelina's image and information? Up until now, I've operated as if I own those rights whenever I'm taking care of her. I now believe that I am wrong. I believe that she owns those rights and that when I'm caring for her I need to be her "advocate" and act only in her best interest. As soon as any child is able to have even an introductory understanding of this specific concept of ownership (research shows that this happens as early as age 5), our social media posts may cause the child to feel that they don't have their deserved level of control over what gets posted about them on social media.

In spite of these bad things, I suspect that JC and I will continue to post photos and videos and information regarding Angelina, mainly because it's a way to keep our friends and family updated and also to let them know how proud we are of her.

But beginning now, JC and I will do the following things.

FIRST, we will discuss this with Kelly and Justen and will adhere to whatever "rules" they offer.

SECOND, we will begin involving Angelina in discussions about posting stuff about her on social media.

AND THIRD, we'll develop a written set of guidelines for our social media postings about Angelina.

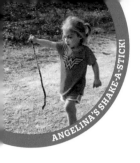

ANGELINA'S SHAKE-A-STICK!

Being Your Child's (or Grandchild's) Champion

"**CAN'T YOU CONTROL YOUR CHILD?**" It's common for autism families to hear such comments and receive strange looks when they take their children to public places. Rather than viewing these situations as things to escape and avoid, they can be viewed as opportunities for advocacy.

Advocacy simply means getting others to understand your point of view and then agreeing with it and accommodating it. Autistic children are usually unable to do this for themselves; families can embrace the responsibility of doing it on their behalf.

Following are five specific areas of advocacy that are appropriate.

IMMEDIATE FAMILY – Parents can be wonderful advocates with the autistic child's siblings. "You know, your brother is autistic and that's why he . . ." "We love you just as much as your brother, but because he is autistic he sometimes requires more of our time and attention."

EXTENDED FAMILY – Families should never simply assume that extended family members "understand." They probably don't. Parents can take on the responsibility of preparing the extended family for holiday gatherings and reunions, and for telling them how to relate to, and what to expect from, the autistic child.

FRIENDS – Families can and should talk about their autistic child and her needs and mannerisms to their close friends and to persons with whom they confide and socialize. There are three reasons for this. First, it educates them and broadens their understanding of the diversity of the greater community. Second, it gives them an understanding of the child and prepares them for encounters with her. And third, it gives them a better understanding of the family's priorities and challenges. Families shouldn't just assume that their close friends already understand. They don't. Families need to speak up. Friends will appreciate and value it.

PUBLIC PLACES – It's normal for autism families to be anxious about exposing autistic children to the general public: parks and stores and public transportation and all sorts of errands and meetings. But every encounter with the public is a potential opportunity for advocacy – for families to educate someone about autism. It's normal for families to avoid such opportunities, but it's sometimes better to embrace them. Almost always when folks understand a challenging situation they are happy to help. It can be as straightforward as, "My child isn't misbehaving, she is autistic. Her brain is wired differently and she has trouble doing . . . I wonder if you could help me by . . ." When persons hear advocacy explanations, they are especially receptive and understanding.

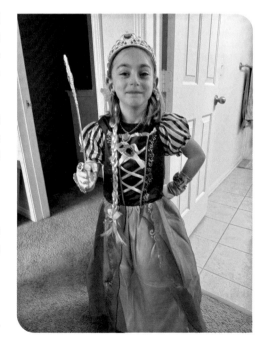

The key to good advocacy with the general public is to plan in advance. What might an autistic child do that will cause the need for advocacy? A meltdown? An encounter with another child? Something dangerous? No matter how "good" the child usually is in public, things that require advocacy will occasionally happen, and it's good to be prepared. What if the child hits another child? What if there is a meltdown in a retail establishment? It's often so much better to say something rather than to simply exit the situation without saying anything. Folks appreciate being able to understand.

Autistic children benefit greatly by being able to advocate for themselves. And families can help them learn to self-advocate. It can be as fundamental as helping a non-speaking child learn to point at the thing she wants or needs. Or it can be as sophisticated as helping her know how to best explain to her teacher that she can benefit from receiving an assignment in a different format.

Autism Speaks has developed a comprehensive "Advocacy Tool Kit" that includes a lot of important guidance regarding advocacy related to legal, educational, medical, financial, and therapeutic purposes. It can be downloaded free from their website (autismspeaks.org).

Superheroes

ANGELINA LOVES SUPERHEROES – and sometimes she strikes the pose as she imagines herself as a superhero. And she enjoys describing her super power. One time it was the ability to stomp really hard like dinosaurs.

I've learned that it's common for autistic persons to relate to superheroes. And I've found a website (goteamkate.com) that has a blog entry that provides a 5-reason answer as to why:

1: Superheroes have an alter-ego.

"Just like children on the spectrum, superheroes live two distinct existences: the one inside their complex brains and the one for the outside world."

2: Superheroes can be solitary.

"Superheroes tend to live a very solitary life. Few Su-

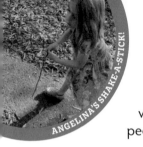

ANGELINA'S SHAKE-A-STICK!

pers can relate to the average person because of their vastly different lifestyles. For kiddos on the spectrum, peers are great, but can be quite difficult to relate to."

3: Superheroes have "special" abilities and/or downfalls.

"This is key. Superheroes have super-sensitive hearing, sight, or strength, among other powers. Children on the spectrum also report many of the same abilities, only the real world application of such powers can result in sensory overload."

4: Superhero language is often scripted and therefore safe.

"Sometimes it can be so hard to know what to say or how to react. Catch phrases such as Buzz's 'To Infinity and Beyond' and TMNT's 'Go Ninja, Go Ninja, Go Ninja Go' can often fill in when the right words just cannot be found. These phrases will often encourage a positive response from others and they are safe and reliable forms of communication."

5: Superheroes are awesome.

"Everyone loves a superhero. So why not adopt the persona of someone that evokes love and adoration from the masses? When it's tough to fit in, our little people have to find a way to stand out and still reach the rest of us."

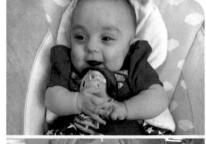

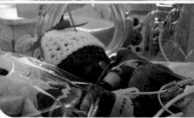

A Wonder Woman doll was Angelina's companion during her long stay in the NICU; when she was released she was finally able to hold it.

[CAUTION: Although I like the website, goteamkate.com, its writer (no information about her/him is provided) is not shy about using "colorful" language: the f-word, the s-word, and probably most of the other alphabet words.]

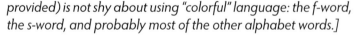

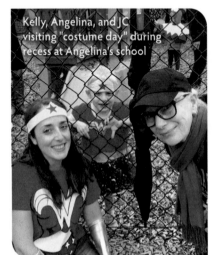

Kelly, Angelina, and JC visiting "costume day" during recess at Angelina's school

In 2018 NBC television featured Lee Bradshaw and his son Jake who is autistic. Lee helped Jake create a superhero comic book series that's still going strong: *JAKE JETPULSE*. The books are easy to read and contain at-home activities that are meant to appeal to autistic kids. I recommend them.

All of which suggests the obvious idea of us working with our own autistic children to develop their own superhero personas along with accompanying stories. I foresee lots of benefits for both Angelina and me.

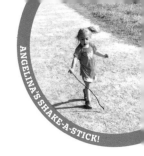

Water Safety and Swimming

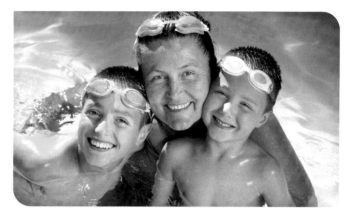

A LEADING CAUSE OF DEATH IN AUTISM-RELATED WANDERING CASES is drowning in nearby lakes, streams, neighborhood pools, and the ocean. And in the general population, 90 percent of childhood drownings occur when the parent is present but is not paying attention.

Water safety skills and swimming safety are two different things.

Water safety skills are analogous to street-smart skills: when to cross the street, looking both ways, no running, etc. Following are the three basics for small children. And it's great if you can practice these skills over and over again at a variety of waters and places.

1:   Don't go near any water without holding an adult's hand.

2:   Always walk (no running, skipping, jumping, etc.) when near water.

3:   Always wear a lifejacket when in any type of boat.

Following are basic guidelines for swimming safety and skills.

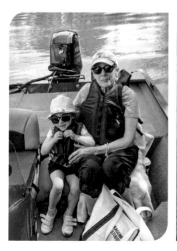 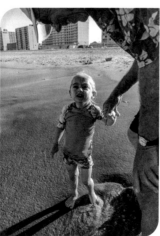

1:   No matter how well you swim, never swim unless a <u>supervising</u> adult is present.

2:   Never jump into unknown water (an unfamiliar swimming pool, lake, pond, or stream). Always wade in slowly.

3:   Don't try to swim in water that is deeper than your shoulders unless you've learned the following skills: able to jump into water over your head; float or tread water for one minute; swim 25 yards without stopping; and exit from a pool without using the ladder.

Teaching your child with autism how to swim AND helping them develop water safety skills from a young age is critical. Water safety and swimming lessons are not the same thing. Water safety describes precautions taken when around any body of water to keep your family safe. Practicing water safety helps reduce the risk of drowning for your child.

Families can do the following to help keep autistic children safe.

1: Enroll your child in autism-friendly swimming lessons. (Here in Richmond, we're fortunate to have a huge and wonderful facility called SwimRVA that hosts everything from Olympic-pool major competitions to shallow-pool children's parties. Although SwimRVA offers autism-specific swim lessons, Angelina took lessons in one of their neurotypical swim classes. The instructors were wonderful! As I write this, Angelina has signed up for one of SwimRVA's week-long summer camp experiences.)

2: Use social stories to reenforce the water safety and swimming safety guidelines listed above. "Social Stories" are pretend stories that simulate given situations: "There was a little girl named Leena who had a swimming pool in her neighborhood . . ."

3: Regularly practice the skills with your child.

4: Use praise to reinforce progress.

5: Stay close to your child when she is in the water.

6: Avoid distractions such as your mobile phone.

7: Learn the signs of drowning: gasping or hyperventilating, mouth at or below the surface, eyes closed, face covered by hair, no leg movement.

8: Learn CPR and first aid.

The bottom line is of course that all types of waters are dangerous. Children are often attracted to water, and parents should give priority attention to water safety and swimming safety.

Waterbowl Activity for Children

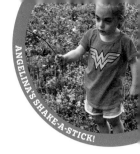

THE WEBSITE WWW.TEACHERSPAYTEACHERS. COM ISN'T FOCUSED ON AUTISTIC CHILDREN, but it does provide links to activities and exercises that were great for Angelina when she was younger. One that is easy and inexpensive is one that I call *"Wet Pom Poms."* I bought all of the required materials at Wal-Mart for just under $15.

Here's the list:

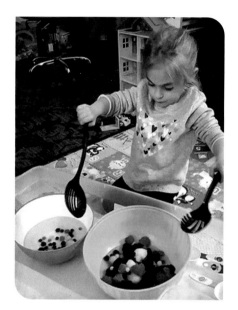

- 2 small bags of multi-size, multi-color pom-poms

- 3 plastic bowls of different sizes

- 3 plastic ladles and/or measuring cups of different sizes

- 1 plastic shoe-storage bin (no top)

The set-up is easy. Put the 3 plastic bowls into the plastic storage bin. Put the pom poms and some water into the largest bowl. Then give the child the ladles and cups and watch what happens.

Angelina would begin by spending time scooping pom poms back and forth from bowl to bowl. This helped develop her hand/eye coordination, manual dexterity, and concentration. Later she would start using her hands to scoop the pom poms and would learn things including how to squeeze the water out of them.

Eventually, I would begin an interactive dialogue that would take any of several directions. For example, I may say, "Angelina, the mommy white pom-pom wants to swim in the small bowl." And my hope (often fulfilled) was that she would find a large white pom-pom and scoop it into the small bowl. Then I might say, "Now the baby white pom-pom wants to swim with her mommy." And she'd find and scoop a tiny white pom-pom. You get the idea.

Or I might say something like, "The yellow baby pom-pom wants to be friends with the baby purple pom-pom," and I'd watch to see whether she'd find and scoop them together. And I might say something like, "Hello baby purple pom-pom. Would you like to go swimming with me?" And hopefully Angelina would scoop both into the bowl that had the water and pretend to talk in the voice of one of them.

I recommend the website.

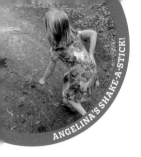

ANGELINA'S SHAKE-A-STICK!

Art and Autism

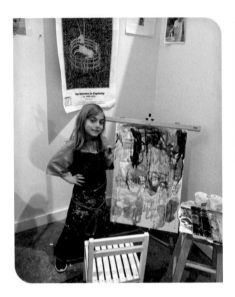
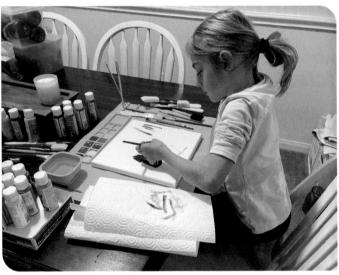

I WONDER HOW MANY FAMILIES OF AUTISTIC CHILDREN HAVE OPPORTUNITIES to expose them to art: giving them a sketchpad and crayons, a tube of paint and a poster board, a glue stick and paper and scissors, and observing what happens?

JC and I are both artists, and JC has a long career as an art teacher of all ages. So we often do art things with Angelina. We've learned that there is abundant research that confirms the widespread value of art-based activities for autistic persons.

Several years ago I visited a music therapy class that resulted in a 15-year-old autistic girl speaking for the first time. Just last month a mother told me about a painting that her 12-year-old autistic son created – a painting that triggered his first verbal communication.

Research points to the value of the arts in enhancing verbal skills, increasing mobility, instilling a positive sense of self, understanding instructions, reducing combativeness, increasing socialization, and so much more. Of course every autistic person is different and there are no guarantees regarding specific art involvements.

JC and I aren't trained therapists, but we can see art's positive impact on Angelina in three areas: dexterity (she is getting better and better in using a paintbrush, scissors, crayons, etc.); attention span (she's progressed from 30 seconds to 30 minutes or more); and an ability to follow multi-step

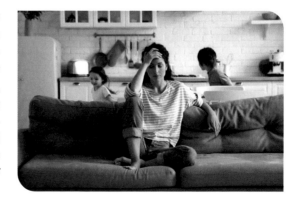

instructions (for example, "Put some glue on the piece of paper and then turn it over and press it down").

Because of JC's extensive experience teaching art to children, she knows what sorts of things work best, what sorts of things best inspire creativity, and what sorts of things enhance a child's pride and self-worth. For example, she never does anything "for" Angelina during an art project; she allows Angelina to do it herself and thus make plenty of mistakes. The end product is always totally Angelina's. When Angelina expresses frustration at not being able to cut things properly with the scissors or squeeze the glue from the tube or anything else, JC will simply encourage her to try again – and will praise her for each step in the right direction.

My methods with Angelina are pretty much opposite of those of JC; I tend to simply give Angelina some art tools (paint, brushes, giant piece of paper) and let her do whatever she wants without any guidance. And when Angelina exhibits frustration, I tend to help her by doing it for her. I'll of course say, "Here's how you do it." I realize that I should encourage Angelina to do hard things by herself, and I'm working on it.

Our arts involvements with Angelina haven't resulted in any epiphanies that we're aware of. And they are not yet activities that Angelina regularly begs for when she's with us. But we do them often and are hopeful that they are contributing to her overall development.

If you Google "art and autism" you'll find lots of information and websites. For example, http://the-art-of-autism.com is an online art gallery and blog. Purevisionarts.org is the website of a New York City studio/gallery for autism and other developmental disabilities. And www.healing-power-of-art.org is a comprehensive website that includes a list of art/autism organizations all over the world.

Stress in Autism Families

WHAT TYPES OF STRESS do autism families experience? And how can grandparents be helpful? Helpful information can be found in a 2009 research study conducted by the Interactive Autism Network. (IAN, now closed, was a partnership between the Kennedy Krieger Institute and the Simons Foundation that conducted research that would lead to a better understanding of autism.) IAN's 2009 "Family Stress Report" resulted from a survey of

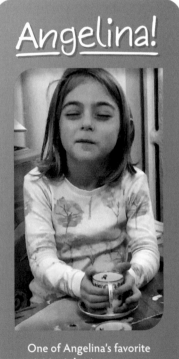

thousands of autism parents. And the Report's findings, albeit from 2009, continue to be relevant and helpful.

The Report has two fundamental findings. First, autism often has a negative impact on relationships between immediate family members, between immediate and extended family members, between family and friends, and on social involvements. Second, autism families can and do show extraordinarily positive resilience.

IAN's Family Stress Report showed that only 25% of mothers and 30% of fathers reported autism's overall positive impact on their marital relationship, while 60% of mothers and 54% of fathers reported an overall negative impact. Both parents identified two primary issues that stood out: division of labor and one parent's denial of the autism diagnosis. Generally the parent who did not work outside of the home reported an unfair and unequal burden of caretaking. And it is common for autism parents to report an inadequacy of "couple time" and intimacy. And when there is an availability of time, often it is accompanied by fatigue and exhaustion that get in the way of the time being productive.

The Report found that autism has a negative effect on the extended family relationships of nearly half of all autism families. This is because autism can be disruptive for family functions and gatherings, and because extended family members usually don't have an adequate understanding of the challenges of autism. Critical comments such as the use of the phrase "a good spanking" are common. And extended family relationships that were always thought to be strong often disintegrate once autism is introduced. Of course the opposite sometimes happens too – weak family relationships can transform into strong ones.

And finally, the IAN Family Stress Report found that 59% of autism families reported an overall negative impact on their friendships and social network. Only 19% reported a positive impact. This is because venturing into the social world can be hard, especially when meltdowns and other problem behaviors occur. And since autistic children often look normal, they don't attract the same type of immediate empathy that children with visible disabilities receive. Thus social interactions are often sprinkled with unkind comments from uninformed and judg-

Angelina!

One of Angelina's favorite activities is having a tea party with JC that includes ancient china from my grandmother and closed-eye meditation.

CHAPTER II: Your Autism Family

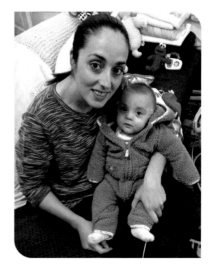

mental persons. Sometimes autism families are asked to leave organizations or groups because of the autistic child's challenges. Parents who had a wide range of friendships prior to autism reported significant strains on relationships. Some closest friends even end friendships because they don't want their own children to interact with the autistic child. One parent said, "I quickly learned who my real friends were." But autism families overall reported finding new friends among other autism families – families who had a first-hand understanding. For autism parents it can be exhausting trying to educate folks.

The Report showed that autism parents often can and do: find pleasure in providing care; enjoy a sense of accomplishment; sense that autism has strengthened family bonds; have a new sense of purpose; have a sense of personal growth; have increased spirituality; and gain a new perspective on what's important in life.

And there is a special value in the Report's final sentence: "A child's diagnosis with ASD may be an end to one set of expectations and dreams, and may lead to the many stresses we have discussed in this series, but it is often the beginning of an inspirational journey as new identities, values, and perspectives are forged."

Angelina's Story:
Home From the NICU, Wires and Tubes

WHAT A DAY IT WAS – finally, after 130 days in the NICU, taking Angelina home. Strapping a new baby into a brand new carseat is hard enough, but when she's tethered to a couple of tubes (feeding tube into her stomach and canula with oxygen into her nose), and a wire (pulse/ox on her foot) it's especially challenging. And then arranging all of that stuff at home . . . "You'll quickly get used to it, and will figure out an easy system . . ." was what the hospital folks told us.

(It would be almost a year later before the word "autism" would enter my mind.)

Kelly, then a single unemployed parent, embraced motherhood immediately and wonderfully. And

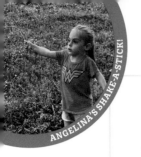

ANGELINA'S SHAKE-A-STICK!

she never complained about the obvious inconveniences and intrusions that were unavoidable parts of living with JC and me in the house where she grew up. What JC and I had to learn – and I think we did so fairly well and quickly – was to keep our mouths shut and let Kelly use her own parenting methods, especially when they differed from ours. (Of course all grandparents throughout history have had this challenge.)

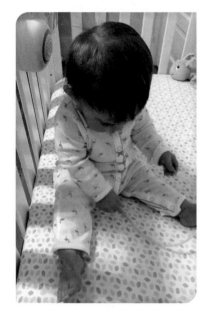

Angelina's physical needs were substantial. All of her "food" was administered via an electric contraption that pumped a milky liquid through a tube directly into her stomach. And the place where the tube entered her body had to be constantly cleaned and bandaged. And the bandages had to be changed frequently due to leakage of yucchy stuff. And every month or two, due to a buildup of stuff that I can't adequately describe, the hole had to be attended to by a physician – procedures that were always painful for baby Angelina. We learned to hate the feeding tube and that hole in her abdomen.

At first the hole was fitted with a sort of flat plastic circle with a hard plastic stem onto which the feeding tube was attached to administer "meals." The stem was two or three inches tall (I say "tall" rather than "long" because it stuck straight out rather than lying flat against the abdomen.) Thus Angelina was never able to comfortably roll over onto her stomach, and all of her onesies (and other clothes as she grew) were punctuated by a pointy thing on her abdomen. At age three she finally got a "mickey" button, and later a "mini" – a no-stem version that wasn't noticeable beneath clothing and didn't prohibit her from lying on her stomach.

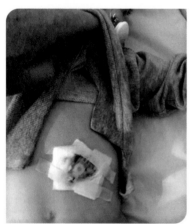

We learned that the "button" could suddenly come out of her abdomen – could work its way out from the wall of her stomach and the two layers of skin, leaving an open, uncovered, exposed hole. The phone rang one day while I was getting ready to start a tennis match: JC and Kelly exclaimed that the button had come out and we had to go to the emergency room fast! I drove home and got us to the hospital where the emergency room doctor was able to replace the button with ease. We subsequently learned to replace it ourselves – a careful, multi-step, sterile procedure. And we had to alert Angelina's "school" (an ABA facility) to be aware that the button may come out. Angelina was the first client they'd ever

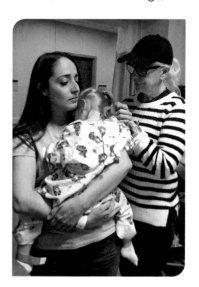

had who had a g-tube.

We hated the g-tube.

We also hated the pulse-ox machine. We had to strap a wire to her tiny foot in just the right way so that it would accurately measure the amount of oxygen in her blood. The wire led to a little machine with lights and numbers and a loud warning buzzer that would go off when the oxygen level got too low. We quickly learned that the buzzer would buzz at lots of other times too – such as when the strap on Angelina's foot came loose or wasn't situated just right. We also hated the wire because at night Angelina would often, no, make that USUALLY – get all tangled up in the wire while she was tossing and turning during her sleep.

We hated the pulse-ox machine.

The third wire/tube – the oxygen canula that fit into her nostrils – was also awful. After placing the plastic ends into Angelina's nostrils, we then had to tape the twin tubes to both sides of her head. They of course led to a big, heavy canister of oxygen with a gauge on top that we had to regulate just right. It was another long tube/wire that always needed attention and into which Angelina usually got tangled at night when she was trying to sleep.

We hated the oxygen tube.

The feeding tube lasted for three years until swallow tests and GI evaluations and weight charts indicated that it was time for the tube to be removed. But first we had to battle Angelina's GI doctor. He at first said he would give authorization for surgery to remove the tube, but as soon as he learned about Angelina's autism diagnosis, he not only reversed his decision, but also recommended an increase in the amount of "food" that we were pumping into her stomach – food that was already causing her all sorts of distress including frequent vomiting. Even though we knew Angelina a lot better than he did, he wouldn't budge, and his authorization was necessary in order to get the surgery. So we switched to another GI doctor who had been highly recommended by friends, and who listened open-mindedly to our descriptions of Angelina's ability to now eat on her own. He examined her, looked at her charts, and after a couple of appointments gave authorization for the surgery: go-to-sleep surgery to sew up a three-layer hole in her abdomen/stomach. We were of course nervous wrecks for that procedure – Angelina's first general anesthesia since the NICU. But it turned out fine, and the nasty-looking post-surgery wound eventually healed wonderfully.

The pulse-ox and canula were jettisoned much sooner.

The absence of tubes and wires allowed for lots and lots of new things.

3

Autism Into and Through Adulthood

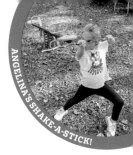

Preparing for Life after High School – Avoiding the Cliff

By Bradford Hulcher

THE INDIVIDUALS WITH DISABILITIES EDUCATION ACT (IDEA) mandates that children with disabilities receive a free and appropriate public education. Few mandates exist once our children exit high school. As an employee of our local Autism Society affiliate for the past 25 years, I have noticed that many families are not aware of or prepared for the "cliff" that awaits once their child exits public education. Families often operate with a very short-term outlook, preparing for each year with an annual IEP meeting to address their child's needs for the next year, without considering or planning for what life holds for their child for the many decades of life after high school.

The purpose of this article is to share the person-centered, long-range approach that my husband and I took with our son, Sam, who is now an adult in his 30s. I won't pretend it was easy. Sam did not have language and had challenging behaviors as a young child; he was a kid who would have been placed in a self-contained special education class. But we wanted him to be afforded the same opportunities and experiences of his nondisabled peers; we received a lot of pushback from educators and administrators over the years. We reminded ourselves that none of the well-intentioned, dedicated educators who expressed their doubts were in this for the long haul; we would be the ones standing beside Sam on his last day of public education, with a lifetime (of what?) stretching before us.

Develop a vision for your child's future; begin with the end in mind. Marsha Forest said, "We create our tomorrows by what we dream today." When your child is young, begin thinking and planning for his life after high school. Will he work? Volunteer? Go to college? Live on his own? As your child matures, provide opportunities for him to share his dreams and goals for his future, based on his strengths and interests. *Our vision for Sam was "an ordinary life," a life that would include friends, community, a job that interested him, and a home of his own; we shared our dream every year with Sam's IEP teams and other community members, including neighbors and our church family. Once Sam was able to articulate his dreams, he shared his desires for a job and community at IEP meetings.*

Provide volunteer opportunities at an early age. Your child will be exposed to potential new interests and gain skills that may transfer to a job someday – taking directions, being on time, working alongside others. *When Sam was in early middle school, he began to volunteer at the SPCA and Foodbank.*

Take advantage of school and community opportunities to expose your child to new interests and build strengths. Most middle and high schools offer a wide variety of electives and special

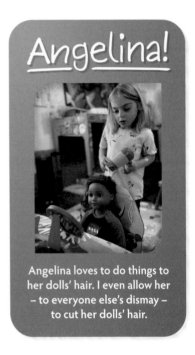

interest school clubs. *Sam was provided the opportunity, with appropriate supports, to explore many electives such as shop, chorus, drama, horticulture, JROTC, and a vet tech program. He participated in a wide variety of extracurricular groups, based on his interests, such as managing the football and soccer teams.*

Angelina!

Angelina loves to do things to her dolls' hair. I even allow her – to everyone else's dismay – to cut her dolls' hair.

Learn about and understand how IEP development shifts to a focus on transition in high school. The IEP team, including you and your child, will develop goals and objectives, including activities and services, that will enable him to reach his goals for life after high school. *Early involvement of our state rehab agency in IEP transition planning provided Sam career exploration opportunities based on his interests, such as interning with a local university football team.*

Explore eligibility for public benefits early. Few mandated public benefits, such as IDEA, exist for individuals with disabilities once their public education has ended. Eligibility criteria for public benefits vary and often have long waiting lists. *Several of the benefits listed below have supported Sam in accessing his own apartment with live-in supports, employment supports, and health insurance.* Your local Autism Society affiliate or ARC chapter should be able to provide guidance for accessing information on these and other public benefits in your state:

- **Vocational Rehabilitation Services** – services to access or maintain employment for people with disabilities

- **Supplemental Security Income (SSI)** – monthly payments to people with disabilities and older adults who have little or no income or resources https://www.ssa.gov/ssi

- **Social Security Disability Income (SSDI)** – monthly payments to people who have a disability that stops or limits their ability to work https://www.ssa.gov/disability

- **Medicaid** – federal/state program that helps cover medical costs for some people with limited income and resources

- **Home and Community Based Medicaid Waivers** – person-centered supports and services delivered in the home and community, funded by Medicaid

- **Housing Choice Vouchers** – assists very low-income families, the elderly, and the disabled to afford decent, safe, and sanitary housing in the private market

Note from the author: Bradford Hulcher is retired from full-time employment, but she is an ASCV staff member: "Information & Referral Specialist." Ann Flippin, ASCV's Executive Director, has told me that

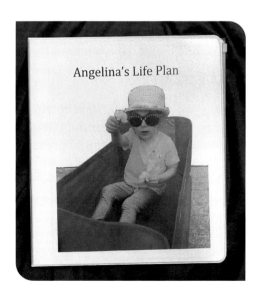

Bradford takes many calls every week from families who need consultation and information. AS-CV's website says this: "Bradford responds to inquiries of any nature, with particular expertise in Medicaid waivers, special education, and resources for adults on the spectrum. Bradford has been affiliated with the ASCV since 1994, first as the parent of a newly diagnosed child, then as a volunteer and Board member. She is a graduate of Partners in Policymaking and a Medicaid Waiver Mentor. Bradford presents workshops on Medicaid waivers, person centered planning, transition to adulthood, and IEP development at local and state conferences. Bradford volunteers on many local and state disability related work groups and advisory boards on behalf of the ASCV.

In her spare time, Bradford enjoys traveling with her husband, Chuck, and spending time on the Northern Neck with her children and grandchildren. Bradford is passionate about providing individuals with autism and their families with vital information to navigate the complex disability systems in Virginia and to maximize each individual's gifts and talents."

The Life Plan

IT'S A GOOD IDEA FOR ALL OF US who have autistic children in our families to develop a Life Plan and then modify it on a regular basis (at least annually) to accommodate changes. Following are the 13 items that are in Angelina's Life Plan. As you can see, it's complex and it takes time and research.

1: MONEY

What are the sources and amounts of money that may be needed to support Angelina for her entire life? Should there be a Special Needs Trust? An ABLE (Achieving a Better Life Experience) account? Will she have the ability to earn money? A professional financial planner can help.

2: LEGAL CONCERNS

Who are the legal guardians for Angelina? What about when/if they are no longer available? Should there be someone appointed as power of attorney, and when might this happen? A special needs attorney can help.

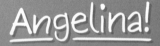

3: PUBLIC BENEFITS

What are the current and future sources of public support and benefits for Angelina? When are the appropriate times to apply? How do you keep up with the various changes that continually happen with public support? Local social service agencies can help.

4: DECISION-MAKING

When Angelina reaches adulthood, will she be legally capable of making her own decisions? If not, will she have a legal guardian who can make good decisions? If she IS capable, should there be a person or group of persons who are willing to help her with her decisions?

5: HEALTH

(This topic is often broad and deep.) What are the details of Angelina's current physical and mental health, including various therapies? What physical/mental health concerns can be reasonably expected for the future? What parts of her health history are important to document? Who are the professionals who currently treat her health concerns, and what is the plan for transitioning to other professionals as needed in the future?

6: ABILITIES/CHALLENGES

What are Angelina's best current abilities and what are her significant challenges? What are the reasonable expectations for the future? How is she currently dealing with challenges (therapy, etc), and what is the plan for the future?

7: DAILY ROUTINE

What is Angelina's school/activity situation and what are the plans for her future – including when she is no longer eligible for publicly-supported school? Is she a candidate for post-secondary education, and if so, what is the plan? Is she a candidate for getting a job, and if so, what is the plan?

Angelina!

Recently I took Angelina to the park so I could get new photos of her shaking a stick. I handed her a multi-color Angelina's Shake-A-Stick, and she proceeded to do everything but shake it: a magic sword fighting dinosaurs, a royal scepter (she was queen and she made me king), an arrow for her bow, a magic wand, a cane as she pretended to be an old grandpa, a rifle for shooting dragons, a mallet that she used to play the park's xylophone-type instrument, etc. She never did shake it.

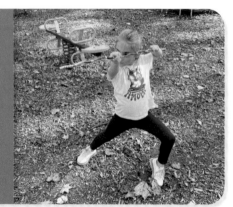

8: GOALS

What are the top few goals for Angelina, and what are the steps for reaching those goals? (For example, one goal might be developing some close lifelong friends. Another might be achieving the ability to do well with transitions – ranging from seemingly small transitions such as getting into a car to huge transitions such as moving to a new household.)

9: LIFE TRANSITIONS

What will be Angelina's significant transitions? (Adolescence, changing schools, ending schooling, changing homes, death of family members, illnesses, etc.) And how can her family/friends continually help her prepare for them and make them as easy as possible?

10: LIVING ARRANGEMENTS

Where will Angelina live during the different phases of her life? (With her parents, independently or in a group home, in an assisted-living facility, etc.) Are there ways to plan and prepare?

11: SOCIALIZATION/INTERESTS

What are things that Angelina enjoys doing with others? Are there additional social activities that she might enjoy, and what can be done to initiate those involvements? Are there things that interest her when she is by herself? What can be done to nurture activities and interests so they can become lifetime enjoyments?

12: LOVE OF FRIENDS/FAMILY

What can be done to assure that Angelina is always – throughout her life – surrounded by persons who sincerely care about her? Is there an opportunity to nurture special friendships with much younger relatives who are not in her immediate family? Are there long-enduring groups or organizations – such as faith-based organizations – that can provide her with a sense of family? And if so, when and how should that involvement begin and be continually nurtured?

13: THE "VILLAGE"

Who are persons who might be willing to be members of Angelina's "Life Team"? (Life Team members are willing to receive updates about her, willing to be called on for special favors and advice and support, and willing to confirm that Angelina is, in addition to members of their own immediate family, someone whom they care about and want to always be willing to help.)

There are additional thoughts about the process of developing a Life Plan for Angelina. First, she should be personally involved in developing and continually modifying the Plan. That might mean asking her opinion about various aspects, and/or simply explaining things as they develop. Second, her Life Plan will be subject to ongoing modification as needed, and a total review at least every year

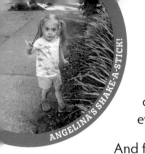

or two. Third, the maxim, "Hope for the best, but plan for the worst," should be in mind with every aspect of the Plan.

And finally, whenever we get a chance, we should seek advice from persons who have aging adult special needs children and ask for their thoughts on what components and strategies can be helpful.

Angelina's Story: Restless Sleep

TWO DAYS AGO I arrived at Angelina's house at 5:30 a.m. to be with her, wake her up, get her dressed and fed, and take her to school while Justen took Kelly to the hospital for early-morning minor surgery. (The surgery went well and Kelly was back home by early afternoon.)

I always raise my eyebrows and shake my head when waking Angelina in the morning and seeing her position in the bed. It's unpredictable: sometimes horizontal, sometimes upside down (feet at the head of the bed), sometimes teetering on the edge, sometimes so totally buried beneath the covers that it appears that she's not there. I never find her in a "normal" position.

When she was a baby and in a crib and living with us I sometimes slept in the room with her (when Kelly was working night shift) and it drove me crazy watching her move and roll and cavort all over the crib. And when she outgrew the crib she'd sleep in the king size bed with me and keep me awake all night with her movements all over the bed. I'd have to keep repositioning her.

Why is she so active in bed? Is this just another manifestation of her need to be continually moving?

Independent Living Skills

SOMETIMES FAMILIES MAKE "INDEPENDENT LIVING" a sort of ultimate goal of success for their autistic children – thus implying that an inability to live independently denotes failure. There are of course lots of neurotypicals who are unable to live independently, the largest category of which is senior citizens who need the support systems provided by "assisted living" facilities.

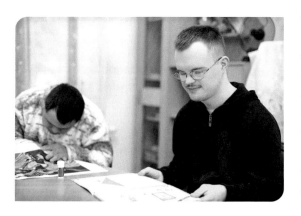

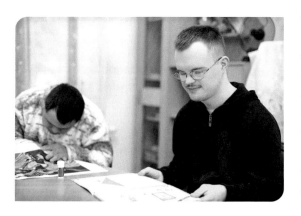 <!-- decorative circle badge top right: ANGELINA'S SHAKE-A-STICK! -->

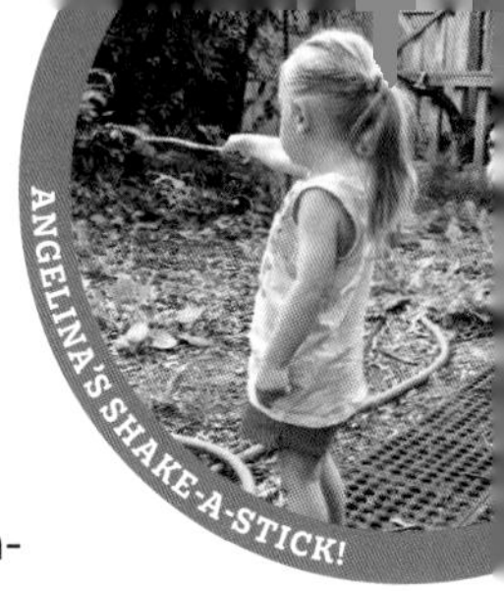

We don't assign the "failure" word to them, and likewise it's not helpful to assign that f-word to autistics who are unable to live independently. Our goal and hope for everyone, autistic or not, should be to provide adequate supports to enable the person to live as happily and productively as possible.

I of course hope that Angelina will continue to be happy and healthy when she becomes an adult, whether she is able to live independently or not.

Independent living skills for anyone, disabled or not, can be grouped into ten categories: health (medication management, sexuality, etc.); safety (at home and in the community); career/employment; self-advocacy; socialization (friends, communication, processing verbal and non-verbal cues, etc.); financial management; community involvement (restaurants, events, places of worship, etc.); transportation (including appropriate behavior); leisure (recreation, team activities, etc.); and household (cooking, cleaning, laundry, etc.).

Although some communities offer actual classes regarding independent living, family members can also be productive teachers. When Angelina is with JC and me, learning opportunities can be found almost everywhere, for example: putting clothes into the washing machine, cracking eggs for cooking, using the remote control for the television, opening an umbrella, inserting the credit card at the store, selecting fruit at the grocery store, and on and on.

There are three guidelines that are important for our relationship with Angelina. One is to use positive reinforcement and congratulatory encouragement – and avoid negative comments. "I'm so proud of you for trying! I bet you'll do even better next time!" A second is to teach the skill in its normal situation. For example, we can do "pretend" purchases with play money at home, but even better is involvement in a real store. A third is to use visual supports such as pictures, checklists, charts, etc. For example, put a star on a picture of a washing machine each time Angelina loads the clothes correctly.

And sometimes we grandparents are better suited than parents for this sort of life skills education simply because our lives can be less hectic than those of our grandchildren's parents. Often grandparents are retired and don't face the normal everyday challenges that confront working parents. We usually care for our grandchildren on a part-time basis rather than 24/7. And we of course have the advantage of wisdom that comes from already having raised children. Parents are usually consumed by three fundamental things: their workplace jobs, the challenges of autism, and the learning curve for being parents.

A final key for teaching independent living skills to Angelina is practice, practice, practice. No matter how many times she practices crossing the street, more practice is still helpful.

Autism Speaks (www.autismspeaks.org) offers a free, comprehensive "Community-Based Skills Assessment" instrument that's available for download on the website. It's for use for persons age 12 and up. It's extremely comprehensive (54 pages), and has graphs, charts, scoresheets, etc. Although the document is way too exhaustive for my use, perhaps it will be a source of productive ideas for your specific situation.

Microboards – The Answer to "What Will Happen When I'm Gone?" Or Not.

FOR MANY AUTISM FAMILIES a major challenge is how to have a support system for the autistic person's life after the parents and siblings are no longer available. Just recently I attended a meeting of a small group of special needs professionals, and when this subject came up I said I wish there were a silver bullet. One of the professionals responded that there is one, "**microboards**," and that she had recently been helpful in establishing some.

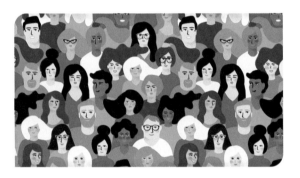

A microboard is essentially a group of persons who together take on the responsibility of doing what is necessary to help a special needs person have a fulfilling life based on that person's aspirations, likes and dislikes, and available resources.

A microboard is a legally incorporated nonprofit entity, members are non-paid volunteers, and the special needs person is a member of the microboard. The microboard's fundamental responsibility is to create and oversee a life plan for the designated person. The microboard adds and/or subtracts members as needed. The membership typically consists of from 3 to 10 persons who are family members and close friends. As a board member, the designated disabled person's voice and opinions receive priority attention. Microboard members not only provide their own skills and networks, but also tap into those of their community connections.

The one very obvious advantage of a microboard is that it is established to be fully functioning and attentive throughout the designated person's entire life. Parents no longer have to wonder what will happen or who will make decisions regarding caretaking etc. after they die. A group of dedicated,

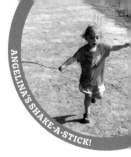
loving, attentive persons will always be in place to assure that the person's life is the best it can be.

Are microboards silver bullets for persons with special needs?

There is an analogy that I am very familiar with: boards of 501c3 nonprofit organizations. These organizations became popular after the passage of 1960s legislation that required nonprofit arts organizations to have 501c3 status in order to apply for federal grants. Today of course there are a zillion 501c3 organizations for all sorts of charitable endeavors and all of them are required to have volunteer boards of directors. Each board's responsibility is similar to that of a microboard: provide oversight in determining and implementing a plan. The theory is of course that a board of directors is just the thing to assure that an organization is strong and worthwhile, following the law, and adhering to best practices.

Now that more than a half-century has passed since the proliferation of 501c3s and their boards, we know that boards, in themselves, are not silver bullets. In fact, almost all executive directors of nonprofit organizations can point to ways that their boards can be counterproductive and even detrimental.

Following are six challenges that 501c3 boards face – challenges that I suggest that microboards also face.

STAFFING THE BOARD'S MEMBERSHIP – Someone has to keep the board members engaged both emotionally and physically. This takes ongoing, person-by-person work. Being on a microboard – like being on a 501c3 board – is a volunteer activity. There is a tendency among all of us to be cavalier about our volunteer activities and see them as far less important than things in our "real" lives.

PAPERWORK – An incorporated microboard is required to submit federal forms, document all sorts of things, send and receive communications, keep minutes of board meetings, etc. etc. There is a need for constant, ongoing work on the keyboard and the telephone. Once a 501c3 organization gets behind, it can be almost impossible to catch up. Ditto with a microboard.

RESEARCH AND KNOWLEDGE – Who on the microboard will have the responsibility of investigating housing? School systems and IEPs? Free public services? The learning curve regarding special needs persons is steep, complex, and challenging.

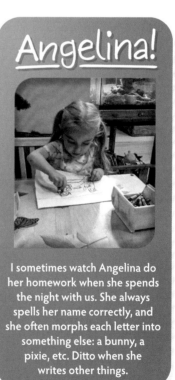

Angelina!

I sometimes watch Angelina do her homework when she spends the night with us. She always spells her name correctly, and she often morphs each letter into something else: a bunny, a pixie, etc. Ditto when she writes other things.

MONEY – When there is a need for money, what is the source? Who determines/approves expenditures?

BOARD MEMBERSHIP – Who should be on the board? Who are prospective board members and what is the recruitment process? What if a board member isn't good? What about board disagreements? (Experience has taught me that it is risky for a 501c3 organization to add any new board member who hasn't first demonstrated three years of love for the organization.)

LEADERSHIP – Nonprofit boards are only as good as the leadership of the nonprofit organization. The same is true for microboards; the leader sets the pace and establishes the tone.

Theoretically, a microboard can help assure that Angelina's entire life will be fulfilling, and that she will always be surrounded by persons who love her and are attentive to her needs. But for now, I'll choose NON-incorporated loving and energetic attention and efforts of friends and family members.

Social Rules, by Jennifer Cook of Netflix's "Love on the Spectrum"

[NOTE: A friend e-introduced me to Jennifer Cook who carved time from her extremely busy schedule to write the following for this book.]

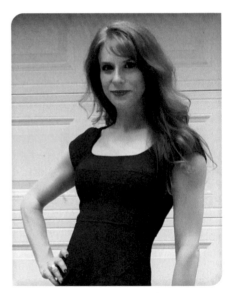

OK, SO THIS CHAPTER IS ABOUT SOCIAL RULES. Only, it's also kind of not. You see, before we talk about invisible, implied guidelines, we first have to understand why on Earth we should devote an entire segment of this book to discussing them in the first place. So while this may seem a bit of a rabbit trail, trust me. I'm autistic. My mind may work in detours, but I'll get you where we need to go.

Imagine you are blind. Perhaps completely. Perhaps just so much that you can see only the brightest of colors or boldest of shapes. But to whatever degree of intensity, you most certainly do not see like most do. That which is obvious to others is, at best, unclear to you. Perhaps you squint and strain. Get a guide dog. Ask for someone to lead you or show you the ropes. Perhaps you don some seriously thick

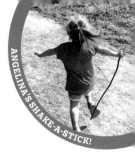

glasses. Great adaptive strategies, all. And. The point, here, is that your lack of acuity is not through fault or lack of effort. It's due to an inherent difference that can be met – and met well – but never completely surmounted.

At the core of the social challenges facing those of us on the spectrum is something which I refer to as "mind-blindness," an inability – or at least greatly affected ability – to step into someone else's figurative shoes, which is something psychologists refer to as "theory of mind" or "cognitive empathy." Neurotypical brains do it naturally. We, on the other hand, are the kind of folks Mary Poppins eloquently described when explaining that sometimes a person we love, through no fault of his own, can't see past the end of his nose. If you can't naturally see past the end of your own nose – that is, naturally step outside of your own perspective – you can't always imagine multiple ways to solve problems, won't swerve to avoid unseen pitfalls, and don't change tactics when causing invisible harm.

I've been around long enough to know that if someone loses a job, they will be upset. If their flight is delayed, they will be frustrated. I understand that certain antecedents lead to certain results, so I can learn to watch for and recognize likely cause and effect scenarios. I observe. I collect information – I read novels, watch for patterns and pay close attention to the description of feelings. I analyze and study psychology and sociology and history to understand people's reactions to various circumstances as well as the explanations of the emotional and strategic motivations behind them. I gather situational evidence. I think all the time – mostly, because I am trying really hard to intuit what I can't.

Cognitive empathy, then, is a concurrently occurring, multiple-perspective awareness. Neurotypical kids aren't super at it – but do grow into it naturally. We don't. We either don't notice or don't understand the thoughts we make others think about us – in fact, we have to learn even to consider that others may have reactions distinct from ours. That what is "obvious" to us, isn't a given for everyone. For us, "remembering to look both ways" does not come naturally. It takes conscious effort. Always. It accumulates slowly, one situation at a time, day upon day, year upon year, and always – always – by intellectualizing. It's never "just there." Eventually, if we are explicitly taught, we can spot patterns. Try to make some generalizations. But there are so many variables between moments and people and circumstances, even those go wrong more often than not.

That's mind-blindness. And I promise you, it is as real as the physical kind.

We can't naturally anticipate how others will feel in response to what we say or do. Again, that's can't not won't. Nobody would punish a blind person for accidentally stepping on his foot, but there's a very different reaction when a "mind blind" person accidentally "steps on your toes." To be fair, though, I understand that we seem unfeeling when we mess up. Uncaring. Aloof. Rude. We relax. Let our guard down. We stop concentrating on those juggling balls....and Bam! We pull the rug right out from underneath our own feet.

Like a physically-blind person might ask a sighted one to "paint a word picture" of what she cannot

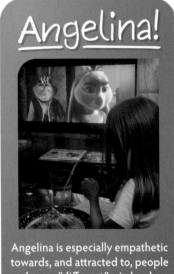

see, mind-blind people need word pictures, too. Typical people easily notice the positive or negative responses to their behavior. It's fairly effortless – as natural as actually hearing someone say "yes" or "no." To them. But not to us. Not only can't we pick up on "subtle" feedback – we don't even know we've missed anything to begin with…not until it's too late, and no one is speaking to us anymore.

Angelina!

Angelina is especially empathetic towards, and attracted to, people who are "different" – in books, movies, and real life. One of her favorite movies is "Chickenhare and the Hamster of Darkness." The protagonist is a chicken/rabbit crossbreed who is bullied by everyone, and who winds up being the hero. (She calls the movie, "ChickenRabbit.")

People on the autism spectrum do not react to many interpersonal situations as neurotypicals expect (and often as experience has taught autistic people to expect, too). That is absolutely true. The big problem for us is that as long as professionals and public mistake perspective-taking "cognitive empathy"/"theory of mind" for empathy in general, we are wildly misunderstood as being cold, shut-off, and uncaring, when nothing could be farther from the truth.

Once we remove the perspective-taking pitfalls, we're talking more about catching feelings than understanding thinking – we're talking "affective" or "emotional empathy." Formally, it's our ability to respond with an appropriate emotion to another's mental state. Informally, it's how we feel and behave if/when we understand what someone else is going through. Largely, it's what we usually refer to as sympathy or compassion – feeling delighted or afraid or concerned or thrilled for someone, doing what we can to alleviate any suffering and securing them in love. That's emotional empathy. And that we've got in droves.

OK, so now back to social rules. When you are mind blind – or at least impaired – you need clear, exacting guidelines. Not approximations. Not fuzzy descriptors. You yearn for concrete explanations and if/then scenarios. Admittedly, the world doesn't always work like that, but please don't blame us when we "bump into" you. We're trying, folks. We really are.

After I was diagnosed, I literally sat back like a cultural anthropologist and wrote an entire book of the "secret" social rules that most neurotypicals seemed to know (although many seem to need some reminders, I'll be honest). For example? Compliments to others aren't insults to you. Everything's hard before it's easy. The best kind of popular happens when someone makes others feel good about themselves. There are levels of friendship. Cooked noodle (flexible) thinking can get you anywhere.

Well, not only did I not expect to publish that book, I couldn't imagine anyone else would need it. How wrong was I? It's now been translated into eight languages and sold over 100,000 copies in En-

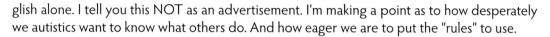

glish alone. I tell you this NOT as an advertisement. I'm making a point as to how desperately we autistics want to know what others do. And how eager we are to put the "rules" to use.

So the next time you're thinking, "I shouldn't have to explain this!" ask yourself if you would say the same to a blind person. Have a little extra patience and consider our perspective. Lend a hand. Be a seeing-eye friend, and walk alongside us. Because with the right support, nobody has to fall.

Jennifer Cook was identified as being on the spectrum in 2011. An autism advocate, on-camera expert for Netflix's triple-Emmy-Award-Winning "Love on the Spectrum US," star of Joey Travolta's "Lights, Camera, Friendship!," and ASD expert for HBO Max, she also consults for companies like Twitch and Amazon. Jennifer is the author of nine bestselling books, available in eight languages – including the foundational The Asperkids (Secret) Book of Social Rules, *groundbreaking memoir* Autism in Heels, *and newest* My Friend Julia: A Sesame Street Book About Autism. *Among her titles are a* Wall Street Journal *Bestseller, Autism Society of America's Book of the Year, a Publishers Weekly "Best Book" title winner, and six of BookAuthority's "Best-Selling," "Best Memoir," and "Top Autism Books of All Time" picks.*

Jennifer is an alumna of Brown and Columbia Universities. She sits on the Autism Society of America's Council of Autistic Advisors, consults for Congress' Autism Research Panel, and is a multi-award-winning international presenter who has spoken everywhere from the White House, to the National Institutes of Health, to royal audiences in Europe. In her work, she helps unzip hidden social rules for neurodiverse people of all ages, coaching them toward more connected, fulfilling lives and relationships. Jennifer is based in Charlotte, NC.

Social Gathering for Autistic Adults

SIGNED UP AS A VOLUNTEER. The e-mail I received contained this: "Our in-person social group for adults with autism … provides opportunities for attendees to engage with other adults on the spectrum encouraging positive social interactions, fostering new relationships, and promoting belonging and acceptance. Volunteers will assist with welcoming and checking in participants as well as supporting participants during activities." The e-mail also contained the link to a video that volunteers are required to watch: guidelines and rules for volunteers. For example, volunteers need to be always alert and vigilant and therefore aren't allowed to look at our mobile phones.

This would be my first in-person involvement with a social gathering for autistic adults, and I didn't know what to expect. What

> ### GRANDPARENT CONFIDENTIAL
>
> *"My grandson, now in his mid-20s, was diagnosed when he was 5. There have been various family problems and estrangements. Now he lives with me in another state."*

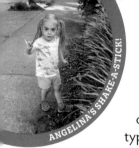

would be their range of support needs? Their range of communication abilities? Their range of intellect? And, even though I'm well practiced and fairly well skilled at engaging with neurotypical strangers, would I be able to engage with a group of neurodivergent strangers?

There were 25-30 participants, mostly in the 25-35-age range, all ambulatory, all verbal, mostly male, perhaps 5 or 6 females. The event was at a community center and was spread among 2 large rooms. One room was filled with all sorts of ways to have fun: Skee-Ball, mini-basketball, full-size PacMan, a giant Lite Brite board, and several card tables on which were games (such as Rummicub). The other room contained comfortable chairs and couches and a pool table.

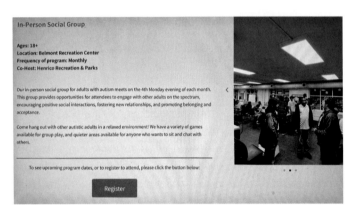

As folks arrived they gravitated fairly quickly to specific activities. I watched as some of them greeted others by name. I had wondered what percent of the attendees would appear to be autistic, that is, whether by observing them I would be able to quickly tell. All of them fit that description. Their vocal patterns, their physical movements, their abilities with the games that I watched them play, etc. were mostly atypical.

I also wondered whether there would be dangerous and/or disruptive behaviors. Meltdowns? Aggressive behaviors? Destruction of property? There were zero instances of any of these – unless you count the guy who spelled a giant F U C K on the Lite Brite board, which apparently nobody noticed or cared about, unless you count one of the event facilitators who quietly whispered something in his ear, after which he dismantled the word, albeit very slowly.

Early on I was standing next to the air hockey machine and one of the attendees asked me if I'd like to play. We played for 15-20 minutes and had fun. He was pretty good at air hockey and obviously neurodivergent. His traits and behaviors? He did odd movements with his hands and fingers each time he scored a goal. His facial expression was neutral both when he scored a goal and when I scored a goal. But after each scored goal, either direction, he'd briefly look me in the eyes. My exclamations such as, "Great shot!" or "I was lucky on that one," caused no reaction, verbal or otherwise.

At one point I smiled and told him that my arm was getting tired (It was.) and he raised his eyebrows and politely said, "Would you like to quit now?" I told him I would just switch to the other arm, which I did. But later when both arms were tired he was graciously agreeable to quitting.

Then, looking at the roomful of persons, I asked him if he knew most of the persons in the room, to which he replied, "Yes, would you like me to show you around?" I said yes and he proceeded to

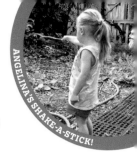

point out a couple of persons and tell me how he knew them. Then he drifted away from me and walked among the activities, briefly pausing here and there to observe. He would be the only person with whom I was able to engage during the 90-minute gathering.

From my vantagepoint there were three themes to the event. First, it seemed that almost all were truly enjoying themselves. Second, it seemed that everyone was perfectly comfortable being among the wide variety of neurodivergent traits and behaviors; nobody's behaviors seemed to bother anyone else. For example, one pool player was perfectly comfortable with the fact that his opponent moved his pool stick back and forth a zillion times before finally striking the ball. For example, everyone seemed comfortable with the Skee-Ball player's procedure of taking each ball and reaching under the protective shield and manually placing the ball in the 100 slot (rather than rolling it up the ramp). And nobody seemed to notice or care that one fellow had put his jacket on with one sleeve twisted inside-out. And nobody thought it odd that one man continually, for the whole 90 minutes, wandered around the room muttering to himself.

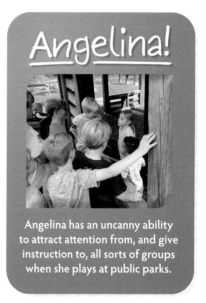

Angelina!

Angelina has an uncanny ability to attract attention from, and give instruction to, all sorts of groups when she plays at public parks.

After air hockey I did try to engage with others. One fellow was at the Foosball table by himself, so I got on the other side and placed the ball in the middle. He quickly engaged by rotating the handles that caused the players to kick the ball. But as I started to twist the handles on my side of the table, it was clear that he was intent on turning all of the handles, even the ones for my team. I sort of played along, but in less than a minute he left.

Then another guy walked to over to the Foosball table and I asked him, "Do you like to play Foosball?" He replied, "Naah," and walked away.

Ditto with basketball and Skee-Ball – both had side-by-side "lanes" that enabled two persons to play independently next to one another. When I'd see someone playing alone with an empty lane next to him, I'd walk over and start playing on the empty lane hoping to start an interaction. I tried this maybe 4 times, each time saying hello, but each time the other person walked away.

I enjoyed looking at a table where 4 women were seated, drawing and coloring and pasting and making art things. One was happily talking about her Friday experiences at McDonalds: the discounts, the Happy Meals, and it costing only $3.37. Another woman had heard my name when I arrived at the event and with her high-pitched, squeaky voice had exclaimed, "John Prine!?" and when I responded that my name is John Bryan, she had smilingly said, "I had thought a star was arriving." The rest of the event whenever she saw me she would grin and exclaim, "John Bryan!"

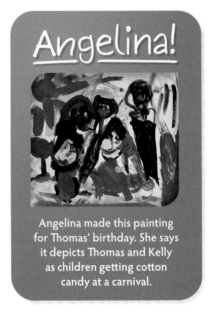

The most incredible person I witnessed was a guy who was shooting small basketballs at one of those small-hooped basketball games that have a sloping net that rolls the balls back to the shooter. There were two hoops and the guy was using both hands and arms to shoot two basketballs at the same time at the two hoops – over and over and over and over, pausing perhaps a nanosecond before each double-shoot. I watched him doing this for a long time, never tiring, always with a huge grin on his face, and never changing expression whether he scored or not. He finally quit when his ride arrived.

There were 3 tables at which folks were playing card games, seemingly knowing what they were doing (although I saw one of the event facilitators explaining things to one player). And at the pool table I observed that folks played happily without adhering to rules and without argument or disagreement.

Angelina made this painting for Thomas' birthday. She says it depicts Thomas and Kelly as children getting cotton candy at a carnival.

The activities would have had different atmospheres if they had involved only neurotypical young adults: there would have been discussions about violations of rules, about whose turn it was, about how someone was hogging a certain game, etc.

I left with two fundamental questions. Why was I unable to engage with folks? (I've read and observed that autistics are more comfortable engaging with other autistics than with neurotypicals.) And does our world appear as different to them as their world does to us?

Postscript: I just now realized that I was the only person wearing a face mask – perhaps a reason why I had difficulty engaging folks.

The Neurodiversity Movement

AS I WAS BEGINNING TO LEARN MORE and more about autism, Ann Flippin (Executive Director, Autism Society of Central Virginia) sent me an article published in 2021 by the *Journal of Autism and Developmental Disorders*: "Neurodiversity and Autism Intervention: Reconciling Perspectives Through a Naturalistic Developmental Behavioral Intervention Framework," co-authored by eleven persons (Rachel K. Schuck et al.).

The article fast-forwarded my knowledge about the neurodiversity movement and its criticisms of autism intervention. The movement says that various intervention strategies (such as ABA) are fundamentally bad. The article provides insights and a bit of history. Following are some takeaways from the article.

In the 1950s autistic children were institutionalized. There were no evidence-based causes for autism, and many professionals thought it was caused by uncaring mothers.

The sixties and seventies saw the emergence of therapies that used rewards and punishments (electric shocks, physical slaps, yelling) to change behaviors such as social interactions, communication, and aggressiveness.

In the seventies autism was recognized as being caused by biology rather than by family dynamics. Also in the seventies various types of drugs and supplements began to be touted as "cures" for autism.

A 1987 landmark study by Ivar Lovaas, "Behavioral treatment and normal educational and intellectual functioning in young autistic children," published by the *Journal of Consulting and Clinical Psychology,* found that 40 hours per week of intensive behavioral therapy (ABA) would greatly help autistic children. (This is what my family was told when Angelina was diagnosed in 2018.) The study is still influential today in spite of increasing criticism of ABA therapy. While ABA does result in "improvement," there is little research regarding its long-term effects into adulthood.

There is now growing attention to non-ABA intervention models that focus on social validity, parent and stakeholder involvement, and positive strategies for behavior modification and acquisition of skills. In addition, most autism research has been on white males; research is needed for diversities of genders and ethnicities. All therapists and service providers should get input from autistic adults that share gender and ethnicity with their clients.

NDBIs (Naturalistic Developmental Behavioral Interventions) are being developed to counter the regimental strictness of ABA – NDBIs that claim to be less stigmatizing and less depersonalizing than ABA. (ABA has become so divisive that some online forums ban its discussion.)

NDBIs follow a strength-based, interests-based approach that maximizes the child's engagement. NDBIs are not confined to controlled learning spaces (as with ABA), but can occur anywhere, such as where the child is playing. The idea is for the child to share a bit of her "language" and guide the therapist into her world.

GRANDPARENT CONFIDENTIAL

"I need help understanding my 7-year-old grandson. His aide in his kindergarten class will let him leave class to go to the playground for hours. I live in a huge city, but it's hard to find assistance. I want to be helpful to my son and his wife because they don't know much at all about autism."

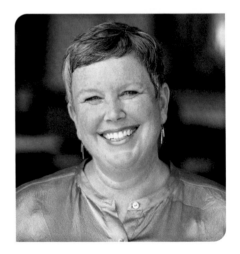

This shift arose out of the autistic advocacy movement (autistic adults speaking out) that blossomed beginning in the 1990s. But there were, and continue to be, many well-established parent-involved organizations that champion therapies and programs that claim to "prevent," "treat," and "cure" autism.

Today there are divergent views regarding what should be considered socially accepted behavior. Negative subjective pathology language is widely used, and there is a need for an overall shift to positive language. (Example: the D in ASD stands for Disorder: a highly pejorative term.)

The autistic advocacy movement insists that neurodiversity is beneficial to society and should be accepted and embraced. But some researchers contest that if interventions (that modify behavior) are applied in a respectful manner and teach useful skills and improve quality of life, then they are worthwhile. Some researchers believe that behavioral interventions can be compatible with the neurodiversity advocacy movement, but they concede that there is a lot of work yet to be done to reach an amicable compatibility.

Flourishing with Autism is Possible: Building the Autism Wellbeing Alliance

By Dr. Patricia Wright, Executive Director, Proof Positive (proofpositive.org)

FLOURISHING WITH AUTISM IS POSSIBLE. Typically intervention efforts for individuals with autism and other disabilities have focused solely on remediating perceived deficits (Fine, 2019). A medical model of treatment has been the approach of viewing people with disabilities as sick or broken, and intervention desires to achieve the greatest degree of normalization, with "normal" being described as those without disabilities (Hahn, 1993; Smart, 2009). While shoring up deficits is warranted and necessary for many, it cannot be the entirety of the strategy to promote flourishing in the autism community. The absence of weakness does not equal strength, much like the absence of acute illness does not equal health. Incorporating the practices of wellbeing into autism services and supports may be able to increase wellbeing for the autistic community.

The Declaration on the Rights of Persons with Disabilities, also known as the United Nations Convention on the

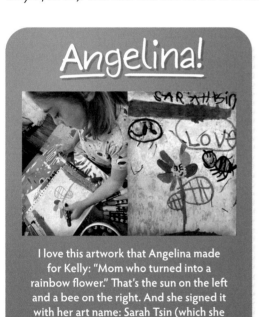
Rights of Persons with Disabilities (CRPD), is an international human rights treaty adopted by the United Nations General Assembly in 2006. It specifically focuses on the rights and wellbeing of individuals with disabilities and seeks to ensure their full and equal participation in society (United Nations, 2006). Nearly twenty years after its adoption, autistic individuals' wellbeing remains below that of the general population in many areas.

Decades of research have demonstrated that individuals who engage in positive psychology practices (e.g., practicing gratitude, utilizing personal strengths, or mindfulness) improve their wellbeing (Lopez et al., 2019). Emerging research demonstrates the effectiveness of positive psychology practices that enhance wellbeing and leverage strengths to promote flourishing for the autism community, but much more work must be done. What might shift if autistic individuals had access to positive psychology interventions and autism professionals benefited from improved life satisfaction, less burnout, and elevated wellbeing? Given the current data for autism demonstrating disparity, including suicidality, loneliness, and mental health, the autism community must be considered, included in, and begin to adopt the practices of wellbeing. Wellbeing must become a focus of autism intervention.

"It is remarkable that emotional wellbeing and the pursuit of it, although being highly valued for every human being, has received so little attention in research on the autism spectrum" (Vermeulen, 2014). The Handbook of Positive Psychology and Disability was initially published in 2003 (Wehmeyer, 2003). This text was one of the first calls to understand the theories (e.g., optimism, hope, and gratitude) and practices (at the individual, family, and systems level) of positive psychology within the disability context. Dykens (2006) expanded this reach into disability by proposing a new agenda focused on the positive internal states of those with intellectual disabilities. The once-perceived notion that the successful development of adaptive skills leads to happiness and thriving for autistic individuals needs to be challenged. Emerging data suggest no relationship between adaptive functioning level and happiness (Vermeulen, 2014).

Positive psychology practices are adaptable and can be accessible to all. Practices such as gratitude can be developed for those across the spectrum. For individuals with strong language skills minimal adaption would be required. A daily schedule reminder could include the prompt to write down three good things an individual is grateful for and create a sentence about why they are grateful for these three things

Angelina!

I love this artwork that Angelina made for Kelly: "Mom who turned into a rainbow flower." That's the sun on the left and a bee on the right. And she signed it with her art name: Sarah Tsin (which she pronounces beautifully).

(Seligman, 2005). An individual with higher support needs can learn about gratitude by sorting and labeling pictures of things they are grateful for and not grateful for in the same way other discrimination tasks have been successfully taught. Once this is learned, they can begin to identify things they are grateful for throughout the day. A picture log of these grateful experiences can be taken to reflect upon at the end of each day. Gratitude is a wellbeing practice with a rich research and applied history of increasing wellbeing. Autistic individuals can access the practice of gratitude with some simple modifications to these well-established practices like "three good things." Gratitude is just one example of an established wellbeing practice; many others exist. With minimal effort, the autism community can incorporate these practices into daily routines and improve wellbeing outcomes.

It is time for the autism community to embrace the idea that wellbeing is a goal. Effective autism intervention must include instruction in wellbeing practices. As the United Nations Convention on the Rights of Persons with Disabilities so eloquently states, people with disabilities, including those who are autistic, must have "full and equal participation in society," which means having the ability to access happiness and flourish.

To ensure that every member of the autism community has access to wellbeing practices, the Autism Wellbeing Alliance was created (Proof Positive, 2024). Membership in the alliance is free. The Autism Wellbeing Alliance ensures the autism community is actively part of the greater wellbeing movement, able to access and benefit from the science and skills of happiness. Together the Autism Wellbeing Alliance works to ensure people are empowered to take control of their own wellbeing and to promote the wellbeing of others.

Join the alliance and ensure every member of the autism community has an equal opportunity to practice the skills of wellbeing and flourish in life!

References:

- Dykens, E. M. (2006). Toward a positive psychology of mental retardation. American Journal of Orthopsychiatry, 76(2), 185–193.

- Fine, M. (2019). Critical Disability Studies: Looking Back and Forward. Journal of Social Issues, 75(3), 972–984.

- Hahn, H. D. (1988). The politics of physical differences: Disability and discrimination. Journal of Social Issues, 44(1), 39–47.

- Lopez, S. J., Pedrotti, J. T., & Snyder, C. R. (2019). Positive psychology: the scientific and practical explorations of human strengths. Thousand Oaks, California, SAGE.

- Proof Positive: Autism Wellbeing Alliance (2024, March 29) Retrieved from: https://proofpositive.org/about/

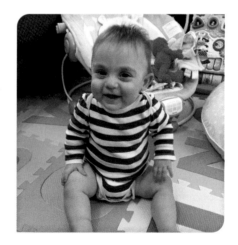

- Seligman, M. E., Steen, T. A., Park, N., & Peterson, C. (2005). Positive psychology: Empirical validation of interventions. American Psychologist, 60(5), 410.

- Smart, J. F. (2009). The power of models of disability. Journal of Rehabilitation, 75(2), 3–11. United Nations. (2006). Convention on the Rights of Persons with Disabilities.

- Vermeulen, P. (2014). The practice of promoting happiness in autism.

- Jones, G. & Hurley, H. (Eds). Good Autism Practice: Autism, Happiness and Wellbeing. (pp-8-17), BILD.

- Wehmeyer, M., (2003). The Handbook of Positive Psychology and Disability. Oxford University Press.

Dr. Patricia Wright holds a Ph.D. and Master of Public Health from the University of Hawaii, and helped design and transform Hawaii's system of support for autistic children. She has had leadership roles for NEXT For AUTISM, was National Director of Autism Services for Easterseals, and has held advisory roles for the Organization for Autism Research's Scientific Council, the Executive Committee for the Friends of the Center for Disease Control and Prevention, Board of Directors for the Association of Professional Behavior Analysts, and the Autism Society of America's Panel of Professional Advisors.

Angelina's Story: Early Challenges

WE THOUGHT THAT ANGELINA MAY NEVER WALK or talk or eat or be potty-trained. She is in great shape on all of that now, but she was significantly delayed. Therapists worked with her a few times each week at our house, and after she was able to walk she had additional therapy at a special "school."

Crawling was a big challenge. A therapist would continually put her in a crawl position and move her little arms and legs back and forth, over and over and over again – weeks and weeks and weeks. Learning to sit without toppling over

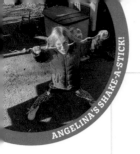

was a challenge. I would put her in a sitting position and then count the seconds until she toppled over. I remember the day she finally stayed up for sixty seconds; I considered it a major milestone. We autism families find real joy in what "normal" families consider minor development things.

It took Angelina a long time to be potty trained. It was as if she was totally unaware that she'd had a bowel movement; she'd continue to walk around and play just as if her diaper wasn't full. When her school said they were going to start her on a potty training regimen, I asked how long it would take. The answer was that it was hard to predict, and that they'd been working with one child for two years. It didn't take two years for Angelina, but it did take a long time.

All this to acknowledge that some persons on the autism spectrum are never able to master even the most basic human functions. Support can be needed 24/7 for a lifetime – more support than you can shake a stick at. I wish I could gift a brightly-painted Angelina's Shake-a-Stick to every high-support family.

Why Listen to an Old Autistic?

"**WHY LISTEN TO AN OLD AUTISTIC** … one old autistic guy yammering about things?" That's how Dr. Jason Nolan began his half-hour presentation for Canada's 2020 AUSOME Conference – a presentation entitled, "Aging Autistically," that I highly recommend and that can be found by searching YouTube: Jason Nolan Aging Autistically.

"Dr. Jason Nolan is the John C. Eaton Chair of Social Innovation and Entrepreneurship, and Associate Professor of Early Childhood Studies, at Toronto Metropolitan University (TMU), where Nolan co-directs the Responsive Ecologies Lab. Nolan is Autistic, and maintains a disability accommodation agreement with TMU. Having just turned 60, Nolan has been thinking about autism and aging for a long time, and has some thoughts to share. Nolan's 'special interests' cluster around sound and musicking, learning with materials, and understanding what makes neuro-normative society tick."

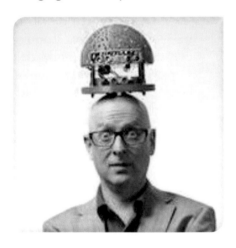

I'd never met Dr. Nolan, but he said yes in response to my e-mail requesting that he look at, and provide feed-

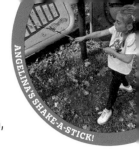
ANGELINA'S SHAKE-A-STICK!

back regarding my written comments about his presentation. Thus, thanks to Dr. Nolan's consultation, the following provides what is meant to be both a teaser for, and a sampling from, his presentation.

I'll start by providing a glimpse at the first and last of Dr. Nolan's concluding suggestions for other autistics. First is, "Find intrinsic interests and motivations … and nurture them." And his last suggestion is, "If you can't laugh at yourself, how can you expect others to?" He follows with, "Laughing and finding joy in life and finding things to be hilarious is an important thing."

And I especially like this: "Let go of your anger and rage and outrage at how stupid everybody else is. Because it's never going to go away … Find lots of places to take quiet rests that are comfortable where other people can't bother you."

Dr. Nolan's path to his current professional status was long and slow and challenging: "I grew up with a general lack of support and encouragement … I was dumb … I wasn't good in school … I screwed everything up, failed at jobs, couldn't get jobs … that was the expectation."

His revelations about his path towards self-understanding are enlightening and profound: "It's really important for autistics to have their sense of self … Why does your family not understand you? … Why do therapists try to fix you? … You have to have a sense of your self and your self-identity … It's not going to be one that other people have thought of for you. You have to figure a lot of this out for yourself. I don't trust other people to tell me what's going on."

I appreciated what he said about the limitations of those of us who are neurotypical. Following are a couple of examples: "Neurotypicals have an impairment that limits their access to autistic thinking … Neurotypicals are insensitive to external and physical stimuli, less sensitive than autistics are." He expounds in an engaging manner regarding this theme.

He advises, "Read books by other autistics, they are weird. There's a lot of different neuroautistic thinking out there that we can be learning from and learning with." (Elsewhere in this book I talk about a few such books that I've read and recommend.)

And he provides his thoughts about "heteronomous conditioning" – "someone else conditioning you through rewards and punishment to do what you're supposed to do." (He includes ABA in this category.) "A lot of autistic young adults and children have been very conditioned by their parents and by therapists in order to help them fit in to have a good life…. Parents and therapists want us to have the best possible life … But at what cost? … What do we lose in order to just be fitting in and be able to act fairly neurotypical?""

He allows that some heteronomous conditioning may be necessary: "How do you get balanced to deal with the external world? … I want my autonomy, but I have to put up with a little bit of heteronomous conditioning in order to get it done."

I very much like Dr. Nolan's obvious absence of any claim to be an end-all authority, including something that he says more than once during his presentation: "These are my opinions. These are not my researched thoughts."

The more I explore the seemingly ever-expanding universe of autism, the more I learn. I am so glad that I discovered this presentation by Dr. Nolan; it has added to my education.

PS – You'll want to watch the entire presentation to learn, near the end, about Dr. Nolan's superpower. And to learn about what I think is a cool term: "free-range autism."

Self-Diagnosis – Could YOU Be Autistic?

ALTHOUGH A PROFESSIONAL DIAGNOSIS OF AUTISM is often required for a variety of benefits and supports, a professional diagnosis requires money, time, and often waitlists. Plus, if you disagree with the diagnosis, additional time, money, etc. is required to seek another professional diagnosis. Thus, it is now common and socially "legitimate" for adults to use self-diagnosis, especially if they are interested in connecting with other autistic adults.

There are many online self-diagnosis questionnaires and I've investigated and participated in several of them. Caution is advised: some let you know AFTER the test that there is a monetary charge; some require too much personal information; and some require subscriptions to various social media things. But I've found one site that I trust and recommend: Clinical Partners (clinical-partners.co.uk). It provides a quick, easily understood test, and it provides an immediate result. When I searched the website of Autism Speaks, Clinical Partners is the only self-test that is provided. And finally, that's the self-test that my adult son used. (See his story, "Thomas," near the end of this book.)

> **GRANDPARENT CONFIDENTIAL**
>
> "*My 6-year-old nonverbal grandson has random angry meltdowns. I don't know what causes them. He eventually calms down and wants to be hugged. I'm confused.*"

4

The Real World

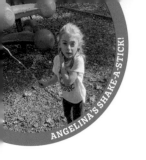
ANGELINA'S SHAKE-A-STICK!

Language and Disability: Words Matter

By Fred P. Orelove

HAVE A BUMPER STICKER ON MY CAR that says "Words Matter." The names we call one another and the way we refer to various groups of people can convey love and respect, or they can reflect overt or hidden prejudices and ignorance.

Over millennia, people who look, think, move, and communicate differently from the majority of society have been discriminated against. For years, most people with disabilities were excluded from public education, kept out of meaningful jobs, and hidden from public view. Not that long ago, women with intellectual disabilities were sterilized without consent. The Nazis singled out people with disabilities for extermination. In ancient Rome, visibly disabled infants were stoned to death. As recently as the early 1980's, until new federal laws were passed, some infants born with Down syndrome had life-saving surgical procedures withheld.

To justify such degrading and discriminatory treatment, professionals coined terminology that rendered individuals with disabilities as second-class citizens. The words used to describe people with intellectual disabilities, for example, have included retard, vegetable, idiot, and imbecile—terms that continue to be tossed around casually.

Even the term "disability" itself has undergone transformation. The landmark federal legislation, IDEA, the "Individuals with Disabilities Education Act," was originally known in 1975 as the "Education for

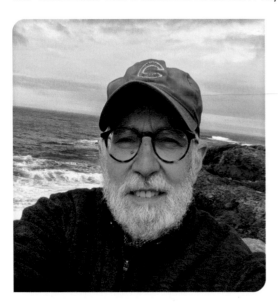

All Handicapped Children Act." The word "handicapped" has mainly gone the way of such terms as "crippled," a term rarely heard today. (Although we still refer to "Handicapped Parking" spaces.) In the mid-1970s, "the disabled" was replaced by "people with disabilities," putting the person, not a single quality of the person, as the defining element.

So-called "person first" language continues to be promulgated by advocates, although the disability pride movement of the past three decades has led to many people with disabilities embracing the term "disabled" as an essential marker of their identity. Similarly, terms such as "crip," "gimp," and "freak," typically viewed as impolite or hostile by the average person, have been taken over by some people, who present their "differences" proudly.

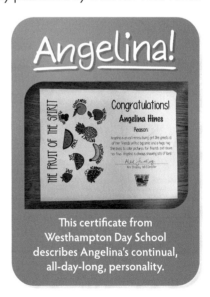

Other terms often used by nondisabled people to refer to individuals with different physical, intellectual, sensory, and learning characteristics include "physically challenged," "differently abled," and "special (or "special needs") people." Those terms are rarely used by disabled activists, who view such language as paternalistic and reflective of a "do-gooder" mentality.

Similarly, disabled people dislike the way they often are portrayed in popular culture and the media. As Joseph Shapiro wrote in his seminal book on disability rights, *No Pity: People with Disabilities Forging a New Civil Rights Movement*, "Disabled people resent words that suggest they are sick, pitiful, childlike, dependent, or objects of admiration—words that, in effect, convey the imagery of poster children and supercrips." Those terms include "invalid," "afflicted with," and "patient," unless, of course, the person is really in a sickbed. Other disliked words are "brave" and "courageous." Most disabled people are not looking to be inspirational.

For a person unable to walk, a wheelchair is an object of freedom of movement. Those individuals are not "wheelchair-bound." They *use* wheelchairs. Similarly, they are *people*, not their mobility devices. I have heard airline employees ask "How many wheelchairs do we have on this flight?" Such use of language is disrespectful.

Language is organic. It transforms over time as common usage and conventions shift, and the speed of change appears to be accelerating. The term "mental retardation" was commonly used by professionals and lay people for a century, only to be replaced by "intellectual and developmental disability." The term "autistic," while still in use, is in flux, joined by "autism spectrum" and "neurodiverse" and "neurodivergent." The way in which a person with a disability wishes to be identified must be respected. As one reader of a recent series of articles on disability published by *The New York Times* noted, "There are two kinds of people in the world: the disabled and the not-yet-disabled." Speak about and to people with a disability like you would like them to speak to you.

Dr. Orelove founded and served as director of the teacher preparation program in severe disabilities at Virginia Commonwealth University from 1981 to 2011. He also served for 20 years as Executive Director of the Partnership for People with Disabilities, Virginia's university center for excellence in developmental disabilities.

Note from the author: My awareness of the importance of using appropriate words when talking about disabled persons was heightened when JC and I got married. Her Down syndrome brother, Tony, became an important part of our lives. He spent a few weeks with us each summer throughout his life. I learned that when there is a disability within your own family, you are often

Angelina!

Congratulations!

Angelina Hines

This certificate from Westhampton Day School describes Angelina's continual, all-day-long, personality.

amused at the ignorance of well-meaning persons regarding which words to use. Our favorite example regarding Tony was when offering his ticket while boarding the ferris wheel at a small theme park, the operator smiled and said, "No charge for the afflicted." Tony's gone now, but all of us still laugh about that word.

Wonderful Legislation – Terribly Underfunded

I N THIS MORNING'S *RICHMOND TIMES-DISPATCH* there is an article entitled, "Mother of special needs son suffers academic setback." The caption below the photograph says, "Wendy Little is the mother of Eryn Little, a 15-year-old with autism. A disagreement over an Individualized Education Program resulted in Little's son being unenrolled for the entire 2022-23 school year with nowhere else to go." The article says, "In these types of cases, records show, the parents rarely win. A FOIA request from special education parents in Fairfax County found that parents only won 1.8% of 1,391 due process hearings between 2010 and 2021."

Those of us who care for children with special needs know about IDEA, the federal Individuals with Disabilities Education Act that mandates a free, appropriate, public education to eligible children with disabilities throughout the nation and ensures special education and related services for those children. The law states, "Disability is a natural part of the human experience and in no way diminishes the right of individuals to participate in or contribute to society. Improving educational results for children with disabilities is an essential element of our national policy of ensuring equality of opportunity, full participation, independent living, and economic self-sufficiency for individuals with disabilities."

Thus far this law has greatly helped Angelina. Her public school is attentive to her special needs on an ongoing basis and engages Kelly and Justen in mutually beneficial ways. But the national overall ability for states and jurisdictions to attend to the goals of IDEA is extremely underfunded. Many localities and schools just don't have the resources. IDEA is a textbook example of a federal mandate that isn't accompanied by adequate resources. In FY2020, according to Brookings, the government provided 20% of needed funds. This of course means that in most cases you need to be a really, really squeaky wheel to get services for your autistic child. And it means that most autistic children are being only partially served, if at all.

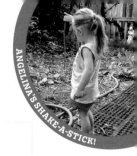

Angelina's Story: Starting ABA

IMMEDIATELY AFTER ANGELINA'S DIAGNOSIS the experts (in person and online) and experienced autism parents all said that Angelina should start getting ABA therapy as soon as possible, the earlier the better, 30-40 hours per week. We visited a couple of for-profit ABA companies in town and selected one.

Angelina cried the first day we left her there (she'd never been away from her family), but she warmed up quickly and by the second week she looked forward to it and would hug her personal therapist each day upon arrival.

We learned that ABA stands for Applied Behavior Analysis. A positive oversimplification is that ABA "teaches" autistic persons to behave in "normal" ways via positive and negative reinforcement systems. A negative simplification is that ABA inhumanely forces autistics to behave in certain ways without any consideration of their own neurological makeup. (I've learned that there are plenty of autistic adults that say that their ABA experiences were torture.)

Angelina seemed to thrive and "improve" with ABA, and we were happy with the company until her therapist left and was replaced by a therapist whom we didn't like. She was frequently late to work (thereby causing us to wait in the lobby), didn't seem to want a warm relationship with Angelina, and welcomed Angelina each morning with odd greetings such as "Hi Angelina, are you ready to hang out?" (Angelina liked her; Angelina likes everyone.)

A serendipitous meeting at a social gathering changed everything. I met Dr. Kathy Matthews who had helped establish The Faison Center in Richmond and who had been there from the beginning, nearly 20 years earlier. Ph.D. from Columbia, nationally networked, and with an autistic brother and an autistic child, she knew her stuff. She invited me for a tour of The Faison Center and I immediately knew that it would be the best place for Angelina – or, for that matter, anyone with autism. The annual cost? Six figures. She told me that the clients' insurance almost always pays for it.

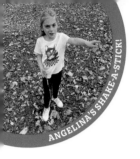

ANGELINA'S SHAKE-A-STICK!

Thinking About Starting a Nonprofit?

By Ann Flippin

CONSIDERING STARTING A NONPROFIT to support your local autism community? Before diving in, heed these essential steps:

Assess the Landscape: Check if similar organizations exist. If they do, consider joining forces to amplify impact. Conduct thorough market research to ensure your organization fills a genuine need.

Seek Feedback: Engage prospective stakeholders to validate your mission. Conduct a needs assessment to gather insights and refine your approach.

Connections: Cultivate a network of individuals and organizations and forge alliances with key players in autism advocacy. The power of collaboration and partnerships cannot be overstated in the nonprofit arena.

Educate Yourself: Acquire knowledge in nonprofit management. Familiarize yourself with legal requirements, financial management, and marketing strategies. Seek mentorship from experienced nonprofit leaders.

Learn from Peers: Tap into the wisdom of seasoned nonprofit professionals, learning from their successes and challenges. Their firsthand experiences offer invaluable insights beyond textbook learning.

Start Small: Begin with localized efforts to test your model and build momentum gradually. Focus on achievable goals and resist the urge to spread resources too thin.

Cultivate Leadership: Recruit board members and personnel who align with your vision. Prioritize competence and commitment.

Evaluate Impact: Regularly assess the effectiveness of your programs and fundraising initiatives. Set measurable goals and adapt strategies based on outcomes. Keep your organizational plan dynamic and responsive – focusing on what is achieving the strongest ROI.

Fundraising Realities: Brace yourself for the fundraising rollercoaster. Understand that securing funding is a formidable challenge. Diversify revenue streams and be prepared for the long haul – securing funding is no walk in the park.

Celebrate Success: Take moments to bask in your achievements. Reflect on the positive impact your organization is making for your community and find moments to appreciate your team's efforts.

Disabilities Studies at Roanoke College

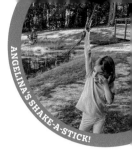

THIS MORNING'S NEWSPAPER has an article entitled, "Professor changing minds through disability studies." The professor is Frances McCutcheon who "spent more than a decade working toward getting a Disability Studies major added to the offerings at Roanoke College." A biology professor at the college, "In her view, every discipline intersects with disabilities in one way or another." The article says that there are 36 similar programs in North American colleges and universities, and McCutcheon says, "The difference between our program and anything we researched" is that the other programs are theoretical and don't provide in-person involvements with disabled persons. "I hate that model. The motto of the disabilities movement is 'Nothing about us without us.'" The program at Roanoke College will include direct involvements and interactions with disabled persons.

All of which reminds me that although I am well-educated, active in my community, and well aware that disabled persons are everywhere, I have been mostly ignorant of their challenges. For example, it was only after I added a wheelchair-assisted man to the board of a nonprofit organization that I headed that I started considering our meeting places through different eyes. Is it barrier-free? What about the restrooms? And it was only after Angelina was diagnosed that I began seeing other persons as unique individuals with unique challenges – usually challenges that aren't their "fault."

Several years ago a colleague told me that when he was in high school he broke his leg and had to use crutches for several months. He said that experience changed the way he sees the world.

One of JC's qualities that I most admire and envy is her natural ability to relate to persons as persons rather than as either abled or disabled, as thin or fat, as young or old, etc. I'm sure this quality was in full bloom in her relationships with her 7 siblings (I have 2), with her Down syndrome brother (I have no disabled persons in my family), with her volunteer work with Little Sisters of the Poor (I did nothing like that), with her fellow students in her Catholic K-12 integrated classrooms (we both grew up in segregated Nashville where my K-12 public schools were all white), and with her fellow students in a huge public university. (I went to a small, all-male, private college.)

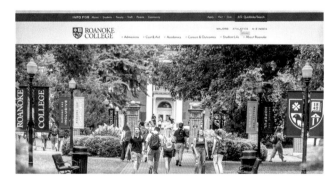

Bottom line: I salute Disability Studies programs as well as all other opportunities to interact with and gain a bit of understanding of persons who have challenges that are different from your own.

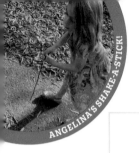

ANGELINA'S SHAKE-A-STICK!

Angelina's Story: Enrollment at The Faison Center

KELLY AND ANGELINA WERE STILL LIVING WITH US when Angelina was accepted into The Faison Center's Early Education Center: 30 hours of ABA therapy every week. Angelina still wasn't talking, but she was walking. And she still had a g-tube. And she hadn't even begun the process of getting potty trained. Kelly had become a full-time nurse by then and her insurance paid for Angelina's enrollment.

Angelina loved The Faison Center. She smiled each morning when we delivered her, and she exited the building smiling each afternoon when we picked her up. We came to know and love the personnel at the Early Education Center, and I even developed a relationship with The Faison Center's administration and was invited to speak to the Board of Directors and was also featured on a promotional video for the Center.

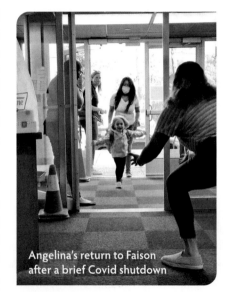

Angelina's return to Faison after a brief Covid shutdown

And Dr. Kathy Matthews (the Faison Center's VP at the time) and I became friends and even did a couple of projects together including establishing the national online group, Autism Grandparents Club (autismgrandparentsclub.com): a free membership club that provided consultation, communication, and an ongoing blog that discussed relevant issues regarding autism. (Carol Vincent runs it now.)

We liked everything and everyone at The Faison Center. And, as far as we were concerned, ABA at Faison was the gold standard.

Only much later did I learn – from autistic adults and others – that there are criticisms of ABA. AND that ABA therapists differ in their styles.

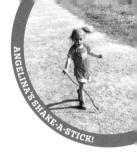

Mind the Gap: Disparities in Care

By Eron Friedlaender

I AM GRATEFUL TO ERON FRIEDLAENDER for writing for this book an extensive, research-cited, academic-ready, article about the disparity of, and need for, a system of coordinated and accommodating healthcare services for autistic children and for their transition to adulthood. With her approval, the article has been herewith edited and shortened to be reader-friendly for the general public. For a copy of her full article, contact me at jbryanfish@aol.com

The healthcare needs of autistic children and adults are largely underdeveloped in practice, research, and policy. Providing healthcare for autistic children is often complex, requiring dynamic organization among multiple healthcare providers within complementary disciplines to support social, behavioral, emotional, and physical needs.

A recent multi-state study found that young children with ASD were significantly **more** likely than peers without ASD to receive most types of healthcare services, but **less** likely to receive preventive services. Receipt of comprehensive care is roughly half as common in autistic children relative to children with other special health needs.

Autistic children depend on emergency departments more than peers for non-urgent needs. Care for autistic patients is less than standard, incomplete, and harder to access. Ameliorating personnel and physical barriers in primary care sites would facilitate more appropriate Emergency Department and primary care utilization. An analysis of the National Survey of Children's Health in 2016 concluded that autistic children were four times as likely to have unmet healthcare needs as children without disabilities.

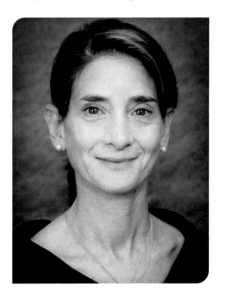

Over 110,000 autistic individuals enter adulthood annually. Formal transition planning to adult medical services and systems is largely inadequate. Autistic adults have higher rates of seizure disorders, low vision, hearing impairments, depression, anxiety, gastrointestinal and cardiovascular illness, and diabetes.

There is a need for developmentally appropriate healthcare settings and healthcare transition planning: a "structured process" to support the shift from pediatric to adult providers. Only 21% of young adults in the United States with autism receive this aid, and there is a largely inadequate quality of

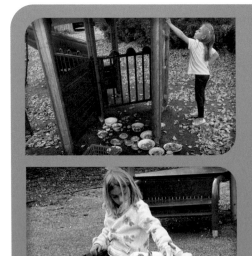
ANGELINA'S SHAKE-A-STICK!

transition services when they are accessed.

High rates of co-occurring conditions, care disparities, unmet healthcare needs, and margin-alization within medical settings contribute to greater morbidity and mortality for autistic individuals. Healthcare staff and providers' inexperience with aggressive or externalizing behaviors, non-speaking means of communication, anxiety, developmental delay, intellectual disability, sensory meltdowns, etc. results in incomplete procedures, restraint, delayed presentations, missed appointments and forgone care. Interventions have focused on providing more visit preparation and support, modifying environmental demands, and provider awareness.

Motivation, planning, sequencing, flexibility, and memory vulnerabilities define autistic profiles, and each skill is required to navigate the business of health. Individuals must also have the personal resources or supports to complete paperwork, follow care plans, maintain insurance, and relate to providers.

Healthcare systems and organizations are largely designed for efficiency and safety. Rigid protocols, long waits, short appointment times, and rotations of providers further tax many people already struggling to plod through a clinic visit or hospital procedure. These experiences are then embedded in a series of physical environments often characterized by chaotic pedestrian movement, limited signage and uneasy wayfinding, bright lights, booming overhead announcements, frequent cries and mournful expressions, monitors and phones chiming, and oppressive anticipation or anxiety. Building in cognitive supports and embedding technology to allow on-line scheduling, telehealth

Angelina!

Our little neighborhood playground has a large container of toys, and Angelina frequently removes the toy pots and pans and plates and cups for a make-believe tea party and meal. The last time we were there, when it was time to leave I asked her to pick them up and put them into the container – a task that a neurotypical brain would have tackled quickly by gathering a few toys at a time for a few quick trips to the container. But Angelina's seemingly impossible method was to fit all of the toys into a single small container and make a single trip to the toy bin. I'm always tempted to say, "It's easier of you do it a different way," but I refrained. As I should every time. We both learn things that way.

options, and communication aids with texting and messaging holds tremendous potential.

There is a need for six priorities for healthcare for autistic persons: 1. A subspecialty for autistic healthcare. 2. Single-location, multidisciplinary clinics. 3. Validated tools for screening and assessment. 4. Collaboration among care teams for patients with similar profiles. 5. Audits of healthcare environments so that they can be made more accessible and usable. 6. Investment in the role of neuroarts including partnerships with autistic individuals.

The means to advance care for autistic individuals of all ages centers on novel cross-disciplinary teaming and cooperation at the intersections of social justice and public health; engineering, technology and the arts; and behavioral, physical and mental health sciences.

Eron Friedlaender, MD, MPH, is a Professor of Clinical Pediatrics at the University of Pennsylvania Perelman School of Medicine and an attending physician in the Division of Emergency Medicine at the Children's Hospital of Philadelphia. Her research has centered on how conditions in the built environment relate to injury risk as well as documenting ways in which individuals with autism are vulnerable within healthcare systems. She leads program development supported by ongoing research initiatives to shape a comprehensive approach to the care of children with autism and related developmental disabilities within the hospital environment. As an advocate for those with autism, she has developed models for community inclusion nationally. She continues to build on her experience as a parent of a child with autism with formal training in advocacy, in collaboration with colleagues at the Center for Autism Research at the Children's Hospital of Philadelphia on community education, and as a medical provider for children in crisis.

Intentional Connections

By Wendy Ross

WHAT MAKES A CONNECTION WORK? Is it a word or a shared gaze? What if you have neither? Does that mean you do not get to connect? So often assumptions are made. If you do not speak, people assume you do not understand. If you do not look, they assume you are not paying attention, or worse, that you do not care. Mental forms are made and people are forced to fit into them.

With the advent of the disabilities movement, curbs were cut to make space for wheelchairs. Ramps were added to stairs. Yet for those with neurodevelopmental challenges like autism, it seems it is often still the person that is responsible for creating their own access. Something that is different in the mind does not seem to get a ramp, even a metaphoric one.

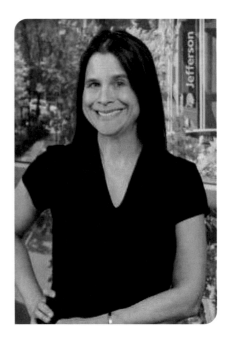

Over time, communities began to make efforts to accommodate the sensory needs of autistic individuals. Stadiums, for example, began to include sensory rooms. Yet so often, families go in the room and never get back into the game. Sensory rooms are a great idea. The problem is that they are often the only idea. Communities then check the box. Inclusion, done.

Inclusion itself has a propriety air to it. I have a space; maybe I will let you in. At Jefferson Center for Autism and Neurodiversity, we believe in belonging. Belonging grows organically. It starts with the people we hope to serve. We ask what matters to them. We ask their family members. We ask verbally when we can, and we ask in other ways as well. When someone cannot speak, their behaviors communicate for them. We listen. We wholeheartedly listen to whole body messages. We do not feel that we have all of the answers (not even close) but we do feel like we are asking different questions and that we are asking them differently.

We start with the autistic community and then we mix in a dash of multidisciplinary and societal perspectives. Speech and language pathologists, occupational therapists, psychologists, educators, nurses, and other clinicians contribute. Different lenses add depth to the picture. We believe that the challenges of the future will be solved by many kinds of minds coming together to share and collaborate. On our team, neurodivergence is more the rule than the exception. In everything we do, there is no single expert.

Bridges are never built with only one side. Information and education must travel in multiple directions. Community resources, education, and accommodations meet on this bridge with participants. Information, feedback, perspectives, and outcomes are shared in an effort to create a best practice from which all can benefit. These outcomes can often drive policy.

Policy creates a place outside of a sensory room; it creates a global space. A constellation of sensory obstacles, communication differences, and social struggles are unique to the autistic population but can impact us all to varying degrees at various times. This is not to say that we are all on the autism spectrum, but rather at any given moment, any one of us could be described for whatever reason as either transiently or permanently neurodiverse. In the same way that someone with a mobility issue, or a stroller, or a delivery dolly might benefit from a ramp created for a wheelchair, the culture shift we create for autistic individuals benefits us all. We all just need to lean in to connect.

Some connections happen with a word or a look or a physical grasp. Others require more intention-

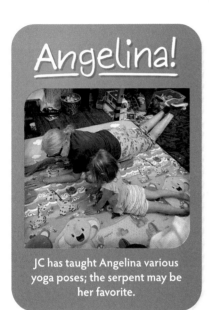

ality. Intentional connections can take time and they can change over time. It is the intention that always leads to us exceeding expectations, especially our own.

Wendy Ross is an American developmental and behavioral pediatrician at Philadelphia's Jefferson Health with a specific focus on autism. Ross founded Autism Inclusion Resources, a non-profit organization to help children with autism participate in everyday activities in their communities. In 2015 she was selected as a CNN HERO: "Dr. Wendy Ross is opening new worlds to autistic children and their families. Her nonprofit, Autism Inclusion Resources, has helped hundreds of families navigate challenging social situations such as sporting events, museum visits and airport travel. She partnered with the Philadelphia Phillies in 2012 to develop a program through which game-day employees learned about autism and how to interact with individuals on the spectrum so that families could feel supported during baseball game outings. Ross is now working with Philadelphia's football and hockey teams. Soon she wants to partner with the city's public transportation agency. 'The hope for Philadelphia is to make it the most autism-friendly city in the country,' she said. Ross helps prepare families for Phillies games by providing booklets illustrating each step of the game. She also escorts families to their first game, and each family is paired with a clinician should additional support be required. 'If you start taking steps outside of your door, your world gets bigger and bigger,' Ross said. 'We just want people to have opportunities.'" Want more inspiration? Watch CNN's video about Dr. Ross (available on YouTube).

Angelina!

JC has taught Angelina various yoga poses; the serpent may be her favorite.

A Space Worth Making

By Sabra Townsend and Wendy Ross

FROM THE AUTISTIC PERSPECTIVE: *Before an interaction or even a hello, the space can stop you. Maybe it is too loud, too bright, too big or too small. You find yourself stuck. You withdraw into yourself, unreachable. Or maybe you move to dull out your surroundings, to better control them. Maybe you run. Regardless of your reaction, you cannot function, and it is not your fault.*

They bring you to a different space but it is separate. It is not why you came, and although you can tolerate it (even enjoy it), it was not the goal. You want to work, to play, you want to be free, and yet the space has stopped you.

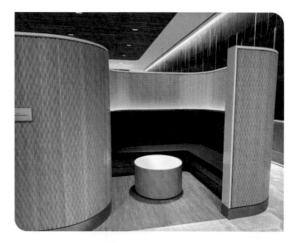

If you could create the space, would the ceilings be higher or lower, the acoustics softer, the lights warmer, the floors bouncier? What would the furniture look like – would it move, spin, squish, or seclude you for a minute? Could you stay in the room long enough to go to school, go to work, or just live your life?

Whether you can speak or not, it is hard to express yourself when you are overwhelmed and before even setting foot in a space, you are done. Your perception has stopped you but it is also what makes you different, gives you the ability to understand or even just see things others may not.

People sometimes think that only the autistic geniuses have something to offer society, but you do too. You see things differently and that matters. You may not express yourself clearly, but you have something to say and it can be significant.

The world is complicated and challenges are everywhere. It will take more than one perspective to solve today's problems. In a world with a lot of static, some things are still clear. The space around you may not suit you and yet you still belong in it. And you are not alone.

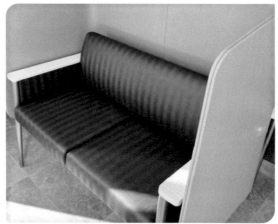

At Jefferson Center for Autism and Neurodiversity, we take the built environment seriously. We believe that places matter for belonging. We include people on the spectrum, self-advocates and their families in all that we do. We believe that cross-disciplinary work is also important. We bring architects, interior designers, occupational therapists, industrial designers, and light artists together with our population to help find the best spaces to promote health and well-being.

Listening sessions prior to project initiation help

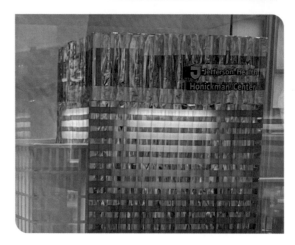

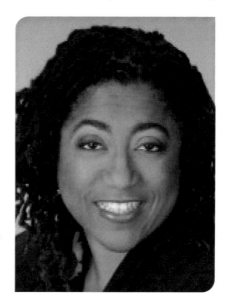

define priorities and interests for making a place. With every iteration, we circle back to check to see if we have hit the mark. When we designed our new line of sensory friendly waiting room seating, autistic individuals of all abilities provided input. If someone was nonspeaking, we videotaped their behaviors and coded their comfort levels to help understand what was working. Incorporating feedback from all kinds of people, even those with any level autism, was integral to the design. Environmental services were consulted to ensure that the final product would be easily sanitized as it was in a medical waiting room. One surprising aspect of this effort was the lack of interest in motion in this seating. Popular features included an optic screen, sensory friendly armrests, and tactile material on the seating and sides.

In addition to the sensory seating, semi-enclosed spaces were created for areas of relative privacy and seclusion.

Jefferson Health works closely with the Jefferson Center for Architecture and the Built Environment to bring students and professionals from all backgrounds together to learn how to apply their craft to a diverse group of people, including autistic clients and consumers. Academic courses including architecture, industrial design, and art culminate in an annual international symposium to share ideas. This hopefully will build enthusiasm for inclusion in the professionals of the future.

Wanting to emphasize autism from a strength-based mindset, we were sure to include art by autistic artist Kambel Smith, who created a sculpture of the building, on display in the lobby.

Over time, we will measure the usefulness and efficacy of these seating designs and likely adjust as needed for the future. Our goal has many parts but one final path – a route to a space worth making.

Sabra Townsend, BSIE, is Director of Operations, Jefferson Center for Autism and Neurodiversity. Prior to Jefferson, she worked in public health, focusing on community service for children with special needs. Most recently, focusing on individuals with intellectual and developmental disabilities, she directed an AmeriCorps national service program, managed medical and nursing students who performed basic health assessments, and provided training to both parents and professionals on topics including special education and everyday strategies for improved life outcomes. She has presented at numerous conferences on issues affecting people with special needs.

Wendy J. Ross, MD, is Inaugural Director, Jefferson Center for Autism and Neurodiversity. Read more about Wendy at the end of her essay, "Intentional Connections" elsewhere in this book.

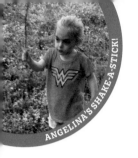

ANGELINA'S SHAKE-A-STICK!

Picturing Autistic Sensory Experiences

By Stuart Neilson

A S AN AUTISTIC ADULT, I find the world anxiety-provoking and full of intense sensory feelings that occasionally cause a panic attack or meltdown. Shared public places can be difficult to navigate because their design seems illogical. I started photographing comfortable and uncomfortable places to illustrate my lectures and articles about sensory issues and social inclusion. I have been developing video processing techniques to capture events that unfold over anything from a few minutes to hours or even days, creating still images of time as well as space. A photograph is a snapshot of a single isolated instant and often fails to convey our rich sensory memories of a place, which are the composite residue of visual experiences and completed actions we observed there. The process of making images is absorbing, calming, and moderates my anxiety. Images are a powerful way to explore my own reactions to the world, and to communicate my reactions and feelings to other people. I am also less nervous of people-watching when I have a camera as a social support, filter and shield.

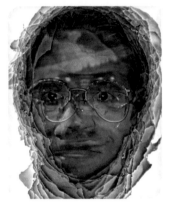

"An enfusion of multiple photographs from birth to now, retaining the areas of the greatest detail from each."

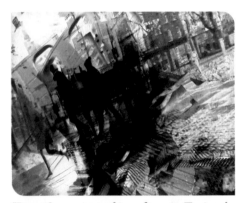

"Daunt Square in sunshine, after rain. The jewel-like reflections off the granite paving, shoppers and the texture of drain covers. I can almost smell the rain and bus exhaust looking at this."

I try to convey my impression of the place, the movement within the place, and the refuges where I might position myself to increase my sense of safety, and reduce my sensory and social anxiety. When my images succeed, I am able to share my sense of place, "cultivating strangeness" for viewers who normally find public spaces so familiar and comfortable that they rarely give its features any serious attention. Cultivating strangeness sets aside that safe familiarity, recognizing how a place may be unsettling or chaotic on first viewing. You can find more of my work at: https://wordpress.stuartneilson.com

Stuart Neilson is an internationally-recognized writer, lecturer, and image-maker based in Cork, Ireland. In 2009, at age 45, he was diagnosed with Asperger's syndrome after many years of ineffective psychiatric treatment. His books include Living With Asperger's Syndrome & Autism in Ireland *(co-authored with Diarmuid Hefferman); his academic appointments have included University College Cork Ireland and Brunel University London where he achieved a Ph.D. in mathematical modeling of inherent susceptibility to fatal disease; and his artworks have been featured in exhibitions including the Venice Architecture Biennale. His images explore autistic portrayals and reactions to sensory stimulus and motion, particularly in public spaces.*

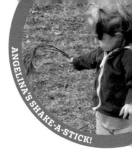

Co-Designing Public Infrastructure and Autistic Equity

By Stuart Neilson and Eron Friedlaender

PUBLIC INFRASTRUCTURE IS UNEQUALLY AVAILABLE to different people in its affordances and restrictions. We live in a world designed by consensus to meet the needs of the majority most of the time. This social contract is, in principle, open to rewriting. Sensory and social overload is a common experience, each of us having a different threshold for tolerating discomfort and negotiating the consequences. For some, avoidance of unease in public places is preferable, and opportunities or experiences are abandoned in the interest of self-preservation. At times it is a personal calculus whether to choose a potentially rewarding experience, despite knowing some individual coping strategies in challenging environments – such as stimming or a sensory meltdown – may be unseemly and provoke negative attention by other people. For many, it is the unpredictable and immutable nature of public and unfamiliar places that stretch our comfort.

To date, sensitive individuals are encouraged to practice tolerance of different social conditions and locations, while advocates call for greater patience and appreciation of differences among us. Despite a global awakening to acknowledge, if not embrace, the blooming autistic populus, disparity in citizenship opportunities (education, employment, socialization, recreation, and independence) remains. This disparity is baked into every aspect of our public space. A pressing imperative, therefore, centers on recontouring the physical elements of spaces and places to enable community mobility and rewarding civic engagement by more people.

Design, in its broad sweep of urban planning or the offhand choice of shape and texture of a door handle, harnesses sway over how a building, park, sidewalk, light fixture or staircase feels, seems, supports, intimidates, obstructs or eases one's experience. Appropriate design enhances our sense of belonging. The same complexities reported by autistic people in interpersonal relationships as well as in complex planning and problem-solving parallel difficulties in navigating the built environment.

Consider circuitous wayfinding, oppressive acoustics, rooms without clear purpose, narrow passageways with unpredictable pedestrian circulation, and limited signage with incomprehensible visual cues. A shared understanding of the influence of design elements on diverse autistic groups promises to acknowledge barriers and privilege facilitators to inclusion. In every place we should ask ourselves "Who is not present?", and how their exclusion can be traced back to funding, expressions of interest and formal design processes.

Participatory parity by autistic individuals drives success; cognitive shifting to make room for non-traditional means of expression strengthens partnerships with autistic collaborators. There is a glowing nexus where the arts meet the sciences if we allow a full range of human expression (spoken and written words; painted, drawn, moving images; musical and vocal sounds; performances) to guide imaginaries of flexible iterations of builds that favor inclusion and accommodation of traditionally unseen autistic populations.

Our greatest collective potential emerges from unlikely partnerships, respecting our limitations with humility to make room for the brilliance of others, unchecked imagination and resilience, and broad assimilation of end-user experience using a range of materials and means to share impressions and expressions of experience. Cross-disciplinary teams representing public health, architecture, and engineering with representation from autistic, minority, disabled, and vulnerable populations and a commitment to shared decision-making is fundamental to a collaborative approach to meaningful inclusion in our communities.

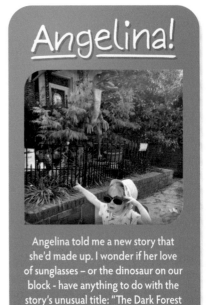

Angelina!

Angelina told me a new story that she'd made up. I wonder if her love of sunglasses – or the dinosaur on our block - have anything to do with the story's unusual title: "The Dark Forest of Day and the Light Forest of Night."

Collaboration across disciplines relies on a common working language across professions and with disabled people at design, delivery and after occupancy, as well as novel tools to measure the impact of interventions. Fundamental to this effort is the urgency to describe group methods through which autistic people may report their needs, a means for designers to workshop ideas with end-users of builds, facility in mapping the accessible environment, and explorations of the cognitive dissonance between disabled and abled people in the same spaces.

Read about Eron Friedlaender at the end of her article, "Mind the Gap," and about Stuart Neilson at the end of his article, "Picturing Autistic Sensory Experiences."

Imagine This – The Healthcare Experience of Autistics

By Wendy Ross and Jane Tobias

YOU HAVE TAKEN TIME OFF WORK to accompany your 21-year-old son to his endocrinology appointment, following up on his pre-diabetic condition. After taking two buses to reach the healthcare center, you arrive only five minutes late due to a delay on the second bus. However, upon arrival, the front desk informs you that the doctor may not be able to see you because

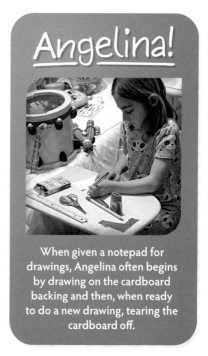

of your tardiness. As you wait in the crowded waiting room, your son's behaviors escalate – he begins to rock and make noises, attracting stares from other patients. Despite your attempts to explain the situation to the front desk, they seem unsure of how to assist you. Growing increasingly concerned that security may be called, you face a difficult decision: should you leave the hospital, knowing that your son will not receive the healthcare he needs today?

Individuals with autism often face challenges in communication, behavior, and social interactions, which can hinder their access to healthcare. This affects them and places additional stress on their families as they navigate everyday life experiences. Perceptions and biases, both conscious and unconscious, further exacerbate these challenges, compounded by a lack of accommodation. The Jefferson Center for Autism and Neurodiversity actively addresses these issues by fostering neurodiverse-friendly healthcare environments. Our journey begins with listening sessions, where we engage directly with autistic individuals and their families to understand their needs and perspectives.

These sessions taught us that difficulties in understanding their condition, sensory sensitivities, and communication barriers are significant healthcare challenges. In response, our team collaborated with families and a multidisciplinary group to develop comprehensive educational strategies across our medical enterprise. These initiatives include direct education in various settings, such as grand rounds, the integration of standardized patients with autism into medical training, and targeted education for medical students to promote a culture of understanding and inclusion.

Angelina!

When given a notepad for drawings, Angelina often begins by drawing on the cardboard backing and then, when ready to do a new drawing, tearing the cardboard off.

Additionally, we have expanded our efforts to encompass all aspects of healthcare interactions, from patient-facing roles to behind-the-scenes operations, ensuring that everyone receives the support they need when entering our facilities. Our educational interventions focus on enhancing knowledge, dispelling myths, and providing practical strategies for inclusive healthcare practices. Through these initiatives, we aim to create a more inclusive and supportive healthcare environment for individuals with autism and their families.

In medical settings, various resources have been implemented to support individuals with autism. Sensory bags containing noise-reduction headphones, fidgets, and sunglasses are readily available to enhance comfort during visits. Moreover, weighted blankets are provided when feasible, further promoting a sense of ease for patients. Visual stories and schedules are utilized to prepare individuals for their appointments, offering a structured approach to reduce anxiety. Practices also prioritize scheduling appointments with extra time and during less crowded times of the day to accommodate patients' needs better. Innovative approaches such as developing patient passports or resumes have

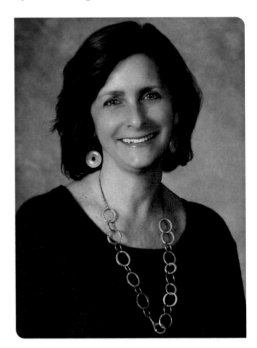

been piloted to enhance communication. These documents consolidate essential information, including preferred communication methods, sensory sensitivities, and other relevant details such as durable medical equipment and guardianship status. By front-loading visits with such practical information, appointments are streamlined, ensuring patients can attend without encountering unnecessary barriers.

Another challenging area involves admitted patients, particularly regarding a need for more understanding of developmental history and trajectory, as well as communication barriers and the assessment of health priorities. A consultation service is being developed, integrating nurse champions across medical centers who collaborate with developmental experts. This initiative aims to equip care teams with essential information to effectively communicate and provide care for this population as situations arise. Such tailored support proves more beneficial than generalized educational sessions, as information may not always be readily accessible when needed most.

As children age out of pediatric care and transition to adult care, many frequently need help with medical follow-up. Adult practitioners often lack the proficiency to involve families in care and understand the holistic needs of individuals with autism. In response, healthcare centers are establishing transitional care programs tailored for individuals with special needs. At Jefferson, the Jefferson Fab Center integrates medical care and social work to assist families in promoting health and accessing other social determinants of well-being in the community, enhancing their overall health status.

Hospital environments can be overwhelming for individuals with autism due to the lack of sensory-friendly spaces. Efforts have been made to create sensory-friendly waiting room furniture, incorporating textured armrests and privacy screens to reduce noise and promote comfort. By prioritizing the preferences and needs of individuals with autism, providing education for both patients and the medical community, and offering on-site support and accommodations, healthcare facilities aim to create more accessible environments for families affected by autism.

Dr. Jane Tobias is Associate Director of Thomas Jefferson University's Jefferson Center for Injury Research and Prevention (JCIRP). She is a Pediatric Nurse Practitioner with expertise in child-adolescent health and organizational structure and governance. (Read about Wendy Ross, a CNN Hero, at the end of her "Intentional Connections" article elsewhere in this book.)

5

Profiles By
and About
Autistics

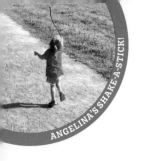

Mia Lynn Abate: First Survive,
Then Thrive.

I N SPITE OF VARIOUS FEDERAL AND LOCAL MANDATES for public services for disabled persons, including those on the autism spectrum, there is only a tiny percentage of funding available to fulfill the variety of needs. Thus, only those families that are persistent, determined, forceful, and continually squeaky wheels obtain attention and services. Following is one example.

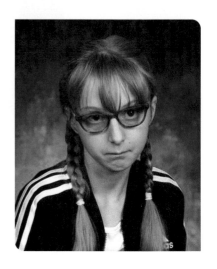

Carol Hinch, now 69, has been raising grandchildren since she was 40. She is smart, compassionate, resourceful, and knows a lot about autism. She greeted the arrival of her multi-challenged baby granddaughter, Mia Lynn Abate (now 13), with aggressive determination along with the watchwords, "Don't underestimate the powers of a grandmother!"

Mia was drug-addicted and was given Narcan when she was born on October 26, 2010 to Carol's son and his girlfriend, both of whom were users, and both of whom were arrested a few weeks later. They entrusted Mia to the girlfriend's dysfunctional parents. Carol scrambled to get custody, and learned that she needed a notarized statement of consent from her son and his girlfriend – which she obtained.

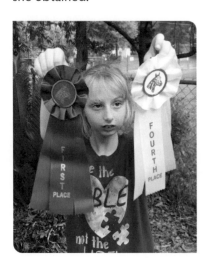

After driving through 14 inches of snow and 22-degree temperature to the house where Mia was living, Carol was given custody of Mia: soaking wet, no sleeper, no onesie, no blanket, no baby food, no medicine, no supplies of any kind. Carol stopped at a store where she bought medicine, special formula (at $55 per can), and basic supplies. During the first week Carol took Mia to two different doctors, both of whom said that Mia was developmentally delayed, was drug-damaged, and that there wasn't much hope for her future.

Mia was a struggle from the beginning. She never slept longer than 45 minutes. She hated to have her diaper changed (perhaps due to a sensibility to the change of temperature). She didn't crawl normally, but moved backwards in a crawl-like way.

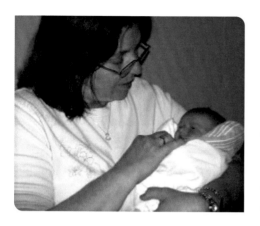

At 6 months she had apraxia of speech. She had gastrointestinal problems – likely due to being a drug baby. She couldn't stand, but would climb anything and would do daring things like jumping off of the back of the couch. At almost 15 months she started walking.

When she was 6 months old, Mia began having therapists in the home 6 hours each day, 6 days a week. And although she didn't talk until she was 4 years old, she learned sign language which she used for a lot of things including for getting potty trained at 17 months.

Carol was eventually able to make appointments for developmental observations of Mia, and finally, at 33 months, she was diagnosed: "severe autism, Level 3." Carol had suspected this diagnosis, but she still cried.

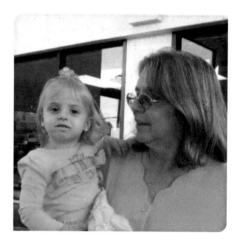

Carol proceeded to engage home therapists including ABA therapy. She tried ABA at a center, but it wasn't productive. The home ABA therapy was good, was never abusive, and continued until the middle of the 3rd grade. Carol also enrolled Mia in Head Start where Mia related well to other kids. (But it was always different with adults. It would take Mia 4 months to establish a rapport with a new therapist.)

At one point, Mia began to have violent, screaming meltdowns – including when Carol would say NO to something. Mia became very good at pointing at pictures of things she wanted, but if Carol didn't have them, there would be a meltdown. Mia could be completely happy and then suddenly transition to violent anger that included hitting, scratching, punching and screaming. This resulted in Carol's neighbors occasionally calling the police.

Meltdowns dominated many days. If Mia could make it to 10 AM without a meltdown, it would likely be a good day. But if there was a meltdown earlier, it would be a bad day. The meltdowns were massive and dangerous, and Carol would put Mia in her room with a gate. Mia would trash the room but for some reason wouldn't climb over the gate.

Carol and the therapists tried various things to remedy the meltdowns, but none worked until they got a tablet for Mia. It worked for both reward and punishment, and it continues to work even now at age 13.

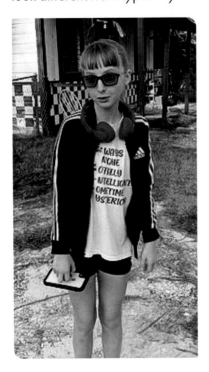

Just before Mia's 3rd birthday she had corrective eye surgery for strabismus (crossed eyes) and severe nystagmus (repetitive, uncontrolled movements of the eyes). (Mia also has astigmatism and enlarged pupils.) After surgery her eyes were black and blue and seeped bloody tears. When Carol and Mia were at a retail store another customer noticed Mia's appearance and called the police. Thankfully the police officer knew Carol and Mia. It was 4 days after surgery when Mia finally opened her eyes, just barely, which resulted in screams. It was 4 weeks before she was able to fully open them. Although the surgery helped a lot, Mia still has some vision challenges, and her eyes look different from typical eyes.

Mia was registered in kindergarten as autistic and nonverbal. But she was highly intelligent, including knowing how to read and how to communicate in sign language. Carol and the school established a 504 Plan for Mia. They also established a communication log that was sent back and forth daily between Carol and Mia's teacher, and a schedule for Carol to have a meeting with the teacher every two weeks. The school provided Mia with a personal aide in the morning and another in the afternoon, but Carol was disappointed that the aides weren't allowing Mia to learn independence; they would carry her water bottle and would even carry Mia.

Mia was well behaved and academically excellent in kindergarten. But she had bad separation anxiety; it was a challenge to get her onto the school van every morning. But finally they learned that Mia liked Hershey Kisses and if Mia was good about getting on and riding to school in the van they would give her two Kisses – one to eat when she arrived at school and one for her to eat later. This worked for several years and enabled Mia to get over the separation anxiety.

But occasionally something unexpected would cause a meltdown. For example, on her birthday the van driver sang Happy Birthday which resulted in a massive meltdown. The driver had been unaware of the note in Mia's documents that explained that Mia hates that song.

During the summer after kindergarten Mia missed the structure of the school day. That was the summer that Carol and a TSS (therapeutic support staff) took Mia to an amusement park for the first time. Mia screamed the whole time they dressed her and screamed and kicked as they carried her into the park. But when the TSS took her on a ride, she had fun. Mia enjoyed the park in spite of having several meltdowns. Later Carol learned the source of the meltdowns: Mia had seen commercials that depicted people swimming in a fake mote to get there, and Mia had thought she would have to swim in the mote.

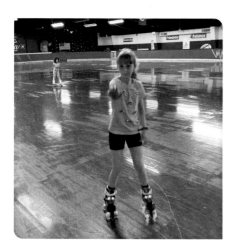

Beginning in the first grade, Medicaid paid for Mia to have a TSS for 40 hours every week: 25 hours at school and 15 hours at home. Mia has ADHD and the TSS was helpful at encouraging her to pay attention at school. The TSS was also helpful when Mia had to go to the bathroom. She not only has issues with privacy, but she also hates and won't use automatic flush toilets – which had been installed in the school's bathrooms. But the TSS was able to locate one bathroom that had a hand-flush toilet. The TSS would first make sure the bathroom was empty and then would stand guard to assure that nobody entered while Mia was there. The school eventually got an orange cone to put at the bathroom's door.

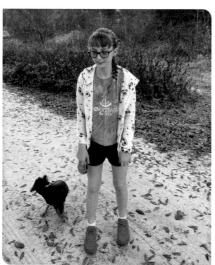

From first grade on Mia has received awards for excellent behavior. And there is always a red folder about Mia on the teacher's desk – a folder that substitute teachers are supposed to read. For example, the folder explains that Mia is allowed to use "fidgets" – things she can manually fiddle with to calm herself. Once during a test, Mia was fiddling with a kneaded eraser, and the substitute teacher grabbed it and exclaimed, "You can't have that!" That caused a major meltdown and the school had to call Carol. They finally caused the meltdown to discontinue by diverting Mia's attention to playing a game with a ball. After that the school modified Mia's 504 Plan to say that only certain substitute teachers could teach Mia's class, and if they weren't available, Mia would be transferred to a classroom where she felt comfortable.

Mia is sometimes bullied, but is often unaware that she is being bullied and never tells Carol unless someone makes fun of her eyes. Carol asks her each day how things went at school and in that way she can sometimes determine whether any bullying took place, and if so, Carol notifies school officials and it usually stops. At one point Mia started arriving home from school each day with bruises on her arms. Carol soon saw for herself that a big girl who sat next to Mia on the school van was punching her on the arms, and Mia's response was to simply cower and not say anything. Carol had to shout at the girl to make her stop. She learned that this had been going on for 10 days. And if ever Carol observes Mia being bullied during a sports event such as volleyball, she has no problem getting the coach to make it stop.

Carol has developed productive relationships with Mia's school's staff and teachers, and is proac-

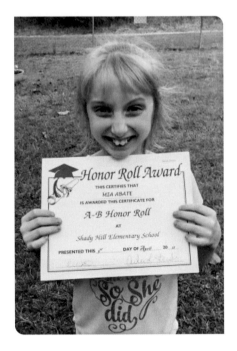

tively involved in all aspects of Mia's education. One result, because Mia is so academically advanced, has been Mia's selection for the school's Cambridge Program – the school district's partnership with Cambridge that provides advanced academics and academic rigor.

An active schedule is helpful for Mia's ADHD; being busy helps to channel her hyperactivity in good ways. Carol has engaged Mia in a variety of activities, both in and out of school. She has played T-ball, soccer, basketball and volleyball which is her favorite and for which she is a great server. She plays volleyball at the YMCA where she has her own membership and is known by the staff. She also plays racquetball there – sometimes with others and sometimes by herself. And she sometimes uses the exercise equipment and sometimes plays pickup basketball games. Mia goes about her activities at the Y independently as long as she knows that Carol is nearby. And at home she has a trampoline and a portable balance beam.

She has tried dance, but was unsuccessful because of her bilateral integration disorder (inability to coordinate both sides of her body together). And she has learned to play the clarinet, and recently even agreed to play Jingle Bells at one of her Church's Christmas services – but from her pew rather than from the stage. She did well and folks congratulated her afterwards.

Mia continues to have some significant autism traits. One is extreme touch-avoidance. Carol can get a sideways hug and can kiss her on the forehead, but not her face. Mia won't hold hands, so Carol has to hold her wrist when crossing the street. Mia can't wear bracelets, and she wears a ponytail so her hair won't touch and bother her. When Carol brushes Mia's hair she will wince in pain if the brush

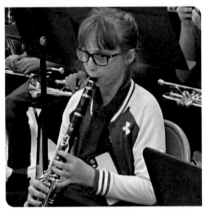

touches her spine in certain ways. If Mia has a nightmare, she will lie in the bed with Carol as long as they don't touch. Mia's doctors can't even touch her. And that, combined with Mia's extreme privacy (she won't dress or go to the bathroom if visible to Carol) will result in major challenges when she starts OBGYN appointments.

Mia continues to receive services from a variety of healthcare providers and therapists including weekly equine therapy, a weekly counselor to help keep her emotions in check (and someone to vent to), a monthly appointment with her pediatrician who monitors her medicines, and a personal home

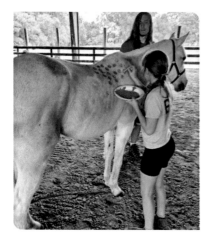

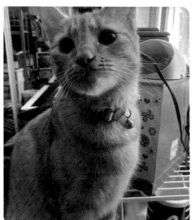

assistant for 20-30 hours each week.

Mia's daily medicines include the following supplements: fiber and probiotic gummies, B-Complex, Omega Fish Oil, magnesium, and melatonin. Daily prescriptions include Hydroxyzine (for anxiety), Keppra, Prozac, Primidone (acid control), Mirtazapine (anxiety), Senokot (laxative), Heptad (nausea), and Quinidine. And Carol keeps the following on hand for emergencies: Zofran (vomiting), EpiPen, and Excedrin for migraines. (Mia was diagnosed with migraines when she was 5, and she uses sign language to say when she has one.)

For a drug baby for whom the medical experts expressed zero hope for her future, Mia is not only a survivor, but also an achiever – including academically, well beyond her grade level. In spite of Carol's attempts to get Mia to call her something else, she calls Carol "Mommy" and says, "She's Mommy. She takes care of me. That's what mommies do."

Also: Mia has three cats including one named Max who is sort of a therapy cat. He gets close to her whenever she is upset, and he sleeps with her every night (not touching her). There used to be another cat in the household that was mean – mean to everyone except for Mia. She continues to miss him. And at equine therapy there is a feral cat that won't let anyone touch it – except for Mia who has made friends with it. Mia is well-versed on everything to do with cats.

Angelina's Story:
The Bad Feeding Clinic

ISSUES REGARDING EATING are common traits among autistic children: aversion to various foods, various consistencies of food, various colors of food, placement of food on the plate, aversion to sitting at a table for meals, even hunger itself.

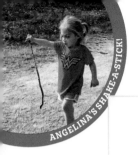

ANGELINA'S SHAKE-A-STICK!

Angelina's g-tube was finally removed at age 3 after a multi-month period of "weaning." I assumed that she would really enjoy the process of eating with her mouth. The opposite was the case. I remember when getting her to swallow even three or four spoonfuls of damp cereal was a huge accomplishment for a "meal." We monitored her weight daily; we rejoiced at every gained ounce and panicked at every lost ounce.

We were told that we should consider enrolling her in a "Feeding Clinic," and we met with a specialist from a highly recommended clinic in our community. The specialist had a little spoon and a jar of some sort of applesauce-looking stuff. She gently offered it to Angelina with no luck. Then she presented it sort of forcefully, pressing the spoon to Angelina's lips in a way that was intended to open her mouth. No luck. And finally, she loudly and commandingly said, with knitted eyebrows and stern expression, "Take a bite!" as she forced the spoon into Angelina's mouth. Which Angelina didn't like at all.

We said thanks but no thanks. Even though the clinic was respected and produced results, we assumed that it might traumatize Angelina in some sort of long-term way. (Autism was new to us at the time and we had no idea whether our instincts were right or wrong. And I suspect that if we hadn't witnessed the brief session in person, we would have enrolled her in the program.)

As I write this, a few years later, I'm glad that we made that decision. And fortunately Angelina learned to eat in her own way, and her weight is no longer a daily-panic concern.

Autism Anglers

WHAT'S YOUR FAVORITE ACTIVITY? My guess is that there's an autism organization or event or group that has your favorite activity as its main priority. (I just now Googled four random activities – bowling, sailing, knitting, and rodeo – and all have autism things.)

My favorite activity since childhood has been fishing, so I was glad to discover the nonprofit organization, Autism Anglers (autismanglers.org). "Autism Anglers exists because of our passion for fishing and a little boy with autism who has melted our hearts. In early 2017 my son was officially diagnosed with Autism Spectrum Disorder (ASD). I have personally spent hundreds of hours researching, reaching out and learning as much as I can about this misunderstood condition . . . Autism Anglers' mission is to bring awareness and acceptance to autism through the sport of fishing. Our goal is to educate a

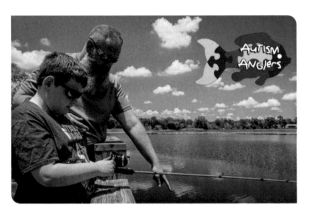

large percentage of the population (anglers) about autism and to use fishing as a calming therapy for those on the autism spectrum . . . Our staff is 100% volunteer."

Don Morse is the founder and president, and his wife Janine provides a lot of assistance. Their son Landon was born in 2012 and by the time he was 2 they had noticed a lack of eye contact, and he was delayed with speaking and walking. And in Pre-K they noticed a big difference between him and his classmates: Landon was stimming, lining things up, and socially different. Shortly before his 5th birthday, Landon was evaluated and diagnosed with autism.

A school counselor told Don and Janine about CARD (Center for Autism and Related Disabilities) which became their wonderful source of information and guidance. CARD is part of the University of Central Florida, is funded by the state of Florida, and provides a wide range of services for 40,000 persons including the Morse family: online classes, support groups, etc. "Our primary focus is to provide individualized, direct assistance to individuals who qualify for our services, including consultative support to their families and those who educate or employ our constituents. In addition to individualized consultation, services include technical assistance and consultation, professional and parent training programs, and public education activities."

"CARD believes that: All people, regardless of their abilities or disabilities, have the right to live as full participants in society; All people have the right to be treated with dignity and understanding; People with disabilities are members of families, and all families have strengths and capacities and have the right to be treated with sensitivity and respect, and as integral members of a person's system of support; People with autism and related disabilities have the right to be regarded as individuals who need services and supports that are based on their unique characteristics."

Landon switched from public school to homeschool when COVID arrived and he continues today with homeschooling. He has several therapy sessions each week (speech therapy, occupational therapy, physical therapy, etc.), and continues to learn how to engage in various social interactions. Forming words is a challenge and he sometimes has hypernasal speech (talking through his nose). He is a grade-level reader, but writing is difficult due to challenges with his fine motor skills (forming the letters).

Landon has sleep issues; he tosses and turns and gets up during the night. And he has daily meltdowns that can be triggered by all sorts of things ranging from weather to food. Meltdowns can include hyperventilating, screaming, and uncontrolled flailing about, and although they usually last

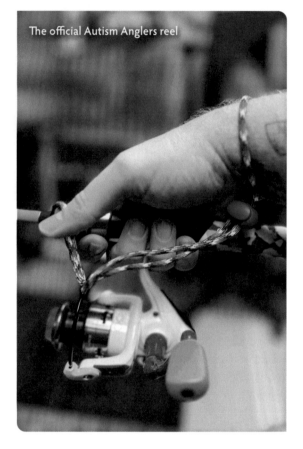
The official Autism Anglers reel

for 5 or 10 minutes, they can last as long as 30 minutes. He doesn't take any medicines; they tried medicines but didn't like that they gave Landon a vegetative personality.

Landon's physical activities include lots of walking, riding a tricycle, and playing in the park (for hours). Landon is extremely outgoing (with kids and adults) and at the park he tries to play with others (although usually nonreciprocal). Landon is not an eloper, doesn't wear any identification, and he knows his family's address and telephone number.

Landon has a few friends, but probably none who would come and just hang out with him. He is active at his church and does various field trips with other kids. He loves theme parks and the rides, drawing, organizing his toys, and shopping. When shopping, he takes his time, looks everything over, and is very polite when asking for assistance. Landon's favorite foods are pizza, mac and cheese, and chicken nuggets. He will at least try most other foods. And he loves Ranch dressing.

Don Morse is one of the few <u>fathers</u> who have started a nonprofit autism services organization. Today Autism Anglers has 10,000 Facebook followers, has engaged supportive corporate partners, and has shipped 4,000 pounds of fishing tackle, at no charge, to persons with autism. A current goal is to engage and train fishing guides who are willing to take autistic persons fishing. Don says he has received enthusiastic affirmation from almost all of the guides he has contacted.

Don has two fundamental recommendations for other fathers (and mothers) who are considering starting a nonprofit autism support organization. First, mentor and partner with an already established nonprofit organization. Second, take some classes to learn about what's involved with running a nonprofit organization.

What about Landon's involvement with fishing? "I've taken him a couple of times," says Don, "but he doesn't really care for it. But I wouldn't change him at all."

Autism and NASCAR – "Rain comes down like the letter i, not the letter j."

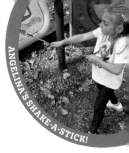

ANGELINA'S SHAKE-A-STICK!

EVER BEEN TO A NASCAR RACE? I've attended just one: the 1995 Richmond race won by Terry Labonte. I had zero desire to go; I went as a favor to a friend who had been pestering me to go with him. And I'll tell you what: it should be a bucket list item for everyone. It's like the Grand Canyon. No matter how many photos or films or travelogues you see, there's just no way to imagine how spectacular the in-person experience is. Just like the Grand Canyon, a NASCAR race is a wide-eyed, open-mouthed, WOW experience. So if you haven't yet gone, my recommendation is to go.

But a NASCAR race is probably the last thing in the world I would recommend for an autistic person. The sensory bombardment is more overwhelming than anything I can think of.

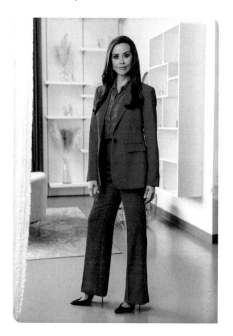

At least that was my thought until I learned about Lori Waran, President of Richmond Raceway. It's of course unusual for a woman to head a NASCAR track, but it's unique, one-of-a-kind, for an autism parent to head a NASCAR track and to be putting in place steps (Lori insists they are "baby steps") to accommodate autistic persons. Richmond Raceway's baby steps include free sensory kits (headphones, fidget toys, etc.) and a sensory room. This is just one part of Lori's community-wide outreach to emphasize Richmond Raceway's open-armed welcoming of diversity and inclusion. She says that Richmond Raceway now has the most diverse audience of all NASCAR tracks.

The title of this section is something that Lori's autistic son, Jackson, now 23, said when he was four. He was riding in the car with the windows down and it started to rain. When Jackson was told that the windows were going to be put up, he protested by explaining, "Rain comes down like the letter i, not the letter j." (And thus each raindrop's vertical path wouldn't allow for curving into an open window.) If you're involved with autism, you know that this is something that a uniquely-wired autistic brain is capable of saying. (Just like Angelina . . . as confirmed throughout this book.)

As this is being written, Jackson Waran is two weeks away from completing a Master's degree in Accounting, after which he has a job waiting for him. But early on, his future was unsure.

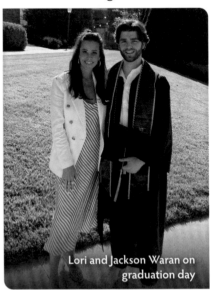

He exhibited strange behaviors as a toddler: wrapping tightly in blankets ("like a burrito"), eating mulch on the playground, biting other children in pre-school, non-verbal issues, extreme sensitivity to loud and abundant noise.

When he was almost three years old, Jackson was evaluated by a professional who gave the autism diagnosis, after which various supports and therapies were begun: physical therapy, occupational therapy, speech therapy, etc. He became verbal quickly. He continued to receive various supports and therapies, as needed, through high school.

Jackson's maternal grandparents, both educators, were extremely helpful and involved from the beginning. They investigated healthcare and schooling, made calls, and provided caregiving. And they were smilingly "amused" by Jackson's quirky behaviors and comments.

Jackson was mainstreamed throughout the public school system, always had IEPs, and also had wonderful support and guidance from a beloved special education specialist.

Jackson's autism presented two special challenges for Lori. First, because she was a first-time mother, she didn't have another child for comparison and was thus susceptive to healthcare professionals telling her not to be concerned about what she considered to be unusual behaviors. And second, because Jackson is, as she describes, "high functioning," it was a challenge for her to be convincing about his need for supports and services.

Jackson has done well in college, has done well with his roommates (who were his high school friends), and now no longer needs supports: he cooks, handles his finances, etc. He calls home from time to time for conversation, consultation, and commiseration. Jackson does have challenges as he interacts with a neurotypical world. For example, even though he can look people in the eyes, and even though he can interact well in social situations, both are exhausting. Lori says that at the family's annual Christmas gathering, after around three hours Jackson needs time to be alone and rest.

One of Lori's goals for Jackson was for him to have at least one friend by the time he graduated from high school. He had three. Another of her goals was for him to have a handful of friends by the time he graduated from college: "He has a couple of handfuls!"

*Note from the author: In 2007, NASCAR's June 3 race at Dover International Speedway was titled, "**Autism Speaks 400 presented by Visa**." A portion of ticket sales went to Autism Speaks. Today Dover International Raceway has a special viewing area designed specifically for autistic persons.*

Lori and Jackson Waran on graduation day

When you go to Pocono Raceway, you'll see that they provide sensory kits, two sensory rooms, and a 5,000-square-foot inclusive playground. (Pocono President Ben May and Lori communicate about their tracks taking steps to accommodate autism.)

Ever heard of Armani Williams? He's the first NASCAR driver to discuss his autism publicly. There's a seven-minute video of his story on YouTube.

PS – Later I'm going to ask Angelina about rain coming down like specific letters of the alphabet.

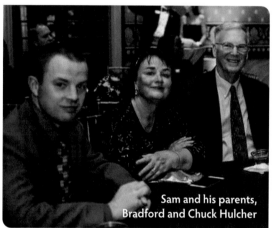

Sam Hulcher – The Author's Introduction to Autism

MY INTRODUCTION TO AUTISM HAPPENED NEARLY 30 YEARS AGO when my friend Gin Robertson introduced me to her 5-year-old grandson, Sam Hulcher. I'd heard of autism but had zero knowledge. Here in Richmond back then, and I suspect in much of the nation, there wasn't much expertise regarding autism. Sam's mother (Gin's daughter), Bradford Hulcher, with encouragement and support from her husband, Chuck, would become one of our city's trailblazing pioneers regarding autism. And Gin Robertson and her partner John Keneski would become role models for autism grandparents.

Recently I interviewed Bradford and used the information to write an article about Sam's life. When I showed the article to Bradford, she provided the following heartfelt and candid response which I greatly appreciated.

"I have been thinking about our conversation and the article that you wrote based on that conversation. There were things I really liked that you wrote, especially the inclusion of Mama and

Sam and his parents, Bradford and Chuck Hulcher

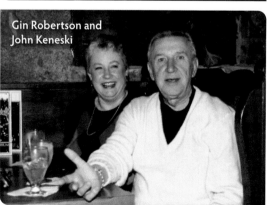

Gin Robertson and John Keneski

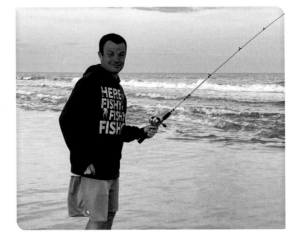

John's impact on our journey and your personal observations of Sam. But something about the article didn't sit right with me; something was missing and I couldn't put my finger on what it was. After some thought, I realized that many of the things that you asked me and that we talked about are not really, in the end, things that are important to our journey or Sam's story; an example would be medications Sam has taken or treatments he has received. Of course, it's your book and your vision and what I am sharing might not track with that. And so I very humbly offer the following thoughts and understand if they do not fit in the scope of your book.

"From a very early age, our dream for Sam was to have an 'ordinary' life, to be included with his typical peers. For many years, we struggled to have Sam included in his school and the greater community and to access opportunities he might not have in 'special' segregated settings. As a child, Sam had high support needs as he had very little language and many 'challenging behaviors;' our vision was not easily grasped by educators or community members. And so we were constantly sharing our dreams for Sam with those who had the power to decide whether he was included and always negotiating the supports that Sam and others would need for inclusion to be successful. Unlike Mama, I have always been a shy introvert and not at all outspoken – until Sam came along. Still, it was really, really hard; it was unrelenting advocacy for 20 years as Sam transitioned from grade to grade, from preschool to high school. This was a huge area where Mama and John's support and encouragement was so impactful to me. They 'got it' and understood what so many others didn't as far as what we wanted for Sam.

"I don't think I conveyed much of this to you as I responded to your questions."

[Following is Bradford's own article about Sam – what she wants folks to know about her family's journey.]

Sam Hulcher has been described as outgoing, a fierce competitor, a loyal and compassionate friend, and a hard and dedicated worker. But Sam hasn't always been seen this way; as a little boy, Sam had many of the classic signs of autism. He could not talk, did not sleep through the night, had daily major meltdowns, and wasn't meeting developmental milestones.

Despite those challenges, my husband and I dreamed of an "ordinary" life for Sam – a life that would include friends, community, a job that interested him, and a home of his own.

We were told by the "experts" that, because of the severity of his autism, Sam would never be able to read, do math, or be around typical peers. Yet, we were determined that Sam be given the opportu-

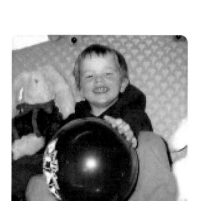

nity to discover his strengths, interests, and talents. It has not been an easy path but Sam, given opportunity, has proven "the experts" wrong.

Sam was a Boy Scout and attended Boy Scout camp. He attended 4 H camp where he learned to kayak and hang glide. Sam was an acolyte at church and joined his church youth group on mission trips to West Virginia and Chicago. In high school, Sam was a member of chorus and drama, performing alongside his peers, in New York City, Nashville, Atlanta, and Orlando. Sam was in JROTC. He managed the varsity football team and the boys' varsity soccer team for 4 years, winning a state championship ring with the team. Sam attended senior prom. He was voted "Most Spirited Dancer" by his class at the annual high school marathon dance. Sam was a well-loved and popular member of his high school.

As an adult, Sam continues to live an "ordinary" life. After a nine-month internship with Project SEARCH and exiting high school, Sam was competitively employed part-time for 5 years at a local hospital. Later, Sam began working at Virginia Commonwealth University's Cary Street Gym, where he realized his dream of employment in a sports environment!

Sam lives in his own apartment with a companion to support him. He volunteers weekly at the food bank, firewood ministry, and SPCA. He participates in local sports leagues with "neurotypical" adults, playing kickball, dodgeball, bocce ball and cornhole. He plays soccer, basketball, golf, and swims with Special Olympics. He attends church and is involved in Bible study. Sam is a sports fanatic and attends every collegiate and professional game he can. Sam was named a model for the 2019 capABLE Campaign and was included in an exhibit at the Virginia Museum of History and Culture.

By God's grace and the opportunities afforded him, Sam has far exceeded the expectations of the professionals who first gave him the label of autism. Sam is not "cured;" he still has autism. But he also has a full and rich life of which we could only, at one time, dare to imagine.

[And following is the article that I wrote after interviewing Bradford – an article that, as you'll see, includes a lot of details that may be helpful to some of this book's readers but, as Bradford says, "are not really important to Sam's journey."]

When Sam was born on July 16, 1990 there were two immediate causes for concern; his head was larger than normal, and he emitted a high-pitched squeal rather than a normal cry – both indicators of possible neurological issues. But an MRI didn't find anything wrong.

As an infant and toddler it was hard to take Sam anywhere. For example, he would start screaming when entering a grocery store. (Bradford now suspects that he had sensory issues regarding the store's lights.) Sam was very tactile-sensitive, he cried a lot and wasn't comforted by being held, he

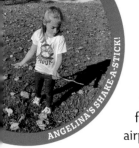

ANGELINA'S SHAKE-A-STICK!

was non-verbal (he began speaking later than normal), and he didn't respond to voices. Bradford thought he might be deaf, but when she saw him look up when there was noise from an airplane flying overhead she realized that he could hear.

When he was 2 the pediatrician said that Sam had PDD – Pervasive Developmental Delay. Bradford found a book in the library that said that PDD often means autism, and the pediatrician concurred. Neither the phrase "early intervention" nor today's commonly recommended therapies were in place back then, so, for example, there were no behavioral therapies for Sam.

Sam went to pre-school categorized as "developmentally delayed." It was then that Bradford met an autism consultant who helped her understand Sam's behavior. Whenever Bradford visited the pre-school, Sam would start crying the moment he saw her; he wanted to be with her. The autism consultant asked Bradford to take her to the school to observe Sam from a distance, but Sam saw Bradford and started crying. Sam's aide started trying to comfort him and Sam said to the aide "Leave Sam alone." The consultant told Bradford to wait and just observe. The aide got closer to Sam in an effort to provide more comfort and Sam hit her. That enabled Bradford to understand that when Sam gets upset, it only makes things worse to try to closely comfort him. His message, "Leave Sam alone," was important.

This was a significant turning point for Bradford's understanding of Sam; she had learned that behavior is a form of communication.

Bradford took Sam to a neurologist who was a disappointment and whom she soon left. (He kept Bradford and Sam in the waiting room for hours, he got them to pay his wife $500 to conduct an educational assessment that said Sam had a low IQ, and he was generally dismissive of Sam's condition.) Of course back then many neurologists didn't have much experience with autism.

Sam was then enrolled in a school that had some expertise with students who were developmentally delayed. The school's IQ test showed that Sam's IQ was average rather than low as per the neurologist. Bradford's autism consultant provided a written recommendation for Sam to have speech therapy 5 days per week as well as extended school year services (schooling for 12 months). The recommendation allowed Bradford to access those services for Sam from the school system. One result of Bradford's aggressive research about autism was her enrollment in a "Partners in Policymaking" program that taught her how to navigate the complex process of getting support for Sam. Her persistence resulted in him also getting speech therapy, physical therapy (to help with toe-walking), and occupational therapy.

There weren't many established medicines back then to address challenging autism problems, but Bradford tried a couple of them. Sam had problems getting to sleep (Bradford had to sleep on the floor in his room until he fell asleep) so he tried taking Clonidine – but discontinued because of side effects. And for anxiety he tried Ritalin, but discontinued because it made him sad, including crying.

CHAPTER V: Profiles By and About Autistics

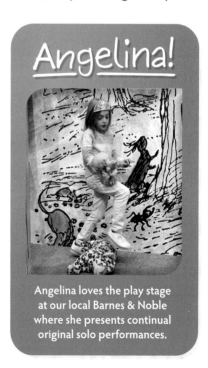

Bradford was aggressive in learning as much as possible, including enrolling in classes and workshops. She recalls the eye-opening information she learned about men's public restrooms; the culture is much different from that in women's restrooms. In men's restrooms you never talk to one another, you never pass toilet paper under the stall to another person who needs it, you go to the urinal that is most distant from any urinal that is being used by someone else, and you never drop your pants to the floor when using a urinal. Autistic children don't just automatically learn etiquette for public restrooms. Sam is very sociable; what if he were to go to a urinal adjacent to someone else, drop his pants to the floor, produce a friendly smile, and start a conversation?

Bradford continued her aggressive research and advocacy and also joined a handful of other parents in meetings convened by the fledgling Autism Society of Central Virginia (ASCV). In the beginning the small group met at Richmond's Children's Hospital and later at a church. As the group grew they started having speakers, started providing childcare during meetings, established a library, held social and recreational events, and held events including a 5K walk/run that has continued to grow and is now a huge annual gathering that includes food and music and a variety of activities.

Sam has grown up to be a happy and engaging working adult. And he has activities almost every night: basketball, church, social groups, etc. He is happiest when he is with people, and they, in turn, light up when they encounter him. He seems to have friends everywhere, including via the sports events that he attends and follows and is very knowledgeable about. (Every morning he buys the daily newspaper to read all of the sports scores and articles.) And he loves the outdoors: especially fishing, crabbing, and kayaking at his brother's home on a tributary of the Chesapeake Bay. He no longer lives with Bradford and Chuck, but he sees them frequently and he sends texts about his activities.

Angelina!

Angelina loves the play stage at our local Barnes & Noble where she presents continual original solo performances.

The only medicines that Sam takes today are an antidepressant and an anti-seizure medicine. Sam had a couple of seizures as a teen, years before he was prescribed with the seizure medication. It was determined that the seizures were caused by severe sleep apnea; once he began using a CPAP he had no more seizures. Sam's current seizure medicine was prescribed few years ago as possible help for some of Sam's behavior issues at work. One result was the cessation of his lifelong bed-wetting. The medicine has no significant side effects, and its continued use has eliminated the bed-wetting, which the doctors now suspect was triggered by nighttime seizures.

At an initial IEP meeting at Sam's first school, Bradford told the Vice Principal about her fundamental goals for Sam's adulthood: to read, to have a job, and to have friends. The Vice Prin-

---

ANGELINA'S SHAKE-A-STICK!

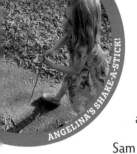

cipal responded that he would never be able to reach any of those goals. Sam has achieved all three.

Sam cares about other persons. He remembers their names. He's compassionate. He's a hard worker. And he loves being part of a team – whether on sports teams or at his paid job or during his volunteer work at the Food Pantry.

I am of course an autism grandparent (Bradford was the first person I called for consultation when Angelina was diagnosed) and I asked Bradford if she has advice for other grandparents – advice based on her mother's involvements with Sam. Bradford offered four recommendations – all of which her mother and her partner John did.

First, they never criticized Bradford, but continually praised her for the good job she was doing with Sam. Second, they kept Sam for a night or two from time to time so Bradford and Chuck could do things. Bradford smilingly recalls once when she and Chuck returned from being away for two or three days there was a stick in the yard with a white flag on it. (Sam had been sick with terrible diarrhea.) Gin and John didn't complain, but rather they laughed about the stick. Third, they celebrated every step of Sam's progress. And fourth, they didn't love Sam any more or less than his neurotypical brother, Clay.

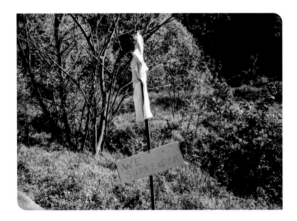

And finally, I asked Bradford if she has advice for new autism families. She advises to interact with and stay connected to other autism parents; they can provide information and assistance that professionals can't. She says to have dreams for your children. She says it's never too early to start learning about transition to adulthood: take classes over and over because it's difficult to absorb all of the information and rules and regulations of what has become an extremely complex system of publicly funded programs and benefits for persons with developmental disabilities,

Gin Robertson, Bradford's mother, introduced me to her autistic grandson Sam, but because she was such a champion for a whole range of diversity and inclusion, I was unaware of her vigorous involvement with autism until now. I've learned that her involvement included hosting the ASCV's board meetings at her home. John became a board member and served as treasurer. And Gin and John together were proud and active advocates.

After Gin first introduced me to Sam I would see him every now and then when he was with her. But after her death I rarely saw him. Prior to Angelina's diagnosis I wasn't involved with autism. I knew Bradford only from having met her a few times with Gin.

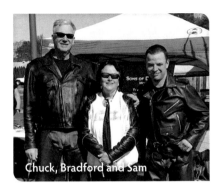
Chuck, Bradford and Sam

These days I see Sam from time to time, including last month when I was a volunteer at a social event for autistic adults. I observed him happily interacting with just about everyone and watched him play pool with two other men – always enjoying the game even when the others bent the rules or perhaps were unaware of the rules. I vote for more of us to have a dose of Sam's characteristics.

[Read more about Bradford Hulcher at the end of her article, "Preparing for Life after High School – Avoiding the Cliff."]

Angelina's Story:
Westhampton Day School

THE FAISON CENTER HAS A PARTNERSHIP with a private, respected elementary school: Westhampton Day School. Westhampton established a second "campus" – a neurotypical pre-K classroom at The Faison Center. The idea was that when Faison students were ready/able, they would be able to walk across the hall, accompanied by a personal aide, and be a part of Westhampton's neurotypical classroom – first for brief periods of time, and then, if no problems, for longer and longer amounts of time.

Angelina made this transition wonderfully and progressed steadily until she was spending most of each day in the Westhampton classroom, albeit accompanied by an aide.

The next step for Angelina, accompanied by an aide, was to transition to Westhampton's main campus that included pre-K through 5th grade. Angelina adjusted well there and was eventually weaned from having an aide, including going on field trips. She was still developmentally delayed – both physically (smallest person in the class) and cognitively – and the recommendation was for her to do another year of pre-K, which she did with no problems.

(All of this was very expensive, but Kelly's insurance along with special scholarship funding from Faison paid for everything.)

After Westhampton, Angelina was ready to enroll in public school kindergarten.

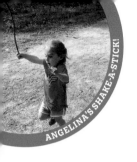
ANGELINA'S SHAKE-A-STICK!

My Double Life as a Parent and a Professional

By Kathy Matthews

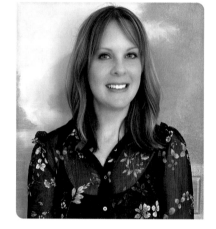

AS A PROFESSIONAL, I'D SPENT ALMOST 20 YEARS supporting individuals and families impacted by disabilities, particularly autism. During that time I served as a teacher's assistant, special education teacher, early intervention coordinator, behavior analyst, and school director, all roles in which I supported and taught individuals of all ages impacted by disability. My work was my passion and my pride. As I was hitting my professional stride, I found myself preparing for my first child, Ethan. I was overjoyed to start this adventure and planned carefully and thoughtfully about how to juggle my career and raise him in the best way possible.

Ethan's arrival was my happiest day. I recall staring at him for what seemed hours at a time. How could someone so small be so beautiful and perfect and how on earth did I deserve this? I captured every moment of his life on my camera, shared it with the world on social media, and involved him in everything I could. His smile, his curls, his willingness to join me in our daily adventures filled me with endless joy. None of this has changed to this day. But what I came to understand about Ethan and our future together did.

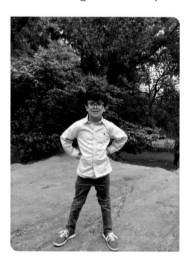

In Ethan's early months and as I transitioned back to work, I noticed things about him that were all too familiar to me. I found myself turning on the kitchen sink faucet to calm him while I prepared his meals. Something about the running water amazed him more than any toy I could find. I watched him spin the top of his yogurt pouch on his highchair tray in a way that no one his age should have been able to. I watched his expressionless face as he moved from my arms to my mother's when she visited. Why didn't he look at my mom when she took him? Shouldn't he notice a new person?

But I knew why. I'd seen signs of it as early as 8 months. He had autism. Autism was my professional world, my work, my passion. In this early stage of his life, I realized autism was crossing into my personal world and about to become my entire life. And just like

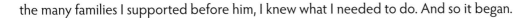

the many families I supported before him, I knew what I needed to do. And so it began.

"Ethan is so lucky to have you."- Ethan and I have had a deep bond since the time of my pregnancy. Just as most parents, those first few months were dedicated to loving, feeding, and caring for him. Loving him was everything I thought it would be. Realizing his autism diagnosis didn't change any of that. But it did change me. Now I was both caring for him and being the professional he needed. The work I did by day was also the work I needed to do at home for him. And, knowing the lifelong nature of autism, his needs might be never-ending. Certainly, as with all children, I expected him to grow and learn and develop. But disability places a giant question mark in the middle of the road asking, will your child be okay when they grow up? I had no idea and this scared me.

As I started on a path to get his official diagnosis and to start early intervention services, I had so many people comment that Ethan was lucky to have me as a parent. They thought he was lucky because I was a professional. What I felt but could never say was that I didn't want to be his professional. I wanted to be Ethan's mom. I knew I had to be both but those roles merged together at this early stage. Everything Ethan did or that I did, I mentally evaluated. Was that the right way to address that? He seems to like that toy, is he liking it too much? Is it possible to like something too much? I was so conflicted about the "professional parent" role I was in that I found myself visiting parks at early hours before most people arrived so that I could work on showing Ethan how to use the playground equipment and not feel weird telling him what a great job he was doing or using physical prompts to assist him. I was no stranger to the side eye from a fellow parent thinking I was being overbearing, without that parent realizing that Ethan didn't know how to do these simple things that their child could do. Autism is such a tricky thing, it doesn't usually have a physical marker, and particularly at this age. Through all of this Ethan was happy and as he learned, he soared. He raced up the steps, climbed the ladders, all with the biggest smile with his curls bouncing around his face.

Around this time and even when I was still pregnant with Ethan, I helped to support efforts in Virginia advocating for insurance companies to fund ABA therapy. I recall sitting at meetings with Autism Speaks and supporting their efforts to help behavior analysts get licensed and to create a pathway for funded Applied Behavior Analysis services. At that time in my role as administrator at The Faison Center for Autism, we were a day school and therefore enrolled students starting at age 5. As a leader of one of the largest ABA centers, it was hard to stomach walking into a building that my own son couldn't attend due to his age. Therefore, I worked to start an early intervention program at our center. I brought Ethan to work for this new program and, given that he was so young and the program so new, after a few hours of therapy, placed him in a playpen in my office for his nap. I had volunteers such as Lynne Faison, help take Ethan from my office to a daycare center where my friend and champion, Danielle Simone, organized an integrated preschool experience for him. Lynne and Danielle were some of my first heroes. I was also lucky to have Jody Liesfeld, Emily Schwab, Rachel Ernest, Jen Weber and so many more who helped, cheered and supported me as a friend and mentor during this time.

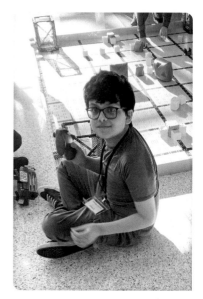

My Quest to Become a Parent – Although I was able to pull together services and supports for Ethan, I was still conflicted in my role. I always felt in charge of his services, I felt responsible for his progress, and I felt the need to bring all the pieces together. How could I not feel that way? I was running the center where he attended. I couldn't separate the role of parent and professional. I was all things at all times. It was so hard to just "be" with Ethan without thinking about all of these pieces, whether everything was how it needed to be, and to consider what else I was missing. Was I doing enough? Was he getting enough help? As always, Ethan was all smiles, full of joy, and despite my worry, progressing. Through this, I was increasingly anxious, conflicted, pressured, and these feelings were taking a toll on my well-being. I can remember taking medication, talking to a therapist, trying to apply self-care routines, but all the things I was doing to help myself were failing, and they were just adding to the list of things that made me feel bad. Something had to change.

As Ethan approached age 4, I decided to circle back to my colleagues in New York, where I learned my profession. They accepted him into their inclusive program and we started a new chapter in life. While in New York, I walked Ethan to school every morning and for the first time was able to drop him off and head back to work. I had no idea how good it would feel to see Ethan walk into a classroom with a team waiting for him, prepared to help, and offering him every opportunity to grow. And more importantly, how it would feel upon dropping him off, to do the thing every parent does after they drop their kid at school, walk away. I began a journey of my own, learning how to get back into a routine of work and self-care, as well as learning how to lean on other professionals. I didn't have to have the answers, I didn't have to feel like I was the one driving the effort. I was instead a key member of Ethan's support team, an advocate for him, a collaborator and coordinator. We spent our weekends at the library, at the park, and at local events. We found friends and we enjoyed every bit of New York. And to this day, I relish every bit of being his parent.

Our family has been back in the greater Richmond area for the last several years and Ethan is thriving. He enjoys school, robotics, takes drum lessons, and loves spending time with this little brother, Andy. There are still challenges but he continues to push ahead and we are looking forward to the future.

Dr. Kathy Matthews, Chief Clinical Officer for All Needs Planning (allneedsplanning.com), has a Bachelor's degree in psychology from Virginia Commonwealth University and a Master's and PhD from Columbia University's Teachers College in New York where she also taught students with special needs from early intervention through high school. She returned to Richmond as an administrator at The Faison Center for 20 years, helping to provide services for children, adults and families impacted by autism.

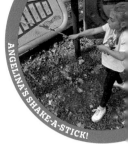

How I Learned to Embrace My Son's Neurodiversity and Celebrate His Strengths

By Kristin Carleton

NOTE: Kristin Carleton (Chief Executive Officer) and Kathy Matthews (Chief Clinical Officer) are friends who have partnered in developing All Needs Planning (allneedsplanning.com) – a company that "provides real world planning for special needs families."

W**HAT WOULD YOU DO IF YOU FOUND OUT** your unborn child had a rare brain condition that could affect his development and behavior? How would you cope if you later learned he also had autism? This is what happened to me and my son John Elijah, and this is our story.

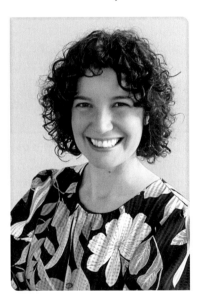

The Diagnosis – I was 19 weeks pregnant when I learned that my son had agenesis of the corpus callosum (ACC), a condition where the band of nerve fibers that connects the two hemispheres of the brain is missing. I had gone to the Children's Hospital of Richmond, using the children's MRI machine because that was the only place they could accommodate me on short notice. In fact, the only reason they worked me in was because I was nearing the time of termination being legal, and my husband and I wanted to know if his condition would cause him lifelong pain. I share this because it's hard. It was the hardest thing I have ever lived through. At the time, I forged ahead – because that is what you do. It is only now that I have started to work through the trauma I felt then. This baby was a baby I had prayed for. I had two miscarriages, and each of those babies I wanted. I felt guilty that my body was not capable of providing them with life. And I felt guilty that somehow I had caused this brain malformation.

I write this because being this vulnerable is hard for me. And healing. And because maybe you, too, have felt these things, and can benefit from knowing that I felt them, too.

I was told that this brain malformation could cause a range of symptoms, from mild to severe, such as intellectual disability, seizures, vision problems and/or blindness, and behavioral issues. I was also told that he might have autism and that this would be a "best case scenario," but that it was hard to tell because autism and ACC can have similar features. I was scared, confused, and overwhelmed, but I also had faith that God had a plan for my son and that he would be a blessing to our family.

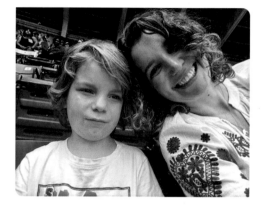

I say "the diagnosis," but like many children with disabilities, it did not stop with agenesis of the corpus callosum. At two weeks old, he had a seizure while in the ophthalmologist's office getting his optic nerve checked (it looks "thin" to this day). A hospital stay and EEG resulted in an epilepsy diagnosis. Soon after that he was diagnosed with septo-optic dysplasia. A further brain ultrasound said that he had no activity in the rear of his brain, and that we should expect him to be unable to process visual images and that he would be severely intellectually disabled. Hypotonia was thrown in.

The Challenges – We threw ourselves into therapy very early. Eli was eligible for early intervention because of his prenatal diagnosis, and I had them come to the house within a few weeks of his birth. This was a phenomenal program for us: family centered, they met us where we were and helped us incorporate his therapies into our daily routines.

When the first therapist (a kind but inexperienced physical therapist who had no direct experience working with babies) told us he was too young to be able to do anything, and reduced our services to fifteen minutes every other week, I had my first real lesson in advocacy, and requested a new therapist. That therapist is someone that we are still friends with today, even though she is not working with my family.

Jenny is amazing. She taught me to look beyond what the world was telling me about the right way for Eli to develop, and to focus on the goal. He would not crawl – this kid literally would not do tummy time, he'd be on his tummy and cry and cry and cry. "Put him on there longer," the specialists would say. "He'll get used to it, eventually he'll get those back muscles going." Nope – Jenny helped us see that there were other ways for us to reach the goal, working with Eli and what he was telling us he needed. So he did not do tummy time, but he did "fly" – on my chest, on my feet, in the carrier – to work on that neck and core strength. Who knows why Eli did not like that tummy time – maybe it was his larger than normal head, or the vestibular input he received from larger than usual ventricles with extra spinal fluid sloshing around. We will never know, and will always be grateful to Jenny for helping us find alternate paths. Eli started walking because Jenny showed him that the independence he gained from walking would help him get what he wanted – and oh he wanted independence. Many people have said "Eli is the most stubborn kid I have ever worked with," and Jenny used that as an advantage.

Jenny is not the only incredible therapist that we have worked with who made a huge impact on our family – there are so many that I am afraid to leave one out. Caitlyn, Sarah, and Becky – Becky, who taught him how to play collaboratively, and scaffolded him so that he developed the confidence to

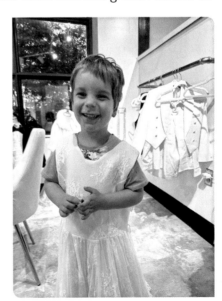

be able to interact with others and again – get to his goal (playing with friends) in spite of the anxiety that came from needing things done in a certain way, or play not meeting expectations. Caitlyn, who walked us through countless sensory strategies, who laughed with me recently about how maybe autism plastic surgery is going to sleep, and waking up with your nails trimmed, hair cut, and fully bathed and fresh – without having to go through the sensory overwhelm of those experiences.

One of the biggest challenges we faced was getting Eli access to services. Everywhere, it seemed, the answer was no. He's not eligible – he doesn't have autism – yes we understand he has the same symptoms as autism, and may benefit from the same supports, but it's not autism. It's agenesis of the corpus callosum, and we don't understand that, we don't have a code for it, we don't have research to support what is needed. The insurance company called the shots.

Getting the autism diagnosis opened up more doors for him. What I was not expecting was the trauma I would feel about receiving it – even though I had actively sought that diagnosis.

Trauma After Diagnosis – I was extremely depressed after receiving Eli's diagnosis. I kept thinking, why does this little boy need to face so many challenges? Why does life need to be so much harder for him? What am I doing as a mom to have failed him? The science part of me said, how do I get those genes to turn off? I was railing at the world. At God. At myself. I was mad. And sad.

I am looking for a therapist to work through a lot of these feelings. It's been almost a year and I still have a lot of work to do. I have been working with a counselor and started journaling my thoughts. Sharing with others, joining a support group, and giving myself some time and grace. I do not expect that there is an "aha" moment where I will suddenly feel healed. No, I expect that this will be a lifelong process.

What I do know is that this little boy is an incredible gift to me, and while it is ok to feel sad about the life that might have been, I focus every day on the life that IS, and the wonder of who he is. Because I was told that this little boy was going to be blind, non-verbal, and not able to walk. Yet here today, he walks, talks up a storm (he is currently interested in space, just ask him about the hottest planet), has incredible vision, and empathy. Yes, empathy. Many think that autism means a lack of empathy but that is simply untrue. If one of Eli's friends is hurt, he is always the first to go over and ask them if they are ok. He asks how he can help, and will rub their back. He may not pick up on the social cues that neurotypical children do, but do not confuse that with lack of empathy.

The Support – When I learned of Eli's diagnosis, I fell back on what I knew. I am a financial planner by trade, so I told myself that he would have the best financial plan that ever existed. I quickly learned that there was so much more to a successful plan for him than simply the investments, savings, and special needs trust. A successful plan was going to need so much more.

I recently learned of the model of a Medical Home – a centralized location where one can access all of the supports one needs, a hub that keeps track of everything and reaches out to all the other aspects of a person's life who has complex medical needs. This model has not been widely adopted, as it is expensive and hard to set up a system of accountability. A good friend and mentor started along that path with his nonprofit, Medical Home Plus, where the Plus is the parents' role and involvement. I love this model with a centralized part, and what I have learned through my degree in Economics and experience as a financial planner is that the best way to ensure supports is to follow the money and make sure it can be paid for. The largest fee that a person usually pays is to their financial advisor, if they are working with one. And so, why not use that fee to ensure that a centralized location can be set up for the support of your loved one? Make that fee work for you.

From that, an idea was born – that families can start to demand that their advisors, specialists, therapists, planners, case managers, CPA, attorney, everyone work together to advance the goals of their family. It's person centered. It's family centered. It is designed to support every member of the family, their goals and dreams. Each person is important.

Too often, a sibling is ignored. Parents put their needs last. Sleep is no longer a priority. One parent has to sacrifice their career. Family centered planning takes everyone into account and looks at meeting each of those needs.

When you are looking to build your own team, I encourage you to first see who will be the hub for the rest of your planning. Will it be you? Is there a company or service or non-profit that you would like to do that for you, who is capable of doing that for you?

Once you have the hub, then branch out from there to find the supporting cast. What do you have in place today? What do you need? How will you pay for it? How will you protect it? What protections will be necessary?

The answer to these questions will then set you on a path towards finding the professionals, family members, friends, and non-profit supports that you will want in your circle. Start with the hub and then fill in the spokes.

I strongly recommend that you start by understanding your own needs. Then look at the spokes. I break things out in three simple steps:

1: Funding – what will you need to fund your own goals? What will be needed to fund your disabled child's goals? Write down what you have now, and different sources you may not have

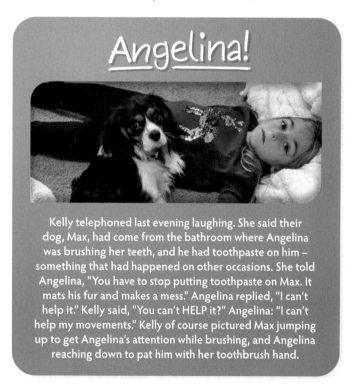

tapped. Working with a special needs planner could help this process, as they can also help you uncover other sources of public and private funding, from government benefits to life insurance, that you may not be utilizing.

2: Legal – from estate planning to decision-making supports to protections for vulnerable individuals, legal planning is more important for families with an autistic family member. Putting those protections in place, while also ensuring things are flexible and allowing each member to reach their full potential, is extremely important. You might start by attending a webinar to get a better handle on the legal tools available. Make sure you find an attorney that specializes in elder law and/or special needs planning, and ensure their training is up-to-date. A lot has changed in the special needs planning legal world in the last few years; an attorney with outdated knowledge may not be serving your family well.

3: Supports – from IEPs, medical advocacy, therapeutic supports, respite, and more, all of us need supports. Autism families have more balls in the air. Writing these down and thinking strategically about what's next can really help you move through this. This is the time to put a care plan in place – what would need to happen when you are no longer here? Do you have all medical records gathered, including diagnosis records and a list of all specialists needed, and how often each specialist is visited? And make sure that your social supports are there too. You need friends. Your children need friends. People that can help fill your cup and keep you connected. Join a support group, find a few other moms, dads, grandparents, going through the same thing and meet regularly. Vent, share notes.

Here are some resources that have been so incredibly helpful to me along the way:

- Joining a Facebook group of other caregivers of kids with disabilities – for both diagnoses that my son has. These other caregivers really got me, and being able to see that I was not alone in what I was experiencing and feeling, before I was ready to share, was so valuable to me.

Angelina!

Kelly telephoned last evening laughing. She said their dog, Max, had come from the bathroom where Angelina was brushing her teeth, and he had toothpaste on him – something that had happened on other occasions. She told Angelina, "You have to stop putting toothpaste on Max. It mats his fur and makes a mess." Angelina replied, "I can't help it." Kelly said, "You can't HELP it?" Angelina: "I can't help my movements." Kelly of course pictured Max jumping up to get Angelina's attention while brushing, and Angelina reaching down to pat him with her toothbrush hand.

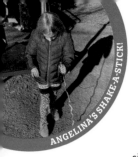

- Finding autism certified or autism friendly vendors. From hairdressers to pediatricians and dentists, finding those who were willing to work with the differences that my son had – from sensory differences, to unwillingness to make eye contact, to extreme anxiety in new situations. Local autism nonprofits can help with this, asking other caregivers, the local Facebook groups, and paying attention to whether it's on the website of the providers is all helpful.

- Finding a special needs planner who can help with financial planning for my lifetime and goals, reflect my daughter's goals, Eli's needs over his lifetime, and understanding the nuances of ABLE accounts, cash flows, funding streams, taxes, and then tying all of that into an estate plan and legal protections for him. I want to be clear. I started a business that does all of those things, and yet I still use a different professional for my own. Because planning for myself is different than planning for others – and I find that it is impossible to separate my emotion or see the big picture in my own life. I encourage you to do the same. Find a professional that can help you work through this. Whether that professional is through the ARC, a financial planning firm, or a disability navigator, find someone that you trust.

- Work with an attorney to establish the legal documents that you need in your estate plan and legal protections. Find someone who specializes in special needs planning or elder law.

- Look into education resources – from IEPs to BIPs, know the language, learn if you need an advocate, know your child's rights, and advocate, advocate, advocate.

- Back up your Mom gut with research, and then stand up for your child. I have had doctors tell me that I know more about my son's condition than they do. Well, sure, I am his Mom, and I want to know as much as I possibly can. There were times where my Mom gut was just plain wrong. I thought my son should develop naturally, and I could sit him on the floor and his reflexes would get him to walking. This was wrong! And his therapist showed me the research and how doing things differently would work. There were also times where I knew what I was hearing was incorrect. Having a doctor read an EEG result and say that Eli could not process visual images, when he could easily navigate around objects, react to things happening across long distances, and point out objects in books told a completely different story.

- Know that you may have to look outside of your local area for some resources and/or professionals. And that's ok. Do virtual as often as you can when this happens.

- Take care of yourself. Arrange a regular babysitter, get a home workout routine going, drink a daily cup of coffee while it's still hot. I found that taking care of myself didn't mean the usual self care – getting my nails done regularly, or getting massages. It meant doing small daily things that gave my brain and body an opportunity to rest.

- My last piece of advice is to take a deep breath. Know that you cannot do everything at once. Both of my children are on therapy vacations right now. They are thriving and need the opportunity to just be kids. Pat yourself on the back.

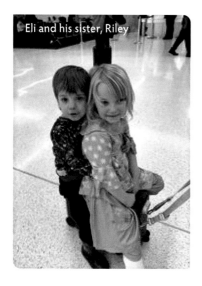
Eli and his sister, Riley

ANGELINA'S SHAKE-A-STICK!

Are you feeling overwhelmed? I did, too. It's actually why I started my business. I felt that my family deserved a team of professionals walking alongside us to help us with all of the details I mentioned above. From financial and legal planning to support strategies, IEP advocacy, and finding the right professionals. And if my family wanted and needed this, other families did too. I wanted everyone to feel they had a team that could provide empathy and expertise in navigating this journey.

Conclusion – My son John Elijah is now 4 years old, and he is the most amazing boy I have ever met. He has autism and ACC, and he is beautiful. He is smart, funny, creative, and loving. He has his challenges, but he also has his strengths. He has taught me so much about life, love, and acceptance. He has shown me that having a diagnosis does not define him, and that he can achieve anything he sets his mind to. He is my son, and I am proud of him. If you have a child with autism, ACC, or any other neurodiverse condition, I hope you know that you are not alone, and that your child is a gift. I hope you find the support, resources, and community that you need. And I hope you celebrate your child's uniqueness and potential every day. I am cheering for you.

Before co-founding All Needs Planning (allneedsplanning.com), Kristin Carleton spent over three years as Vice President of Financial Planning and Investments at James River Wealth Advisors in Midlothian, Virginia. She was also a founder and director of the special needs planning organization Eli's Village in Richmond, Virginia. Before that, Kristin worked extensively in the financial services field as both an advisor and a Registered Client Service Assistant, among other roles. She has dedicated her life to building plans to help ensure that every family, regardless of their situation, can enjoy fulfilling and capable lives.

Ross Lipstock

NOT MANY PEOPLE KNEW ABOUT AUTISM IN 1982 when Ross Lipstock was born. He progressed well from birth, but before he was 2 his mother, Joan Babich Lipstock, noticed that he was different from the others in a play group; one difference was that he didn't socialize well.

Ross had a good friend in his neighborhood, but one day the friend's parents started making excuses why he couldn't go to Ross's house when invited. And Ross stopped getting invited to birthday parties in the neighborhood. Years later Joan learned that a new couple that had moved into the

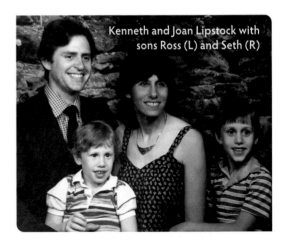

Kenneth and Joan Lipstock with sons Ross (L) and Seth (R)

neighborhood – a child psychologist and a social worker – had told the other neighbors that it might harm their children if they interacted with Ross.

In nursery school Ross played mostly on his own. Joan would see him pacing around the perimeter of the playground with no attempts to include him with the other children. One day the school told Joan that Ross had had a bowel movement in his pants and therefore wouldn't be able to attend the school anymore. Later Joan learned that it was a lie; he hadn't had the bowel movement.

Joan enrolled Ross in a county preschool program that served children with disabilities. Joan says the program was a "catchall" for all sorts of disabilities, even blindness and deafness. When Ross entered elementary school he was labeled "noncategorical" and he was placed in a class with other developmentally delayed children. These classes changed school locations every year, because it was easier for the transportation department to move this smaller number of kids. With different classrooms and different schools, it caused additional challenges for Ross such as getting lost in the hallways. Ross wasn't making friends in the program, and he sat alone at lunch. Joan therefore started driving Ross back and forth for lunch at a small religious school where he could sit with others and experience a bit of socialization and attention. It was around this time that the diagnostic criteria for autism widened, and almost overnight Ross' diagnosis of "noncategorical" went to being on the autism spectrum.

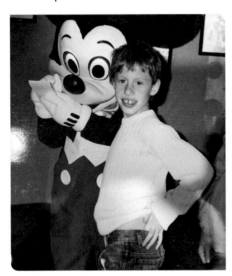

Ross was different from neurotypical students, but he never exhibited poor behavior or aggression. In middle school they put him in regular classes and provided an aide for him. But, unknown to Joan for months, the aide was there only for the first few weeks, and Ross was left to learn without assistance. He would try hard to do his homework, and sometimes his dad or mom would find him up at his desk still working at 3 AM. His teachers told Joan that Ross was very attentive, was taking notes in class, and was working hard. Finally one teacher noticed that during class Ross was doing make believe writing so that he would appear to be doing his work.

Joan realized that the county school system wasn't able to provide the supports that would enable Ross to get

CHAPTER V: Profiles By and About Autistics

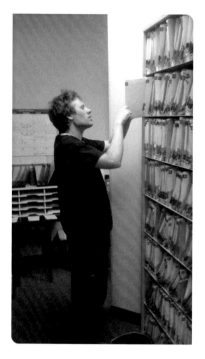

an education – supports that are guaranteed by the federal Individuals with Disabilities Education Act (IDEA), so she asked the county to pay (as IDEA required) for Ross to attend a school that could provide the needed support. Ross' teachers were supportive, but the county said no, so Joan filed a lawsuit. The Lipstocks lost the case and got minimal funding. Nevertheless they enrolled Ross in an hour-distant private boarding school for those with learning disabilities. At this new school with smaller classes with other kids with a variety of developmental delays, Ross began to blossom. His parents were surprised to learn that he had creative writing skills that seemed to have come from nowhere. Ross still had his quirks like picking teams to play on by the color of the outfit and whether it had buttons or not. But he played on teams!

This school only went through middle school, so Ross began another adventure in a high school in another state. The students, all with learning disabilities of various types, came from across the U.S. and from abroad. The Lipstocks soon learned that Virginia was the only state not fully funding the students at the school. While there, Ross continued to thrive and grow in his studies and social interactions. That is not to say that Ross' learning difficulties, shyness, and social awkwardness did not sometimes take its toll and that often these difficulties were overlooked by the staff. For example, one time Ross was scheduled to learn adaptive skiing. He was the only one in his dorm scheduled to go. Ross had never learned how to set an alarm clock. Nobody knew this since Ross would take cues from his dorm mates as to when their alarm clocks went off in the morning. This time no alarms went off and Ross missed the bus. The counselors were shocked; they had no idea that this 15-year-old did not know how to set the alarm. But they were impressed at his coping skills.

After he graduated from that high school, Ross spent a year at an out-of-state vocational school that was part of a community college, which the high school had recommended. While there they directed Ross to skills that were a poor fit for him. His parents decided to bring him home and have him enroll in a vocational program for people with learning disorders. It was at this school that Ross found a good vocational fit. Ross started in the field of clerical assistant and he has never looked back, having worked for the last 20 years at his dad's medical office.

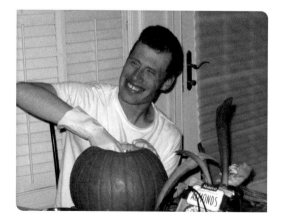

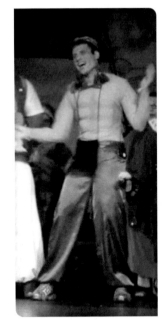

Ross also enrolled in a special program for those with disabilities at a local restaurant. After the program was completed, the ownership liked Ross' work ethic so much that they hired him as a busboy. He worked there two nights a week for seven years while also working at his dad's office. Since Ross doesn't drive, he depended on the CarVan – a bus service for persons with special needs. The problem was that it rarely ran on time, and often Ross was left outside after the restaurant closed at 9pm waiting for the bus until 10 or 11 o'clock. Eventually he simply had to quit. At one point Ross worked at three jobs. At the third he took apart computers for recycling at a business owned by a family friend who was a wonderful mentor to Ross.

Ross continues to be a very valuable member of the team at his dad's office, although guidance from staff and job coaches have been essential. Ross still has little concept of time, and difficulty with practical math, but he has developed skills in the office that others rely on every day.

NOTE: One of Joan's most endearing volunteer projects has been Dreamers Theater which she and 2 other volunteers started in 2003. Ross loves music, and the idea was to provide a program that would enable Ross and others with neurological disabilities to perform publicly. The first performances were vaudeville type events. Eventually Dreamers Theater began presenting full musical plays, all original, some written by Joan. The subject matter of the plays evolved into plots that addressed real-life experiences of the performers – with the most recent plays based on the performers' experience with bullying. Dreamers Theater attracted the attention of Richmond's public television station which produced a documentary that was picked up nationwide by 130 television stations. (The documentary can be viewed on the landing page of dreamerstheater.org.)

Profound Autism – "Jack Matters, Too: A Mother's Perspective on Her Son's Place in the Autism Community"

By Judith Ursitti

This article was first published on the website of the Association for Science in Autism Treatment (ASAT – asatonline.org) and is republished here with permission from Judith Ursitti, Cofounder and President

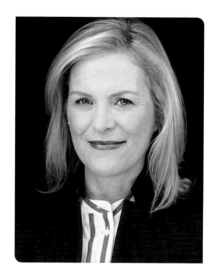

of the Profound Autism Alliance (profoundautism.org). Its website says this about Judith: "She became immersed in autism advocacy in 2005 when her son, Jack, was diagnosed at age 2. Since his diagnosis, she has worked on the passage, implementation, and enforcement of autism insurance reform as part of the team that passed legislation in all 50 states."

LOVE THIS YOUNG MAN WITH ALL OF MY HEART. I worry about his future. He has so much to offer this world. But frequently, I read things that seem like they deny the realities of valuable humans like him.

He's not a savant. He doesn't type. He gets up in the morning and gets ready for school. He works hard every day, striving for connection and independence, supported by a team of loving therapists.

Speech, OT, PT, ABA,… All of it aimed at empowering him. He runs and swims after school. Exercise is such great medicine. He's not into TV or movies, really. He spends no time on the Internet. He loves listening to music on his iPad. Lately, it's been Katy Perry and Kanye.

He was diagnosed with autism at age two. He was diagnosed with a severe intellectual disability at nine. A diagnosis of OCD came a little later. This combination of alphabet soup brings a lot of pain and struggle. He's hurt himself. He's hurt me. It can be hard.

He loves and is loved. He likes to swing as high as the swing will go. He loves to go to the store. He loves to go to Outback Steakhouse and eat wings. He loves his sister and is sometimes annoyed with her. He likes to hang close. He also likes to be left alone.

He hums and rocks and paces. He laughs. He enjoys looking in the mirror and making goofy faces. He screams loudly over and over and laughs and laughs and laughs. He is authentic. Refreshingly so.

He is not the prom king. He is not represented in research or the media very much. It's very hard for researchers to include people like him in their work. His sensory challenges, his inability to read or write or speak leave him on the periphery of autistic representation.

I have many autistic friends with various profiles. They are some of my favorite people. Truly. The truth is his severity makes him really different than them. I'm not even certain that the shared diagnosis is accurate. But hey, I'm not a scientist.

But I do think this is such a compelling reason to work really hard to conduct research for people like him. Individualized supports and services can really help human beings like him.

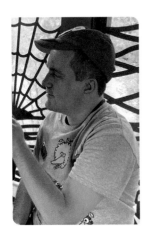

What's the point of my rambling? Please just know that when you hear the word autism, or you read something by autistic authors representing the autism community, it's generally not inclusive of people like my son. This needs to change. His experience matters.

He and so many others like him need inclusion, acceptance, and support, particularly from their own community. They desperately need research to provide answers and to improve their quality of life.

The ongoing balance of joy and pain is part of the human experience. But his version of it weighs heavily on him. He deserves peace. Please don't forget about people like him.

Jamie's Story

By Ann Flippin, Jamie's Sister

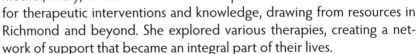

RICHMONDER JAMIE MILLER, A 33-YEAR-OLD AUTISTIC ADULT, is a natural people person. Outgoing and friendly, he finds joy in a multitude of activities, from savoring meals at local restaurants to exploring the aisles of Target. Jamie also enjoys spending leisurely afternoons in the park, reveling in the sights and sounds around him, and finding solace in the rhythmic motion of riding escalators. Above all, he thrives in the presence of others.

Jamie falls towards the extreme end of the autism spectrum, qualifying him for extensive support services including round-the-clock assistance with daily living tasks and housing.

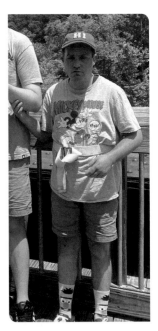

His journey began with a typical infancy and early childhood, but at the age of two, he experienced a sudden regression, losing speech, social interaction, and exhibiting distress through high-pitched screams. Determined to unlock her son's potential, Jamie's mother, Mary, embarked on a tireless quest for therapeutic interventions and knowledge, drawing from resources in Richmond and beyond. She explored various therapies, creating a network of support that became an integral part of their lives.

Jamie's struggles with aggression, self-injury, and communication have been persistent obstacles. His family has navigated these challenges with

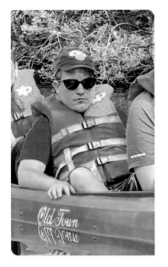

resilience, relying on a constant stream of therapists who became like extended family members. Throughout his education, Jamie encountered both successes and setbacks in finding suitable support systems within public and private schools, leaving an indelible mark on Richmond's autism education community.

Medical complexities have further complicated Jamie's journey, from dietary restrictions to early puberty and multiple life-threatening hospitalizations. Despite these hurdles, he currently resides in his own home in a supportive environment with round-the-clock care.

While Jamie's cognitive and physical abilities resemble those of a toddler, his love for social interaction and his vibrant sense of humor shine through. He also delights in reminiscing about loved ones, finding comfort in memories of his late father and grandmothers.

Through the complexities of his journey, Jamie's resilience, vibrant spirit, and unwavering connection to those around him serve as a testament to the power of love, support, and human connection in navigating the intricate landscape of autism.

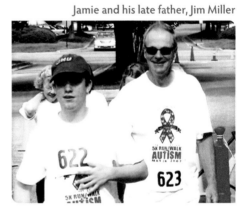

Jamie and his late father, Jim Miller

NOTE: A few years ago, Ann wrote the following about Jamie during Autism Awareness Month:

I have learned many valuable things on our journey together, through its many stages, twists and turns. While my personal autism journey has felt quite challenging and overwhelming at times, it has also been extremely meaningful and transformative.

My brother has taught me:

- the importance of patience

- to have great compassion and empathy for others

- about resilience and never giving up no matter how hard it can get

- to celebrate the little things, and also to not sweat the small things in life

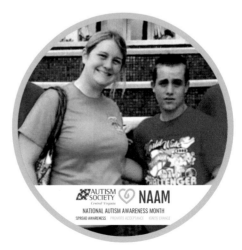

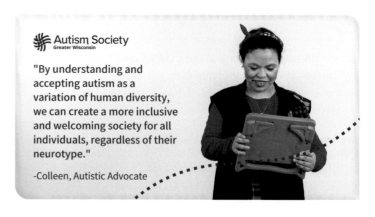
ANGELINA'S SHAKE-A-STICK!

• just how strong the power of unconditional love is

My brother and our journey together have made me into the person I am today, and without him I know I would not have this incredible and rewarding life!

Colleen McCluskey – Wisdom of an Autistic Self-Advocate

I am grateful to Colleen McCluskey and the Autism Society of Greater Wisconsin for their permission to reprint the following article that has been featured on ASGW's website (autismgreaterwi.org).

APRIL IS AUTISM ACCEPTANCE MONTH. While acceptance and inclusion are year-round efforts, the Autism Society of Greater Wisconsin recognizes April as a special opportunity to seek out and amplify a range of autistic experiences and perspectives.

Colleen is an autistic advocate in Central Wisconsin. She recently shared with us her perspective on acceptance in our community:

ASGW: What do you wish the community knew about Autism or acceptance?

Colleen: Many autistic people, myself included, often wish that their communities knew that autism is a natural neurological variation. Often, autism is stereotyped as being inherently negative due to autistic people's inherent difficulty with allistic communicative practices and tendency towards forms of expression that don't resonate with societal norms. In my opinion, autism itself is a neutral quale, with its own set of strengths and challenges. For example, while many autistic people may have difficulty with social communication and interaction, we also tend to have exceptional memory skills, intense focus, and great attention to detail. Similarly, autistic people's unique way of processing information can lead to new and innovative ideas. By understanding and accepting autism as a variation of human diversity, we can create a more inclusive and welcoming society for all individuals, regardless of their neurotype.

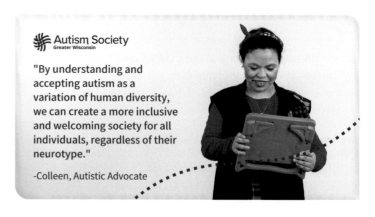
Autism Society Greater Wisconsin

"By understanding and accepting autism as a variation of human diversity, we can create a more inclusive and welcoming society for all individuals, regardless of their neurotype."

-Colleen, Autistic Advocate

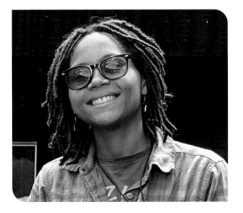

ASGW: What does an accepting community look like to you?

Colleen: A community that accepts autism would be one that values and celebrates the diversity of all individuals, including those on the autism spectrum. Such a community would ideally respect my communication style and sensory needs and make an effort to understand them. It would also be a place where individuals of all neurotypes would be included and embraced in community life, without being stigmatized or discriminated against. Finally, an ideal community would prioritize accessibility and accommodations to ensure that all individuals have equal opportunities to participate and thrive.

ASGW: How does Autism acceptance affect your quality of life?

Colleen: Autism acceptance positively affects an autistic person's quality of life in many ways. When individuals on the spectrum feel accepted and valued, they are more likely to have positive self-esteem, a sense of belonging, and greater opportunities for social connection. They are also more likely to have access to accommodations and support that can help them succeed in school, work, and other areas of life. Additionally, when society embraces autism and neurodiversity in general, it can lead to greater awareness and understanding, which can help to reduce stigma and discrimination against not only those on the spectrum, but against marginalized populations as a whole.

Rachel Pretlow

Rachel Pretlow is the Community Engagement Manager for the Autism Society of Central Virginia and Co-Chairs the Society's Self-Advocate Council. ASCV's website says this about her: "As a Community Educator, she is focused on expanding and enhancing our educational programming by supporting the development, implementation, and evaluation of community trainings. She also assists with the execution of tasks associated with grant-funded programs and initiatives. Rachel has experience in habitat restoration, farming, education, and positive youth development. She is passionate about cultural preservation and indigenous healing modalities. Rachel holds a Master of Health Science degree from the Johns Hopkins Bloomberg School of Public Health. She enjoys exploring, swinging, dancing, and making traditional crafts."

I first encountered Rachel when she was ASCV's facilitator for a Zoom viewing and discussion of the movie, "The Reason I Jump." A few days later I emailed her and asked if I could

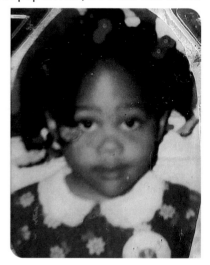

interview her for this book. She agreed and asked that I send my questions in advance, which I did. Later I discovered and listened to an online podcast interview with her and also watched an online video of her presenting her "Autism 101" talk – both of which helped me learn more about her.

Communicating with Rachel has enhanced my own knowledge about, and understanding of, autism. At my request, she wrote the following profile about herself:

WAS DIAGNOSED WITH "AUTISM SPECTRUM DISORDER- LEVEL 1" when I was 30 years old. I believe that some individuals who were to see me in my current state of non-speaking, rocking, and extreme sensitivity to light, sound, and touch would be surprised that I was identified as Autistic during adulthood. However, several aspects of my identity contributed to this later-in-life diagnosis, including that I'm Black and Native (Nottoway, Saponi), and I'm a woman.

Many assumptions that may come to mind when you read those things about me are true (e.g. low socioeconomic status family, Christian upbringing, limited access to resources). Those factors also led to me finding out during adulthood that a reason why I have felt like a peculiar creature for so long is because I'm Autistic.

I learned the necessity of masking well before I knew anything about Autism because of the realities of being Black. My parents had to teach me that in order to increase my chances of staying safe, I had to be quiet and well behaved. An Autism diagnosis would not have helped me much in the context that I grew up in; I still would have been expected to comply without question or consideration of its impact on my well-being. I was considered to be fine because I did not cause trouble, at least outside of my home.

I think that for many individuals with marginalized identities, statistics can be haunting and motivating. Yes, I check the Black/African American box when I fill out paperwork, BUT I'm one of the "good ones" who works, doesn't rely on government assistance, and stays out of the criminal justice system. When I realized in my late teens that I fit the profile of someone with what was known at that time as Asperger's, I continued applying the same expectation that I always had of myself: to be one of the "good ones." This meant pretending to be my closest version of a White neurotypical. Defy the odds. Earn respect.

For those who believe in the false, linear notion of the Autism spectrum, they would consider me "high functioning." I have typically been able to mask well enough for long enough that most folks are not able to tell that I'm Autistic. This is a privilege that has allowed me to access many things, including attending a prestigious college and university, being invited into social spaces, and maintaining employment. In each of those contexts,

CHAPTER V: Profiles By and About Autistics

I have experienced people who for some reason make it a point to disparage Autistics, and I manage to keep smiling through the inner pain and disappointment. Outward proximity to neurotypicality still tends to be viewed as a desirable achievement and a goal for several commonly "prescribed" therapies for Autistics. So then I'm a success story.

However, focusing on external displays of behaviors (or a lack thereof) fails to acknowledge the actual experiences of a "Level 1," highly masking Autistic person. It is true that I attended a prestigious university. However, during my studies, I was forced into a leave of absence after inpatient psychiatric hospitalization and an attempted restraining order. It is true that I have had a job consistently since I was 18 years old. But there is a pattern to my employment. I easily impress interviewers with my education, diverse work experience, and highly practiced speech and charm. I demonstrate myself as an ideal employee for about a year. Then I succumb to the Autistic burnout that started about two months into the job that I'm successfully able to ignore until I implode. So I quit the job, take a few weeks to find a new gig, and repeat the cycle. A few years ago, I moved back in with my parents because I could no longer force myself into the Western cultural expectation of working AND living independently.

I currently work for an organization that provides programs and support for Autistic people and their families. In my position at this job and as a leader on the organization's council of Autistic adults, I am adamant about uplifting the voices of those who are the most marginalized in our community. Even in this space, where I'm openly Autistic and advocate for myself and others, I'm still sitting here writing this passage (with sunglasses on, earplugs in, and a pencil strapped to my hand) because I have been unable to go to work on this ninth straight day of burnout. I've been committed to avoiding the oft-quoted statistic of Autistics who are unemployed or underemployed. After everything that my Ancestors fought for, how could I *still* end up as a janitor? But I'm experiencing burnout more frequently; my demand threshold has lowered. So I have to change something.

With the help of my therapist, I have recently shifted my priority to embracing my authentic self. My life goals are to homestead and simply be happy. Last month, I received a scholarship to purchase a tablet to upgrade my AAC access and express myself authentically. I'm also in the process of restructuring my engagements to prioritize my interests. I'm not sure how I'm going to acquire the land and resources that I need to achieve my goal of homesteading, especially if I have to alter how I earn an income. However, while factors like being raised in a Black, deeply religious family may have been detrimental in some ways, like potentially denying me access to services that could have helped me at a young age, they have also helped me be resilient and rooted in my faith. I believe that I can be myself completely AND have my needs met. I know that God has the final say. Amen and Asé.

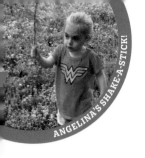
ANGELINA'S SHAKE-A-STICK!

Michael Bishop, AKA The Berserker Blóthar

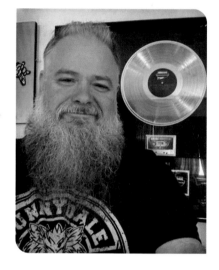

ANGELINA LOVES MUSIC AND LOVES LIP-SYNCH-ING AND PERFORMING INTERPRETIVE MOVE-MENTS. *Her favorite music source is Kidz Bop Radio – the antithesis of GWAR. I haven't yet exposed her to GWAR, but I definitely will when she's a bit older and can appropriately appreciate its importance. I got to know GWAR's Michael Bishop a few years ago and he's not only helped me on a couple of projects, but is also generous with his fishing news – an interest that we share. And considering that neurodivergence is a major theme of this book, I asked Michael if he (because of GWAR's divergence from just about everything that's neurotypical) would be willing to write an essay on neurodivergence. Following is what he wrote – not at all what I was expecting, but surprisingly akin to what some autistic adults have told me about their own lives. (Michael's not autistic.)*

"In a word, my work is digressive, and it is progressive too,—and at the same time." —Laurence Sterne, *The Life and Opinions of Tristram Shandy, Gentleman*

I have stories to tell, but I struggle to tell them coherently. My thoughts race ahead of my ability to articulate them, leading to unfinished sentences and convoluted digressions. I'll start narrating an anecdote, only to lose interest in my own train of thought because I've already mentally followed it to some conclusion or tangential inquiry. Often, I forget my thoughts aren't audible, and I trail off into private reverie without realizing I've stopped speaking in the middle of a story. This digressive, disjointed communication both amuses and frustrates my loved ones. But it's more than idiosyncrasy – it's a manifestation of my life-long struggle with ADHD.

This essay chronicles my experiences as a child labeled "hyperactive" and an adult finally diagnosed with ADHD and processing speed deficits. I'll also argue that the modern age of digital distraction and fragmented attention spans present possibilities for greater recognition, empathy and accommodation of neurodivergent ways of knowing. Technologies like AI could make space for alternative cognitive styles to thrive.

As an elementary student, I was diagnosed with "hyperactivity" and prescribed Ritalin for my restlessness, distractibility and impulsivity. But the medication only treated my symptoms and did not

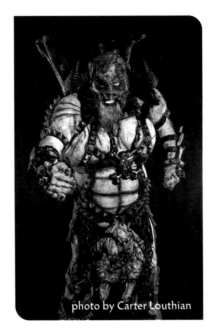

ANGELINA'S SHAKE-A-STICK!

GRANDPARENT CONFIDENTIAL

"My 11-year-old grandson is high functioning. Does that mean high or low on the spectrum? His only interest is trains."

address underlying cognitive differences and the social adjustment issues they caused. Despite a medical explanation, I was constantly punished and shamed for being "irresponsible," "careless" and "disorganized." I forgot school assignments, lost jackets, shoes, even bicycles, and arrived late for everything from Sunday School to baseball practice. When I was in school, I was a cut-up, attention seeking, always acting out.

This chaos echoed my mother's own struggles. A loving, intelligent woman, she too was plagued by losing things. "I hate keys and mess..." she'd lament, with tears of frustration in her eyes. We were both judged to be ditzy and careless, despite our good intentions. Over time, I internalized these messages, and I came to feel fundamentally flawed. Still, my mother believed in me and was convinced I was a talented and bright child who was simply misunderstood. I think actually that the diagnosis of hyperactivity made her feel better—that my struggles were neither her fault or my own.

At school, while my behavior left much to be desired, testing revealed I was "gifted" with advanced language abilities. Somehow, the same testing revealed I was also "learning disabled" and severely challenged in math. Seeking to creatively interpret an IQ test through narrative and drawings rather than formulaic answers, I inadvertently "bombed" the gifted class assessment and was removed from the program, dashing my mother's hopes that I was a genius bored by a mundane curriculum.

As I grew older, the "hyperactivity" label faded, but cruel new descriptors took its place – "irresponsible," "lazy," a "bad student," and just "bad" in general. These labels overlooked how I thrived in extracurriculars leveraging expressive talents for acting, forensics, the school newspaper, writing original poetry, fiction and plays. More than anything else though, I loved music. I led songs in church, and I taught myself how to play piano and was writing my own songs by the time I was 9 years old. By adolescence, I'd left religion behind and discovered punk rock as an alternative community embracing societal outcasts. It was perfect for me. At 16, I formed my first band and by 18 I was putting out records and touring internationally as a professional musician.

For over a decade, I lived the lifestyle of a touring rock musician. I had easy access to drugs and alcohol, and I used them prodigiously to escape my racing thoughts and restlessness. Many of my peers also self-medicated this inner chaos through

photo by Carter Louthian

addiction, and I grieved several friends who died trying to silence the noise of their minds.

At 30, newly married and feigning responsibility, I returned to academics, seeking to avoid "real work." But my ambition to go to community college and transfer to a four-year school ran up against difficult math and science requirements. It wasn't until a professor recommended testing for learning accommodations that I discovered I wasn't just "hyperactive" and a chronic screw-up, I had ADHD and cripplingly slow processing speeds.

Upon receiving this diagnosis, years of pent-up frustration poured out. My perpetual difficulties with time management, focus and cognitive processing finally made sense. I remember crying in the parking lot when it hit me what the diagnosis meant. For the first time, my lifelong challenges crystallized into a legitimate medical explanation rather than personal failings. While processing speed troubles can be conflated with ADHD, the two are distinct, and I have both. The inability to complete tasks in a culturally expected timeframe generated upheaval and trauma for me my entire life, leading to sorrow and lost opportunities. But this diagnosis also empowered me, allowing educational accommodations like extended test time that transformed my academic performance. I eventually earned a PhD in Music.

GRANDPARENT CONFIDENTIAL

"Our 6-year-old granddaughter was diagnosed when she was 3, and I took care of her a lot until I had to quit recently because of a health issue. She's smart, but she is bothered by loud noises, bright lights, and crowds of people. She never gives me trouble, but she screams at my son and my husband and behaves negatively towards them. I need to learn more about autism."

Today's digital era of constant connectivity and fragmented attention increasingly mirrors the restless, non-linear thought patterns of the ADHD/neurodivergent mind. As we all struggle against doom-scrolling spirals, the overstimulation and cognitive detours I've grappled with my entire life are becoming a universal human experience.

Far from rendering us obsolete, rapidly evolving technologies like AI writing assistants offer tools to compensate for neurodivergent challenges. By vocalizing trains of thought and leveraging AI's organizational capabilities, I can wrangle my ideas into cohesive narratives that previously evaded me. AI doesn't write for me, but when I put my thoughts down, it helps me to sort through them and provide an outline of a narrative, something that has always been a struggle for me. I don't need it. I can always abuse myself into productivity. I even managed to squeeze out a doctoral dissertation, all without the ability to make an outline. But AI has the effect of liberating my ideas and allowing me to put them in boxes and get them out of my mind.

AI presents an opportunity to expand our conception of "normal" cognition and create more inclusive space for neu-

Angelina!

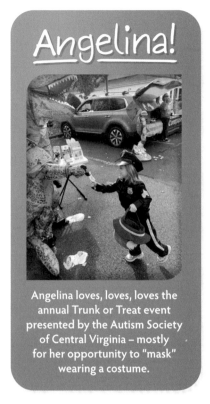

Angelina loves, loves, loves the annual Trunk or Treat event presented by the Autism Society of Central Virginia – mostly for her opportunity to "mask" wearing a costume.

rodivergent ways of thinking and creating. I am hopeful that by constructively integrating these technologies, we can help destigmatize perceived cognitive shortcomings and open new pathways for neurodivergent individuals to achieve focused productivity when needed, and more fully express our unique creative potential. Our perpetually distracted present may inspire long-overdue empathy and accommodation for neurodivergent people who see something familiar in our culture's increasingly fragmented and digressive cognitive landscape.

Michael Bishop is the lead vocalist and a principal composer, lyricist and writer for the legendary shock rock band GWAR. He is also the vocalist and songwriter for the Richmond, Virginia post-punk band Kepone, and the co-founder of Misery Brothers, a project combining soul and country music with narrative theatrical performance. Bishop holds a PhD in Music from the University of Virginia and has worked as a lecturer in popular music history and performance studies. His research interests include popular music and regional identity, the history of rock music performance, aesthetics, the gothic, film music, and ethnographic approaches to music.

Michael began working as a professional musician, performer, and writer at the age of 18 when he joined GWAR as the band's bassist. He played the role of Beefkake the Mighty, and worked as a musician, composer and lyricist on the band's first four albums between 1987 and 1994. As part of Slave-Pit, the art collective that produces GWAR, he also performed for and helped write the group's stage and film productions. During his tenure, GWAR toured extensively establishing themselves as innovators in the world of punk and heavy metal with an outrageous and irreverent narrative stage show blending comedy and cartoon violence with rock performance. Michael helped create three long-form videos and numerous other video projects including the Grammy nominated "Phallus in Wonderland" (1992) before leaving GWAR to pursue his own projects in 1994. He rejoined the band as the vocalist after the death of the band's original lead singer in 2014, and has recorded two albums and an EP with the band's current lineup.

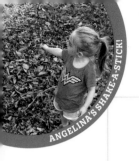
ANGELINA'S SHAKE-A-STICK!

Angelina's Story:
The Note from School

A S FAMILIES OF CHILDREN ON THE AUTISM SPECTRUM know (no matter where on the spectrum), even the tiniest bit of "progress," even the slightest amount of improvement of challenging behavior, even the most modest glimpse of joy can be cause for tear-producing celebration. We had one of those yesterday concerning Angelina.

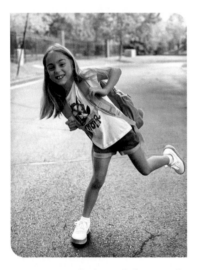

You have to realize that our family is well past that day in the NICU when Angelina finally reached two pounds, well past the day when Angelina amazed us by actually crawling without her therapist moving her legs back and forth, well past the swallow test that allowed the removal of her g-tube, well past when she finally began to babble, and when she, and when she, and when she . . . Among autism families, these tell-everyone celebrations can happen frequently or far between, and while often unremarkable to families of neurotypical children, they are special to us.

The cause for yesterday's celebration? A letter that was sent home from school in Angelina's backpack – a letter regarding the special assistance she has been receiving to help with her reading abilities. The letter included this: ". . . Angelina has made sufficient progress and no longer requires this additional intervention." Justen texted us a photo of the letter as soon as he read it. And when Kelly got home from work she texted it to us too, along with her tears.

JC's and my two children, Kelly and Thomas, aren't disabled, and while they were growing up we of course celebrated and marveled at lots of things such as saying their first words, awards and performances at school, creating special artworks, passing their driving tests. But such achievements were expected. Only during the past 8 years with Angelina have we discovered a whole different and more amazing type of celebratory joy – even akin to the celebration caused by those first three words that Neil Armstrong spoke, "One

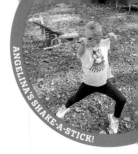

small step . . ."

We are so lucky that these types of celebration have been steady and frequent during Angelina's life – but of course also sprinkled with occasions for concern. But right now is celebration time.

(Kelly's follow-up text read, "She's struggling in math a bit. Last night I found a website called Adapted Mind, and Angelina and I worked on math problems together.")

Onward and upward.

Elizabeth Bonker – Champion for Facilitated Communication

MET ELIZABETH BONKER FIRST VIA E-MAIL and later via a telephone conversation with her mother, Virginia Breen. I was seeking permission to reprint Elizabeth's nonspeaking presentation that is featured on the website of Rollins College, along with some introductory information that I'd written about Elizabeth and her organization. Elizabeth said yes and also provided some helpful editing for my introductory information:

Of the more than 30 million nonspeakers with autism worldwide, there are approximately 5,000 who communicate by typing. One of the very best representatives is Elizabeth Bonker whose 2022 valedictorian commencement address at Rollins College went viral. You can find it easily on YouTube.

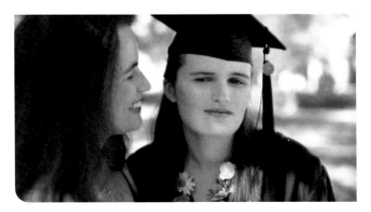

Elizabeth has founded a nonprofit organization, Communication 4 ALL (communication4ALL.org), with the mission to ensure all nonspeakers with autism have access to communication and education. In 2023, Communication 4 ALL launched C4A Academy, a program of internet-based instructional videos to teach nonspeakers how to type, free of charge. Students first learn to point

to letters and then press them on a keyboard to express their wants and needs as well as their hopes and dreams. C4A Academy includes free written lessons to implement the program, a Facebook group, supplies, and other resources like "Ask an Expert" that will help families.

Elizabeth's mission is to change the way the world understands nonspeaking autism; it is a neuromotor disorder, not a cognitive one. Please visit Communication 4 ALL's website to learn how you can take action and help nonspeakers gain communication equality.

The Autism Society of America's website says this: "She has given dozens of published interviews and keynote addresses including at the Stanford Medical School Neurodiversity Summit, the Neurodiversity in Business in London, and the India Inclusion Summit in Bangalore. Elizabeth's story has been featured in three documentary films: SPELLERS, Understanding Autism, and In Our Own Hands. Elizabeth is a 2022 graduate from Rollins College's Honors Program and her valedictorian commencement address went viral with 4 billion media impressions propelling her mission onto a global stage. Elizabeth is a member of Autism Society's Justice Center Task Force and Public Policy Committee. In 2024, Elizabeth was elected to the Board of Autism Society of Florida."

And here is Elizabeth's speech, as featured on the website of Rollins College:

I was born healthy and could speak as a toddler. Then, at 15 months old, my words were inexplicably taken from me. My parents took me to Yale Medical School, where I was diagnosed with autism. Despite what the doctors said, my parents never gave up on me. They recognized that I was a thinking person trapped in a silent cage.

It was only when my grandmother happened to see an episode of *60 Minutes* that things started to change. The show aired a segment on Soma Mukhopadhyay, the creator of a system called the rapid prompting method (RPM) designed to help autistic non-speakers communicate. My mother reached out to her, and we were off to Texas. I was 6 years old, and we had found my Annie Sullivan.

GRANDPARENT CONFIDENTIAL

"My grandson is nonverbal, but he's smart and can write alphabets in different languages and can redraw things he sees. I want to learn more about autism."

Now, I communicate by typing on a keyboard. But when I first started, I spelled out words by pointing to letters on a letter board. People with non-speaking autism often have difficulty initiating movements, so learning to type is tedious. With months of practice, I made progress, and the world began to open up to me. I started writing poetry because it allowed me to say more in fewer words.

By the time I was a teenager, I'd published my first book, *I Am in Here*, a collection of poems. Now I've just released my first two songs of an album, also titled *I Am in Here*, a collaboration with The Bleeding Hearts and Tom Morello of Rage Against the Machine, who brought my words to life with their beautiful music.

Deciding to attend Rollins was easy because the College's focus on community engagement and social innovation supported my life mission. Rollins had also shown great kindness to my older brother, Charles, who is affected by autism and graduated in 2019 with honors.

I majored in social innovation with a minor in English to help build the skills I would need to be an effective changemaker and writer. One of the best things about Rollins' liberal arts program is that it provides students with the flexibility to take courses across disciplines. I took classes in sociology, statistics, anthropology, education, political science, and more. Every professor invested the time to get to know me and help me think about how to apply their field to my mission. My law and public policy courses helped me advocate on Capitol Hill in summer 2019, and my film and English courses have made me a better storyteller.

While at Rollins, I found a community of like-minded social justice advocates in the Pinehurst Organization. I have been deeply inspired by their passions and dedication, whether it was weaving blankets for the homeless, cleaning up Lake Virginia, or volunteering for Second Harvest Food Bank. My fellow Pinehurstians are my friends and cheerleaders.

When it came time to develop a plan for my senior honors thesis, I decided to take the knowledge and skills I'd garnered at Rollins and put them into action. The result was the April launch of my nonprofit, Communication 4 ALL, an organization dedicated to providing communication resources for all non-speakers so that they too can be freed from their silent cage. I owe a huge debt of gratitude to my thesis advisor, anthropology professor Rachel Newcomb, and my thesis committee members, communication professor Anne Stone, sociology professor Matt Nichter, and social entrepreneurship professor Josie Balzac-Arroyo, whose mentorship will continue to be invaluable.

Everything I aspire to do relates back to Rollins' ethos: Life is for service. My journey hasn't always been easy, but I believe that a life of service is a marathon rather than a sprint. And I

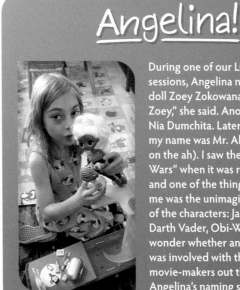

Angelina!

During one of our LOL play sessions, Angelina named one doll Zoey Zokowana. "She goes by Zoey," she said. Another name was Nia Dumchita. Later she told me my name was Mr. Akiahko (accent on the ah). I saw the movie "Star Wars" when it was released in 1977 and one of the things that amazed me was the unimaginable names of the characters: Jabba the Hutt, Darth Vader, Obi-Wan Kenobi. I wonder whether an autistic brain was involved with those names. To movie-makers out there: I volunteer Angelina's naming services.

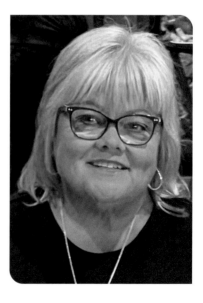

am celebrating the small victories along the way as I work to give a voice to my brothers and sisters who suffer in silence. Non-speaking autism is so poorly understood – it's not a cognitive disorder – and I believe every non-speaker with autism can learn to communicate as I do.

I am delighted to be one of five valedictorians representing the class of 2022 and am honored that my fellow valedictorians selected me to give the commencement address. As I prepare to graduate, I reflect on the questions I first had when I came to Rollins: Would I fit in? Would people take the time to get to know me despite my slow typing? Happily, I've been embraced by my professors and fellow classmates, and I have cherished being treated like every other student. I hope Rollins has also been impacted by my time here in some small way, in seeing the potential in students who don't look and sound like everyone else.

Note: I've read the bestselling book by Elizabeth and Virginia, I Am in Here, *which features front- and back-cover praise from Tom Brokaw, Temple Grandin, and Robert F. Kennedy, Jr. One of the book's significant themes is Virginia's relentless research and efforts and hopes that Elizabeth " . . . will be healed by God or by science or a combination of the two . . . " The word "healed" is key to Virginia's thinking. Another theme is Virginia's certainty that within Elizabeth's head-banging, verbal silence is a 166-IQ brilliance that produces profound thoughts and observances and speeches via facilitated communication.*

Isaac

By Carol Vera Vincent, Isaac's Grandmother

NOTE: Carol Vera Vincent, a nurse, has two autistic grandchildren: Isaac and Cormac. (Cormac's article follows this one.) I met Carol first via the Autism Grandparents Club (autismgrandparentsclub. com) and then via her Facebook group: Grandparents of Children on the Autism Spectrum, which has hundreds of members and continues to grow and which convenes frequent Zoom meetings. Carol has become a good, trusted, friend – not only to me but to others in the Facebook group.

SAAC WAS BORN ON SEPTEMBER 3, 2012 following an uncomplicated pregnancy. About six months after birth, Isaac was diagnosed with torticollis (defined by an abnormal, asymmetrical head or neck position, which may be due to a variety of causes) for which he received physical therapy with good results. He walked before he was a year old, and met his gross motor milestones.

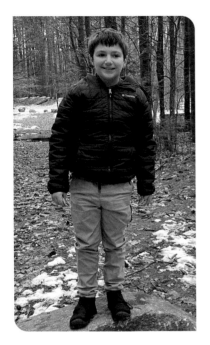

Within the first year, his parents noticed non-typical behaviors. He lined things up and would frequently run back and forth across the room. His speech was delayed, and he was often echolalic, repeating lines from his favorite movies. When this information was brought to the pediatrician, it was dismissed.

By the time Isaac was 18 months old, he knew all his letters and the sounds they made as well as all of his numbers. Wherever he was, he looked for (and found) letters. It was when his parents signed him up for a YMCA gymnastics class that they first realized how different his behavior was than peers in a structured setting. He would run up close to the mirror, laugh and skip back and forth looking at himself while his peers had an easier time following directions.

Again, they brought it up with the pediatrician who finally agreed to refer him to a developmental pediatrician. The wait for an appointment to be evaluated was eight months.

Once given an autism diagnosis, Isaac started early intervention which included ABA therapy for six months, occupational therapy (OT) and speech therapy. At age three he started preschool which was a structured group in the classroom. He received OT, physical therapy and speech therapy. His parents considered ABA as additional therapy, but waitlists were long and some ABA agencies urged them to take him out of public school. They were uncertain about this, especially since that recommendation was made without an evaluation. Ultimately they decided the individualized program at school was better for him.

Isaac has attended public school since preschool. He has always been in a Special Education classroom with inclusion built into his day. He does better in the smaller class, but is brought to the general education classroom for certain subjects (with supports). His parents and school team are always evaluating to make sure his time is spent in a meaningful way. He attends extended school year in the summer. Isaac currently has an IEP that is reviewed frequently by his team at school, his parents and his advocate. The public school system has not been perfect and there have been many frustrations along the way, but his parents continue to feel it is the best path at this time.

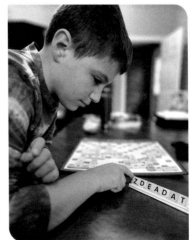

Isaac made great strides with his speech, and outgrew echolalia.

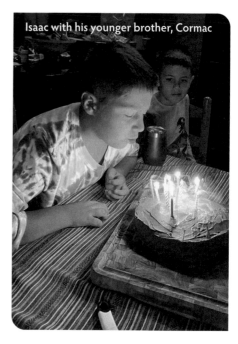

He also made enough progress that he no longer was considered to have a speech delay. He is verbal, and has made big progress in communicating his needs and wants, but doesn't often engage in long conversations.

As he now approaches middle school, the focus is shifting toward more independent life skills. At home he is slowly taking on more responsibilities helping with chores and fixing simple snacks or meals for himself. He takes great pride in accomplishing tasks on his own.

Isaac with his younger brother, Cormac

Routines are important to Isaac. He does best when he knows what to expect. He likes to have a calendar to keep track of upcoming events and is very emotionally invested in the world around him. As a young boy, Isaac became overwhelmed in noisy settings which often led to meltdowns. Over the years however, he has learned strategies to cope and can often be found in a quiet room if things get overwhelming. He is pretty good at recognizing when he needs to relax and reset.

Isaac moves through life in his own unique way. As a baby, he was snuggly, but didn't engage in most other social behaviors. Today he is happy and comfortable with who he is. He enjoys spending time with his cousins, especially sleepovers, but still doesn't engage in many social activities. He likes to be with other people, but generally does his own thing.

When Isaac wants to accomplish a new skill, he is persistent and practices until he gets it. He celebrates his achievements with a "good job Isaac" and shares them with everyone. Isaac likes to do things for himself and has been known to politely decline help by saying "No, I've got this."

Isaac brings so much to the lives of others, simply by being himself. At eleven years old, he exemplifies what really matters in life. He speaks honestly and from his heart, and this is one of his most endearing qualities. If more people were like Isaac, the world would be a better place.

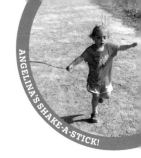

Cormac

By Carol Vera Vincent, Cormac's Grandmother

FOLLOWING AN UNCOMPLICATED PREGNANCY AND DELIVERY Cormac was born on November 22, 2015 weighing 7 lbs. 13 oz. He was a typical baby in many ways, but was not a good sleeper. Despite recommendations to have babies sleep on their backs, Cormac would only settle on his belly. He loved to be held and snuggled. He was a happy baby and met all of his fine and gross motor milestones. Cormac was very socially engaged and enjoyed interactions with other people. He was always sensory seeking and curious.

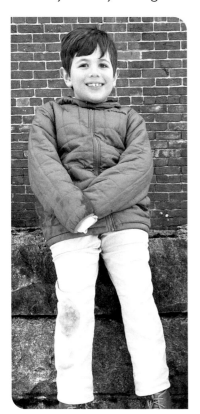

Because his brother had recently been diagnosed with autism, Cormac's parents knew there was an increased chance that he too would be on the spectrum. Due to the long delay (8-9 months) in getting his brother evaluated, Cormac was placed on a waiting list at about one year old. He was finally evaluated at 21 months, and was found to have a significant speech delay. At the initial appointment, the developmental pediatrician was leaning towards no autism diagnosis. Not too long after though, she called back saying that she did see enough and that he would benefit from the services he'd be eligible for. This has proven true over the years as Cormac has received critical services, underscoring the importance of understanding the unique needs of an individual regardless of how their presentation fits into the common definitions of autism.

From age 2-3, Cormac was enrolled in an early intervention program that provided ABA, speech and occupational therapies. He was in a structured classroom program to prepare him for school. At 3, he went to pre-school at the local public school where he received most of his therapies. Cormac also did ABA at home for a year, but the experience was disappointing. His parents felt it wasn't directly addressing his individual needs. There was too much staff turnover, lack of understanding of what Cormac needed and repetitive "cookie cutter" strategies to change his behavior.

Cormac has been in public school since pre-school. He did well initially, but in first grade when he was expected to sit quietly at a desk for extended periods of time, he began to struggle. He was diagnosed with Attention Deficit Hyperactivity Disorder (ADHD) which helped explain his difficulty in meeting the teacher's expectations. Additionally, the classroom supports outlined in his IEP were not in place. The school team began reporting behaviors that his family never saw at home. Cormac was acting out aggressively and struggling to fit in with peers. This was uncharacteristic behavior for him as he always played well with other children outside of the school setting. At present, his parents are trying to figure out what it is about the school environment that triggers him. They suspect it is a combination of the academic expectations and the large number of peers that are causing his anxiety, resulting in unexpected behaviors. His parents, along with his advocate and the team at school, have recently agreed that Cormac's needs would be better met in a different setting. They are in the process of determining exactly what that will be.

Cormac has always been very social. He has frequent playdates and sleepovers with cousins and thoroughly enjoys this time. He is quick witted and loves to make people laugh. Typical of boys his age, he is amused by the occasional "toilet" joke.

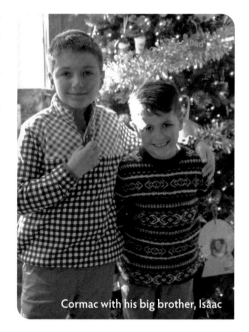

Cormac with his big brother, Isaac

Anxiety and ADHD are his primary challenges. He struggles to accurately read social situations and frequently talks when quiet is required. His struggles with anxiety are evident in his concern that others are staring at him and judging him. He often says that he just wants everybody to love him. According to his teachers, he is well liked by his classmates, and when a task requires working together, many of his peers want to work with him.

From an early age, Cormac has been very inquisitive. His interests are varied and he wants to learn as much as he can about everything. He likes to read and is currently enjoying the Dogman graphic novel series. Cormac also writes and illustrates his own graphic novels. He recently received a camera as a gift, and has been making and editing short videos with the help of his father. Like most eight-year-old boys, he also enjoys playing video games. Cormac likes to play outside where he can use his imagination to the fullest. He is especially fond of hiking and swimming when weather permits.

Cormac is a kind-hearted boy who brightens the lives of all who know him. He is creative and contemplative beyond his years.

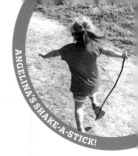

Angelina's Story:
Thanksgiving

THANKSGIVING WAS A BLUR. JC and I entertained Angelina and four little cousins (ages 6, 8, 11, and 13) from Alabama whom she'd never before met. Angelina was in Heaven; she loves interacting with other children. The cousins are neurotypical, and an uneducated observer wouldn't have noticed anything different about Angelina. Autism-savvy persons may have noticed a few things. Angelina toe-walks much of the time. She is always on the move, walking from one place to another, climbing on furniture, etc. (her type of stimming – rather than flapping her arms and such). She continually switches involvements (playing school, playing doctor, playing store, etc. "You be the customer and I'll be the storekeeper." Three minutes later, "Now YOU be the storekeeper and I'll be the customer.") And she is extremely empathetic. If someone falls down and gets even the least bit hurt, Angelina is there to put an arm around their shoulder. If someone scrapes a knee, Angelina wants to get a good look and asks for a bandage. If someone is upset and starts crying, Angelina is there with comfort. Neurotypical kids can be empathetic, but Angelina's version is more intense, and sometimes we have to ask her to back away if it's with a kid who is a stranger on a playground. Personal space limitations don't compute in Angelina's empathetic brain.

On Thanksgiving day everyone (17 persons, 2 dogs) met at my niece's home. Angelina and the cousins were relentless as they commandeered the fun places of the house. And again, most persons wouldn't have noticed anything different about Angelina. And during the set-ups for the various versions of family photos she cooperated as well as, or better than, the other kids.

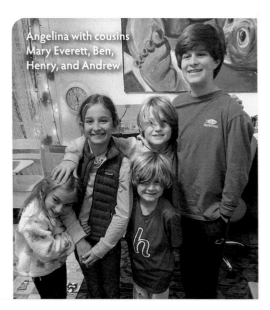
Angelina with cousins Mary Everett, Ben, Henry, and Andrew

My few years of exposure to autism suggest that Angelina, although her brain is definitely wired neurodivergently, is unusual in her lack of noticeable autism traits. But throughout this book I provide examples of the workings of Angelina's amazingly and amusingly neurodivergent brain.

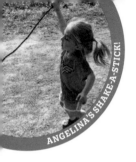
ANGELINA'S SHAKE-A-STICK!

UNmask Autism – Kellie Vanella and Jacob

A NEUROTYPICAL PROFESSIONAL FRIEND INTRODUCED ME TO KELLIE VANELLA. I would have never guessed that Kellie is autistic nor that she continually confronts the 24/7 challenges as described here. The blogs that she has written for her company's website, www.unmaskautism.com, have given me a greater understanding of autism. The website says this about her: "Kellie Vanella is an Autistic Self-Advocate, Mother, Board Certified Advocate in Special Education, VBCPS SEAC Member, COPAA Member, 2023/2024 Partners in Policymaking Participant, Blogger & founder of Unmask Autism, and Author of the disability journals: 'Unmasking,' 'The Longest Goodbye,' and 'Beyond the Looking Glass.'"

In early 2018 Kellie considered that her six-month-old son, Jacob, might be autistic. He was intently playing with something and he wouldn't look up when she repeatedly called his name. Later that day while nursing him she realized that he didn't do typical nursing things such as looking at her, playing with her hair, etc.

Kellie's knowledge of autism was textbook only, and she felt a lot of fear at the thought of her son being autistic. She resolved to just wait and see. It would be ridiculous to tell his pediatrician that he is autistic; nobody gets diagnosed at six months.

At Jacob's 15-month checkup, one of the assistants mistakenly handed Kellie his M-CHAT-R (20-question assessment for autism) – and later realizing the mistake, the assistant took it back and said that it was a document that would be provided at Jacob's 18-month visit. But Kellie's quick look confirmed a probable autism diagnosis.

Shortly after his 15-month checkup Jacob was in his highchair eating dinner when his head suddenly slumped down. Then his head, torso, arms, and eyes started making seizure-like movements. After a few minutes he recovered and smiled. Kellie had videoed it, and suspecting something serious, she and her husband took Jacob to a children's urgent care facility and showed the video – which led to an EEG and other tests and assessments.

Kellie hadn't yet shared her autism suspicion with her husband, but told him that the "seizure" might be a type of stimming (repetitive or unusual movements or noises). Her husband wasn't familiar with that term. She explained about stimming, but didn't mention autism; she had an intense fear of saying that word to anyone.

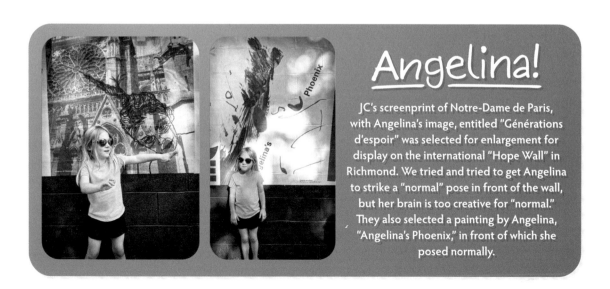

Jacob's initial EEG didn't show anything, but a subsequent 6-hour EEG showed something in the left temporal lobe. Kellie knew that's where language is processed and it may have explained why he wasn't yet speaking. An MRI was negative, thus indicating that there was no tumor.

At Jacob's 18-month checkup they gave her the M-CHAT-R and asked some follow-up questions. The doctor concluded, "Okay, well we have some concerns; let's get him started with early intervention. This doesn't necessarily mean he's autistic . . . let's just wait and see." But given the negative MRI and the M-CHAT-R results, Kellie was now 100% certain that Jacob was autistic and she insisted that an ADOS (Autism Diagnostic Observation Schedule that allows trained evaluators to use observations to assess children's communication skills, social interaction, and imaginative use of materials) be scheduled.

She was referred to a neurologist who specialized in autism and who observed Jacob running around the room, not talking, etc. The doctor provided a diagnosis of Autism Level 3 (level that requires the most support), a folder containing autism pamphlets, and a recommendation for 40 hours per week of ABA therapy. Two weeks later Jacob's ADOS also resulted in a diagnosis of Autism Level 3.

Kellie already knew what ABA is, and behaviorism had always given her a bad feeling: a system that uses drills and rewards to train and condition autistic children. A workweek of drills and training was a big weight for a toddler to carry. She didn't trust some stranger sitting at a table drilling and conditioning Jacob without her observation. But a respected doctor had recommended it.

Kellie interviewed various ABA providers and even briefly considered going back to school to get a BCBA certification (Board-Certified Behavior Analyst), but decided not to because she simply didn't agree with the premise. She had already engaged a few early intervention therapies for Jacob to help

Angelina!

JC's screenprint of Notre-Dame de Paris, with Angelina's image, entitled "Générations d'espoir" was selected for enlargement for display on the international "Hope Wall" in Richmond. We tried and tried to get Angelina to strike a "normal" pose in front of the wall, but her brain is too creative for "normal." They also selected a painting by Angelina, "Angelina's Phoenix," in front of which she posed normally.

with motor skills, etc.

She joined the Facebook group of her local autism services organization, but quickly became uneasy with the social aspects of the group; she just didn't fit in with the other parents and didn't agree with the services that they were using. At one point she posted, "Has anyone ever questioned the use of ABA?" There was silence – except for one private message that included a video of a mother who, years later, strongly regretted making the decision *not* to have her child receive ABA therapy.

Kellie stayed in the Facebook group but didn't participate. She disliked the continual postings of negativity: "Autism won today." And she didn't enroll Jacob in ABA therapy.

As this is written, Jacob is now six years old and has started a half-day schedule at a Montessori School. He is fully talking (he abruptly began one day when he was three and a half) and is at grade-level with his vocabulary. He engages and plays with his peers, is very outgoing, makes friends, and gets invited to birthday parties. He sometimes has social misunderstandings because of difficulty interpreting things.

Kellie openly discusses autism with Jacob; he knows he's autistic and understands that he's different.

Jacob has never experienced any of the types of severe meltdowns that are common with autistic children. He may get upset for a minute or two when he is unprepared for a transition, but nothing else. Regarding eating, he had some sensory preferences during his toddler years, but now he eats fairly well – a few challenges but not severe like those of a lot of autistic children. And he has always slept all night long, even as an infant.

Regarding stimming and sensory issues, Jacob is sensory-*seeking*. He enjoys crashing, tumbling, gritting his teeth, and full-body stuff including crashing into other persons' bodies. Kellie can often anticipate a body crash and she greets it with a big squeeze. And she has a weighted blanket that can provide bodily pressure for him.

Jacob is generally happy and devotes a lot of time to his special interests which currently include Minecraft, Angry Birds, and Transformers.

It was during Jacob's diagnosis process that Kellie began to consider that *she* may be autistic. She eventually posted the following on the Facebook site: "Has anyone been diagnosed AFTER their child?" She received this response: "Look at MASKING." (She learned that masking means memorizing and doing and saying things that look and sound "normal" – even though it's not the real you.)

Kellie was born in 1979 and struggled a lot as a child. Her parents were diligent about trying to help and they compiled information about Kellie's struggles – written information that Kellie discovered after Jacob was diagnosed and that led to Kellie's own diagnosis at age 42.

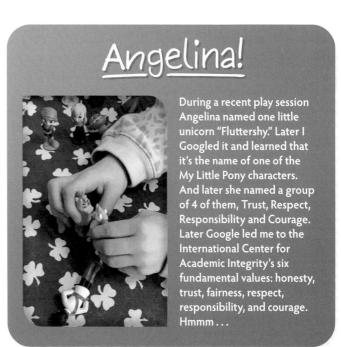

She has mixed feelings about being diagnosed later in life. Having the autism label in the 1980s would have stigmatized her, and appropriate support wasn't available then. The challenges she faced as a child are still part of her adult life: socialization, recognizing facial expressions, daily interactions, back-and-forth conversations, eye-to-eye contact, sensory overload, etc.

Masking and scripting (using memorized and prepared words and phrases that are appropriate for various situations) are her constant companions. She hates this, but realizes that it not only helps her avoid social blunders, but also keeps her safe in some situations and ensures that she is taken seriously in professional and medical settings. Her diagnosis carries a lot of harmful stigma. But in casual social settings she masks less and is open regarding her neurology.

Masking and scripting began when she was a child. She would use her tooth-brushing time to prepare for the school day – such as planning how to respond to various things the teacher might say. She would often almost miss the bus because she spent so much time on this.

Her wealth of past experiences has now populated her mental file cabinet with enough information that she appears highly competent. But she still sometimes misses things, and this bothers her a lot with enormous guilt. She has to constantly extend grace to herself.

Kellie has to do a lot of preparation to appear competent for various interactions and experiences. For example, she knows that whenever she has a medical appointment she has to prove her competence because of the stigmatizing diagnosis on her chart. She has to use scripting and masking and can never be herself because she'll be rejected and criticized.

Another example happened just recently. A life insurance broker informed her that she had been denied coverage because of her autism diagnosis. In order to get insurance she was forced to share things about herself that other people do not have to disclose to get insurance: her 21-year parenting experience, her level of education, her professional accomplishments, her goals, etc. She was essentially asked to prove her competency in order to be considered for coverage – in spite of being

Angelina!

During a recent play session Angelina named one little unicorn "Fluttershy." Later I Googled it and learned that it's the name of one of the My Little Pony characters. And later she named a group of 4 of them, Trust, Respect, Responsibility and Courage. Later Google led me to the International Center for Academic Integrity's six fundamental values: honesty, trust, fairness, respect, responsibility, and courage. Hmmm ...

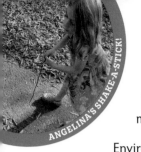
ANGELINA'S SHAKE-A-STICK!

healthy and not a medical risk. This example confirms why she has to exhaust herself using masking and scripting – which she continues to hate.

Environments that include a lot of sensory stimulation are especially challenging. She can't be in a room with flickering lights or with clanging dishes. Sometimes a lot of background noise causes her to have to read the lips of persons with whom she is talking; all of the noise sounds the same. She can't comfortably drive at night because of all of the lights.

And all of this, especially masking and scripting, is wearing and she has to give herself frequent breaks.

Kellie had these same challenges as a child during the school day, but she held it all inside. She was perceived as shy. But when she would get home she would release all of it with severe meltdowns, sometimes for hours: falling on the ground screaming, flailing, banging her head, totally out of control. Any attempts to touch her would make it worse; she is touch-avoidant.

Kellie now has her own business, Unmask Autism, that provides services for parents of autistic children. Kellie still feels pressure and anxiety when talking with a new person, but she has developed scripts and she tries to stay one step ahead of where the conversation might go – constantly trying to have the right responses ready (selected from her mental file). Back and forth conversations are a challenge and she has to pay close attention to when it's her turn to speak. She has trouble reading pauses and facial expressions and she sometimes has missteps that she later realizes. It is awkward and distressing for her when she doesn't respond correctly.

But Kellie is extremely organized and structured, and is very creative and a big planner. She finds her own clients, mostly by networking. Networking is of course not her strong point, but she knows how to do it. She recognizes her personal challenges and has learned how to compensate – especially with the use of masking.

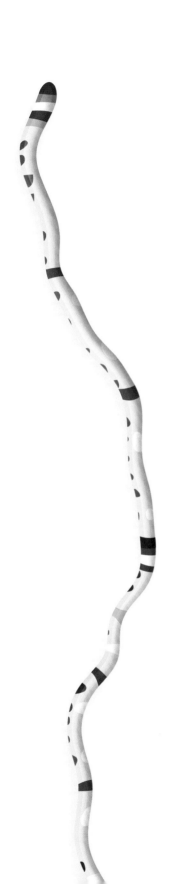

6

Books, Movies, & TV Shows

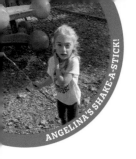

I Will Die On This Hill

IF YOU LOOK AT MY COPY OF THE 2023 BOOK, *I WILL DIE ON THIS HILL,* by autistic advocate Jules Edwards and co-author Meghan Ashburn, you'll see a lot of dogeared pages – more such pages than in any of the many autism books I've read. And this book, perhaps more than any of the others, has caused me to rethink my thinking on lots of issues.

Meghan Ashburn is a neurotypical parent of two autistic children. Jules Edwards, also an autism parent, is autistic herself. I agree with two of the reviews that you'll see on the website of the publisher, Jessica Kingsley Publishers. Nikki Walker: "If you work with autistic children or have an autistic child in your family, *I Will Die on This Hill* is the very next book you should read, and maybe the most important book you'll read in your life." Marcie Alvis Walker: "Ashburn and Edwards' honest and unsentimental book will make you a better human being and, therefore, a better neighbor, better educator, better family member to Autistic adults, Autism parents and the children who need us all to do better."

Here's what Jules says on one of my dogeared pages: "The first thing I ever learned about autism was that autism is bad. Children with autism are unsalvageable, incurable burdens that are a waste of life." On another dogeared page Jules explains why it's wrong to say things such as "I love my child but hate their autism," "Autism is not a disability, it's a different ability," and, to an autistic child, "You can wipe your own ass," and/or, "You don't smear poop."

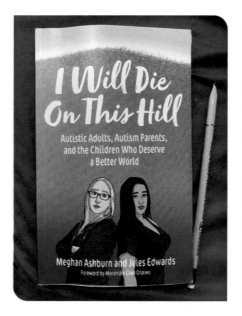

A dogeared page of one of Meghan's sections of the book tells what's wrong with encouraging parents of newly-diagnosed children to go through the various stages of grief. How would any child/adult feel if they knew that their parents experience grief about their existence? On another of Meghan's dogeared pages she shares her thoughts about large, online forums: "They're too public, too negative, and too harmful."

Jules isn't shy about sharing her thoughts about behaviorism and ABA: "It seems to be the hill everyone is prepared to die on, whether for or against." She is critical of ABA specialists who say that ABA therapy is especially important for Black autistics and other marginalized ethnicities – because ABA will help mask their autistic behaviors and traits and therefore make them safer when encountering such things as police involvement. She sums up her opin-

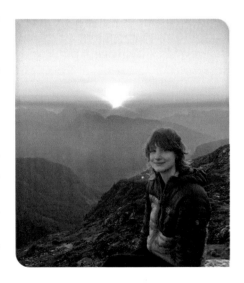

ions like this: "I can say with 100% certainty that this is complete bullshit – not to mention racist."

I've mentioned negative comments by the authors, but the book contains lots and lots of warm, positive, loving content: personal experiences, guidance and advice for parents, and plenty of hopes and good expectations for all of us as our communities live with and embrace autism. "When we find that space to value and treasure one another beyond the transactional model of 'working' spaces then we find a brilliantly beautiful level of understanding and support."

Plus, the book offers continual recommendations for other good books about autism. This book goes at the top of my "must read" list. Find Jules Edwards on her website, autistictyping.com, and Meghan Ashburn at notanautismmom.com.

"Extraordinary Attorney Woo"

A Review by Autistic Self-Advocate Olivia Visser

(This review was first published by The Peak and is reprinted here with permission from Olivia Visser and The Peak.)

NETFLIX K-DRAMA *EXTRAORDINARY ATTORNEY WOO* FOLLOWS THE LIFE OF A YOUNG AUTISTIC ATTORNEY, Woo Young Woo, who lives in Seoul with her father. The series is dramatic and charming, while respectfully addressing serious social issues like mental health, labor rights, and sexism. Many western media outlets have attempted to represent autism on screen with little success. I was pleasantly surprised to find that *Extraordinary Attorney Woo* effectively captures the many challenges of adjusting to adulthood as an autistic person who just wants to fit in. I could really connect with this sense of isolation depicted on screen.

It was emotional to see a show articulate the social aspects of disability so well. Many series pathologize autism by using tropes that focus on "symptoms" or treatment rather than the autistic experience. Shows like *Atypical* and *The Good Doctor* medicalize autism by frequently showing their autistic characters in therapy. Autism is more than just a disability – it comes with considerable social stigma and isolation. Fitting in at work and even just engaging in simple conversation is a challenge for Young Woo, and she works through this with her friends and family instead of therapy – everyone's different.

Part of what made the show more authentic for me was its honest portrayal of autism. Young Woo is far from perfect – she has a lot of difficulty with interpersonal relationships. She often finds herself hyper-focused on particular topics like whales and law, and ends up overlooking how other people feel when she has a goal in mind. Like everyone, autistic people have flaws. This series portrays Young Woo's flaws as natural instead of demonizing her. At the same time, it celebrates her quirks and mannerisms as differences that can make life more enjoyable.

The problem with autism's media representation is that it's targeted towards neurotypical people, who *see* autistic people's behavior but lack an understanding of what goes on inside our heads. TV shows like *The Good Doctor* and *The Big Bang Theory* try their best to make autistic people seem aloof, unreasonable, and unrelatable. Because of this, I rarely find myself enjoying shows with autistic characters. *Extraordinary Attorney Woo* was enjoyable to watch because it often reminded me of myself. Young Woo's introspective remarks about feeling unfit for society were tear jerking at times.

Genuinely relating to a character is something you nearly never experience as an autistic media consumer, since you have limited *and* poor representation. Young Woo's relationship with Lee Jun-ho was familiar and touching to watch, and I appreciated that this show highlights some of the difficulties of navigating relationships as an autistic person. Young Woo repeatedly finds herself more interested in discussing law than her relationship, which hurts Jun-ho's feelings. She forgets that many people like to be asked about themselves at times, while Jun-ho doesn't understand that info dumping can be its own love language. It particularly stood out to me when Young Woo expressed frustration with the restrictive nature of her thoughts: "All my thoughts tend to center around me, so I make people close to me lonely. I don't know when or why I do that. And I don't know what I can do to stop it."

Extraordinary Attorney Woo has its own flaws, despite being one of the more tasteful shows with an autistic character. I had to overlook some blatant clichés like Young Woo having a high IQ and photographic memory. You don't need to portray autistic people as hyper-intelligent for a show to be interesting! It also has a few content warnings to watch out for: ableism, abuse, suicide, and sexual assault. The most significant criticism comes from those who say Young Woo should be played by an autistic actor. This argument is important. Media representation should start with the hiring process, not with the fictional character we see on the screen. Multiple autistic actors auditioned for *Atypical*, but a neurotypical lead was hired. *Extraordinary Attorney Woo* doesn't have any known autistic cast members, which is a shame.

That being said, I don't think we should write the show off as unwatchable. It's important we continue making strides to expand our neurodivergent representation, even if that means we fail at times. I would love to see *Extraordinary Attorney Woo* return for its second season with an autistic actor, but more importantly, I hope neurodivergence becomes a normality in television rather than being an exaggerated trope.

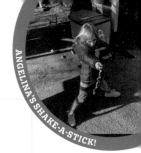

Angelina's Story:
Neurodivergence and Christmas Gifts

ANGELINA, KELLY, JUSTEN AND JUSTEN'S MOTHER, LYRAE, CAME TO OUR HOUSE on Christmas day to eat dinner and open presents. As I've said, persons not familiar with autism would likely think that Angelina is neurotypical. But on Christmas I found it interesting to observe how Angelina's brain works in a neurodivergent way. No neurotypical brain would ever have the ability to think like Angelina.

For example, one of her gifts was a pair of left-handed scissors. (She's left-handed and of course has difficulty making clean cuts with right-handed scissors.) I told her they were left-handed and so she gripped the scissors in her left hand, but upside down. That is, the blades pointed down rather than up. I had to show her that they were to be held exactly the same as right-handed scissors.

She then got a present that had a tightly tied ribbon around it. We told her to use her scissors to cut the ribbon. So she cut the last inch of the straggler piece of ribbon that dangled from the bow. Then she cut another inch and then started cutting the loops of the bow – never attempting to cut the part of the ribbon that constrained the wrapping paper. We eventually showed her which part to cut.

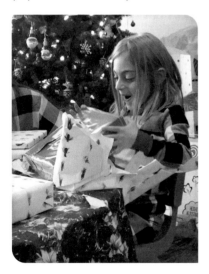

The gift was a fancy van for LOL dolls. LOL dolls are cute little dolls that come in those plastic surprise balls that include lots of accessories. It seems like all little girls, including Angelina, love them. Angelina was appropriately enthusiastic about the LOL van. But she was far more enthusiastic about the next gift: a pink fleece blanket just her size. She hugged it while jumping up and down and screaming happily as if she'd won the lottery – and didn't stop.

But now, each time she comes to our house she beelines it to the LOL van and says, "Let's play LOL! LOL! LOL!" Which I do. I get to be one or more of the children, never the mother or the aunt. (And she doesn't mention the pink fleece blanket.)

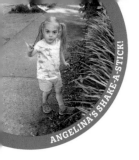

ANGELINA'S SHAKE-A-STICK!

Books About Autism

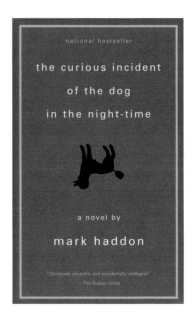

national bestseller

the curious incident

of the dog

in the night-time

a novel by

mark haddon

"Gloriously eccentric and wonderfully intelligent."
— The Boston Globe

RECENTLY A FACEBOOK FRIEND IN ANOTHER STATE WHO IS A SPECIAL EDUCATION TEACHER and whose students include persons on the autism spectrum e-mailed me to say that he'd seen a wonderful play; he recommended that I read the book from which the play was written: Mark Haddon's *The Curious Incident of the Dog in the Night-Time*.

I'd already read it a few years ago when I was an autism newbie. And at that time I recommended the book to others by writing and saying things like this: "While this book focuses on only one specific person, it does help you understand that an autistic brain is often wired in ways that the rest of us can neither understand nor comprehend."

But I was guilty of promoting autism stereotypes. *The Curious Incident of the Dog in the Night-Time* has received lots of praise and honors – both as a novel and as a play. I liked it very much. But this book as well as several other popular books and movies and television features that focus on autistic persons can and do result in their audiences arriving at opinions about autism that are based only on the featured persons. Even today when autism is getting so much more public attention, when many members of the general public hear the word, autism, they assume that it's just like the Dustin Hoffman character in the movie, "Rain Man."

All of which begs the question, How should I respond when folks ask me about novels or movies or television shows about specific autistic persons? My inadequate answer is that it depends, case by case.

My favorite review of *The Curious Incident of the Dog in the Night-Time* is written by Serena Shim, who writes, "I am disappointed that novels like these, along with the media, have popularized many stereotypes that people with autism have to overcome," and, "Many in the autism community believe that the novel and the play helped spread more awareness of autism spectrum disorders to more people. I hope that we can all work together toward spreading a better understanding of what autism is about and increase support in our communities."

There are now probably thousands of autism books, and more being released continually. Where do you start if you're new to autism? If you're a many-years veteran? If you're a parent or family member? If you're an educator, therapist, healthcare specialist? If you're an autistic adult? Although

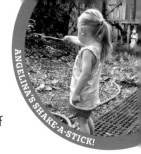

I've now read a bunch of autism books, they're not even the tip of the tip of the iceberg. So in this section of this book I'll tell you where you can find lists of books and I'll also provide brief comments about some of the books that I think are important.

If you Google "Good autism books," you'll find lots of lists. Following are four of my favorite lists (alpha order): Autism Society of America (autismsociety.org, list of books for children), Autism Speaks (autismspeaks.org), That Au-Some Book Club (notanautismmom.com), and Living on the Spectrum (livingonthespectrum.com).

And following are brief looks at some of the books that I've read.

All Cats are on the Autism Spectrum, **by Kathy Hoopmann** – I bought this book because I'm a cat person and because I'm aware of the saying that autism is like being a cat in a dog's world. The book has real photos of real cats accompanied by brief text such as, "When they are spoken to, they may refuse to make eye contact." Of course the word "refuse" implies something that's not the case with autism. The book is a clever idea, but it sometimes misses the mark on both photos and text.

An Early Start for Your Child with Autism, **by Sally J. Rogers, Geraldine Dawson, and Laurie A. Vismara** – When Angelina was diagnosed, an expert strongly recommended that I get this book and begin using it as soon as possible. At just over 340 pages, it's extensive and exhaustive. And although the book's content is great, my thought is that it's a rare autism parent who has time or energy to plow through this tome and its step-by-step regimented processes.

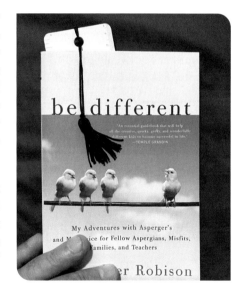

Be Different, **by John Elder Robison** – This is THE book that I suspect will be most beneficial for autistic adults. I agree with Mark Roithmayer's liner on the book's back cover: "A fascinating and unique guide for young people who may be struggling with autism and feel 'out of sync' with the world around them."

Chasing the Intact Mind, **by Amy S.F. Lutz** – One of the nation's foremost experts on severe autism and a parent of a severely autistic son, Amy Lutz confronts some of autism's hottest issues that have emerged with the rise of autistic activists. Is facilitated communication real? Should we really "presume competence" in severely autistic persons? Should all autistic adults be able to administer their own affairs? She presents her cases with scholarly, research-based cases and studies alongside personal examples. Not an upbeat book for sure (after all, its theme is that often the search for an intact mind is fruitless), it's nevertheless important for a real understanding of the severe end of the spectrum.

College for Students with Disabilities, **by Pavan John Antony and Stephen M. Shore** – Published in 2015, ". . . this book explores the current situation for students with disabilities in higher education. It highlights what works, what the challenges are, and how things can be improved." The book has plenty of autism-specific information.

Hidden Brilliance, **by Lynn Kern Koegel and Claire LaZebnik** – I agree with a review on goodreads.com: " . . . explains ways to identify your child's strengths and abilities and then use them as a tool for social communication, improved learning, and overall growth." This 2023 book is praised with statements like "groundbreaking" and "long overdue."

Ido in Autismland, **by Ido Kedar** – (discussed elsewhere in this book)

In a Different Key, **by John Donvan and Caren Zucker** – This is THE book to learn about autism – from its beginnings to today. The book is long – over 600 pages – but its beautifully written style and amazing stories make it continually compelling and intriguing. This book is singular in fulfilling its subtitle: "The Story of Autism." Put it at the top of your reading list.

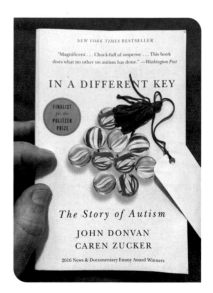

I See Things Differently, **by Pat Thomas** – A wonderful book for children who have siblings or classmates or friends who are autistic. It not only helps them understand autism, but also encourages them to be kind and inclusive.

I Will Die On This Hill, **by Meghan Ashburn and Jules Edwards** (discussed elsewhere in this book)

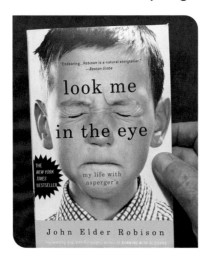

Life, Animated, **by Ron Suskind** – This 2014 bestseller by a Pulitzer-winning journalist is about the author's autistic son, Owen Suskind, whose memorization of Disney movies translated into his profound observance of, and communication with, "normal" society. It was later made into a documentary film that just last month was screened in a Zoom meeting by the Autism Society of Central Virginia – a meeting that included a post-screening, real-time discussion with Owen. The book and the movie are among my favorites!

Look Me in the Eye, **by John Elder Robison** – One of my very favorite top-shelf books, this is the bestselling autobiography, written when he was 50, by a now-67-year-old autistic professor at the College of William and Mary. A brilliantly engaging

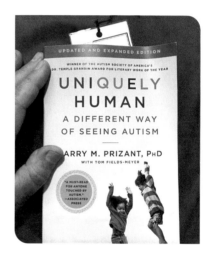

writer, Robison shares the intimacies of the challenges of his youth; his very interesting quest for jobs and careers (including being THE electronics wizard for KISS in their heyday, rigging their Les Paul guitars to spit fire); and his continual efforts to relate to "normal" friends and colleagues. (He is SUCH a good writer!)

Safeguarding Your Child with Autism, by Jack Scott – ". . . describes the scope of safety issues, how the presence of autism contributes to an elevated risk, and the strategies and tools which can be used to minimize the hazards and consequences at home, school, and in the community."

Start Here, by Autistic Self Advocacy Network – This is THE starter book that I recommend for autism parents. Even with their 24/7 challenges, parents will be able to quickly digest and benefit from this slender (48 pages), easy-to-read, guide. The book fulfills its back-cover promise: "We'll talk about how to support your autistic child as they learn and grow."

The Curious Incident of the Dog in the Night-Time, by Mark Haddon (discussed elsewhere in this book)

The IEP from A to Z, by Diane Twachtman-Cullen and Jennifer Twachtman-Bassett – Just what the title says – a great resource for getting appropriate and effective IEPs in place.

The Reason I Jump, by Naoki Higashida – I read the book and saw the film – both moving and compelling. BUT, this is another book (like *Ido in Autismland* and others) that claims to reveal the "voice" of an autistic person who can't speak and who shows no evidence of a level of cognition sufficient to "write" the complexities of the text. To believe or not to believe? See the section of this book that discusses facilitated communication.

Uniquely Human, by Barry M. Prizant – Another of my top-shelf autism books, I love both its title and its theme: "Autism is not an illness. It's a different way of being human." It provides a wonderfully revealing understanding of autism's differences. I agree with *Chicago Tribune's* assessment: "Required reading for anyone touched by autism."

Visual Thinking, by Temple Grandin – (discussed elsewhere in this book)

And one Magazine: **"Autism – A New Understanding," a publication of VeryWellHealth (verywellhealth.com)** – I was recently searching for autism magazines at Barnes & Noble, and this was the only one they had. And it was well worth the $14.99 cover price. Just short of 100 pages, the magazine provides excellent articles on just about everything anyone would want to know about autism. I highly recommend it. But the caveat is that I can't find anywhere to order it online. Amazon says it's not available, and I don't see an opportunity to buy it on the publisher's website.

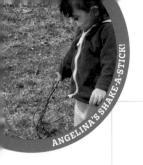

ANGELINA'S SHAKE-A-STICK!

Angelina's Story:
Always Moving – "I Can't Help It."

WE WERE IN CHARGE OF ANGELINA ALL DAY YESTERDAY – took her to school, picked her up afterwards, and brought her to our house to stay until Kelly and Justen picked her up at 8pm after they got off work from the hospital. I had an event to attend, so it was just JC and Angelina for a few hours – during which JC learned a couple of poignant things.

Angelina is always active, both talking and moving, so it can get tiring continually talking with her and continually keeping up with her movement – not flapping arms or any common stimming traits, but simply going from place to place, in this case in our living room which has a variety of stuff for her: an old-timey school desk, a Peppa Pig house and accessories, some notebooks and drawing pads, a box of pretend cooking/meal things, a toy cash register and fake money, etc. You get the idea. Angelina typically goes from one thing to the other and engages us in "pretend" scenarios. "You be the customer and I will be the store owner," she'll say and then will welcome us to her store and proceed to offer us merchandise. Or, holding a notepad and pencil, "Welcome to my restaurant. May I take your order?" And on and on.

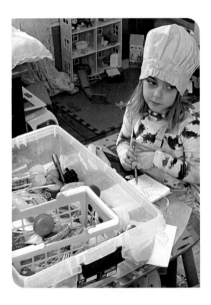

There is a television in the room and she loves to watch those YouTube videos of people playing pretend with dolls. You'll see a hand holding and "walking" a Barbie and talking for the Barbie. Then another hand holding a Ken and responding. And all sorts of other similar videos: Bluey, Elsa and Anna from Frozen, Peppa, etc. When Angelina is watching these on television, she doesn't just sit still. She keeps moving: climbing on the back of the couch, walking around the little table in front of the television, etc., and it will tire you out just watching her do this. At one point last evening JC said to her, "Angelina, why don't you just stay still for a few minutes?" And Angelina's reply was poignant: "Meme, I

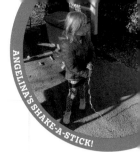

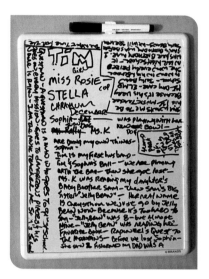

can't help it." JC almost teared up as she realized that such movement is an ingrained part of Angelina's makeup, that she needs it.

The other poignant thing was when Angelina was setting up a pretend story with character parts for her and JC, and JC asked Angelina if she'd like to write the story (Angelina knows how to write, albeit very slowly and with slightly contorted lettering) on a dry-erase board. Angelina declined, so JC asked Angelina if she'd like for her to write it on the board as Angelina told it. Angelina liked that idea, so they spent the next 15 minutes or more with Angelina dictating and JC writing. JC said Angelina loved, absolutely loved, doing that, and that it would have continued if there had been more room on the board. JC learned that Angelina is willing to dictate her creative storytelling for JC to transcribe – not just "willing" but happily excited. That process enabled her pretend storytelling to be even more enjoyable and creative for her.

I'm looking forward to my turn to be the scribe.

"Love on the Spectrum"

"OVE ON THE SPECTRUM" IS A NETFLIX REALITY SERIES that chronicles the dating lives of a few autistic adults – from 20s to 50s – who are searching for true love. The series has been well-received by neurotypical viewers, but there are some notable criticisms.

My favorite review of the show was written by Sara Luterman who is autistic.

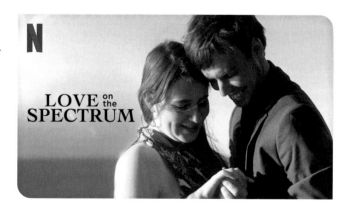

Here's the final paragraph of her review: "'Love on the Spectrum' probably won't educate anyone about autism, or even about the realities of autistic dating. It isn't science. But if you want to watch a dating show in which everyone is treated with kindness, you might want to add it to your Netflix queue."

All of her review is similarly well-conceived and written. Early in the review she says, "Unlike most reality television, the production crew isn't trying to stir up drama. No one gets voted off the island. No one is told to pack their anime figurines and go. Although I was not completely pleased with 'Love on the Spectrum,' it is kind, and I respect the creators' good intentions."

Throughout the review she confirms that the problem (as with virtually all shows and books about specific persons with autism) is that the show will cause viewers to believe that these specific persons accurately represent autism, when, in fact, autism is different in everyone.

And she points out some of the show's embarrassing and incorrect implications: "In one particularly galling moment, the production staff ask Sharnae and Jimmy, an autistic couple who are moving in together, if they have 'consummated their relationship' – to which they sort of laugh and confirm that they have. They are a couple in their 20s. They are moving in together. They sleep in the same bed. For any readers in doubt, I can assure you: Autistic people have sex, just like anybody else. Jimmy and Sharnae have had sex. It was a bizarre question and supremely uncomfortable to watch."

There are three ways that JC and I can possibly be helpful to Angelina when she starts to discover love and romance.

First, we can understand that it's common for autistic persons to yearn to have a loving, life partner – and that it's common for them to see this as a major challenge.

Second, we can continue to educate ourselves about this topic, including via the information on the following four websites as well as others: autismspeaks.org, spectrumnews.org, researchautism.org and raisingchildren.net.au

And third, without revealing confidences, we can keep Kelly and Justen informed about our involvements as confidants for Angelina.

Romance, usually intertwined with sex, is of course like hunger and thirst. It's an extremely compelling biological force within almost everyone who has reached adolescence, including autistic children. It doesn't go away, it's usually not readily discussed, and it can be emotionally consuming. Our job will be to provide comfort, understanding, and wisdom – sometimes in a way that parents can't – for Angelina.

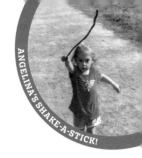
James Prosek and Temple Grandin's
Visual Thinking

THE FULL TITLE OF TEMPLE GRANDIN'S WONDERFUL 2022 BOOK is *Visual Thinking – The Hidden Gifts of People Who Think in Pictures, Patterns, and Abstractions*. I was halfway through it when I happened upon a YouTube video of James Prosek's 2018 TEDx talk at Yale and its amazing kinship with a fundamental theme of *Visual Thinking*: brains that think in pictures (rather than in words) have extraordinary abilities to understand things. Grandin's book explores many aspects of this theme – especially the observance that mainstream schools and mainstream workplaces are mostly unaware of, and mostly marginalize, the potential productiveness of persons whose brains think in pictures rather than in words.

In his TEDx talk James Prosek (who has never identified as autistic) says this about himself: "I draw, therefore I think." And he also says, "It took me a while to realize, but it's actually the failure of words and language that helped bring richness and purpose to my life . . . to help find a way to fill the spaces in between – where words couldn't go."

I met James years ago when he donated a written article and an edition of signed, 4x6-inch prints (he's a notable artist and writer) to help raise money for conservation in conjunction with a book I was writing. We didn't use all of the prints, and I have kept the remainders hoping to find another good use for them. After I saw his TEDx talk, I called James and asked for his permission to use the remaining prints, in conjunction with this book, to raise money for the Autism Society of Central Virginia. He was unaware of Temple Grandin's *Visual Thinking*. But he was intrigued and he said yes. The signed print is from his giant, life-size painting of a bluefin tuna.

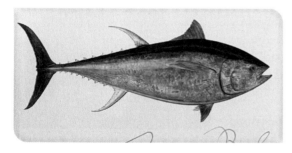

So, with special thanks to James Prosek (Google him; you'll be amazed!), readers of this book can get one of the signed, James Prosek prints by sending a charitable gift to the Autism Society of Central Virginia. See this book's "One Last Thing" section for details. (I'll personally send you the signed print along with smiling gratitude from all of us!)

James Prosek is an artist and writer, including features in such publications as The New York Times *and* National Geographic Magazine, *more than a dozen books, and artworks exhibited by such establishments as London's Royal Academy of Art, The Smithsonian American Art Museum, and the Philadelphia Museum of Art.*

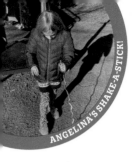
ANGELINA'S SHAKE-A-STICK!

Shelley Rotner – Must-Read Children's Books

I wish Shelley Rotner's widely acclaimed books had been in my children's library when they were little. Only since Angelina's birth have I discovered them. Rotner's books, especially Lots of Feelings *(also available in Spanish) and* Every Body – A Celebration of Diverse Abilities, *are great for those of us who have reading sessions with autistic children. (She's also an artist, photographer, and photojournalist, whose work has been featured in such publications as* Time Magazine, Outside Magazine, *and* National Geographic's World Magazine.) *I sent her a message through the "contact" button on her website (shelleyrotner.com) and asked if she'd be willing to write an essay for this book. She said yes! Here it is:*

HAVE THE UNIQUE OPPORTUNITY AS A NON-FICTION CHILDREN'S BOOK AUTHOR and photographer to represent kids – real kids. My books are photo-illustrated. I want all children to be able to see themselves in my books. My books share a common thread of inclusivity and diversity.

While all kids are different in many ways there are more similarities. Kids just want to be kids—to learn, play, love and be loved. Some kids have more challenges, but everyone brings their own uniqueness that enriches and deepens what these differences may bring. It is my hope that my books help kids navigate their world, cultivate empathy, and become better friends to others.

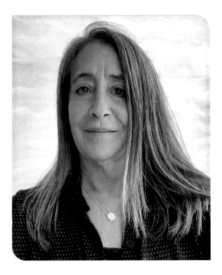

Everyone, kids and grown-ups alike, has been challenged by stressful times with a significant break in our communications affecting how we connect to others. How do we "read" how someone else might be feeling? How do we show and express our feelings?

This is certainly challenging for all, but especially for young children just learning to understand their "inner" emotional world and trying to figure out how to translate these feelings to others. It is even more challenging for kids that have inherent issues in the way they process and connect to others.

I have seen these compromised communications working directly with children, educators, parents and caregivers. In a fast-forward world we run the risk of failing to have truthful and meaningful

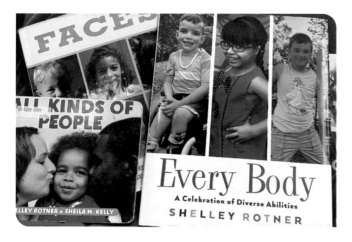

connections.

When the pandemic first started, I asked my 5-year-old granddaughter who was in kindergarten then, how she knew how other kids felt since everyone was masked. Her answer was that she learned to read their eyes. As difficult as that was, it was also transformative. It was like learning another language. It made kids slow down, and really look at others since their feelings were less apparent. As it turns out, that's a useful skill to have. It's a valuable non-verbal way to "read" how someone else may be feeling and helps everyone to communicate, interact, and connect. I hope there's a lot to "read" in my books without reading the words by looking at my straightforward photographs of kids.

Another example I witnessed while I was with my 4-year-old granddaughter recently, was an exchange at a playground. Her friend, a 4-year-old boy on the spectrum, was pushing her on a tire swing rather energetically and a bit too high and strong for my comfort zone. I suggested slowing down a bit. His response was, "I can see she's smiling so I think she likes it. I think it's okay." He was probably right. He knew how to "read" how someone was feeling.

Along these lines, I think my book, *LOT'S OF FEELINGS*, reinforces that we all have lots of feelings but also, how do we express them and interpret how others feel too. Photographs of kids help to simply, and directly convey this.

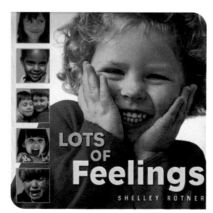

My book *EVERY BODY* celebrates children with all abilities. This book gave me the opportunity to portray a diverse range of kids in a valued and loving way so that they can be seen and heard. Once again, because they are photographs, I think the readers can see themselves and/or develop a greater understanding of others and a different way of being in the world.

In the wide world, with a diverse spectrum of humans, we all need to respect, share, and love our unique way of being. With this diversity, we can gain a deeper and meaningful perception of how to grow and become bigger by collaborating on a grander stage.

Everyone has lots of feelings…

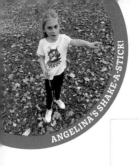

ANGELINA'S SHAKE-A-STICK!

Angelina's Story:
River City Inclusive Gym

JC AND I RECENTLY TOOK ANGELINA FOR AN ASCV-SPONSORED SESSION at River City Inclusive Gym. Their mission: "Improve the lives of individuals with disabilities through fitness and fun!" Their vision: "Give each athlete the opportunity, time, courage, and confidence to show their strengths and build their self-esteem." Their Core Values: "Always adaptable, always approachable, always having fun."

Angelina had a great time. There were 8 autistic participants (up to age 8) and each was paired with a "coach." There were all sorts of physical contraptions, each designed to be both fun and challenging. Angelina loved all of them and continued to excitedly jump up and down when going from one to another.

Physical movement – the more energetic the better – is Angelina's version of stimming. She doesn't flap her arms or rock back and forth or chew pencils or twirl her hair or any of the other common stimming behaviors. She just likes to stay on the move. I wish every community had a River City Inclusive Gym.

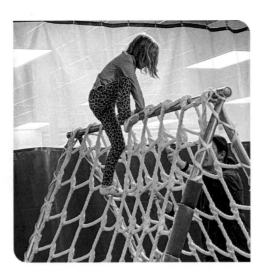 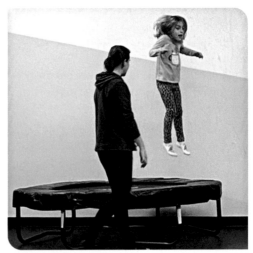

7

Controversies and Viewpoints

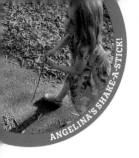

ANGELINA'S SHAKE-A-STICK!

Controversies – #!*X*%#!

"**YOU'LL FIND THAT THERE ARE SO MANY DIFFERENT PERSPECTIVES** and articles out there, with many polarizing opinions." – Ann Flippin, Executive Director, Autism Society of Central Virginia

When Angelina was first diagnosed I didn't know much about autism, and I had zero awareness that there are autism controversies. But it doesn't take long for autism families to be confronted with at least a few controversies – some of which may find family members on opposite sides. And both sides are always well-meaning.

The three fundamental reasons for autism controversies – many of which are heated – are that the manifestations of autism are diverse, the needs for research are diverse, and the fundamental opinions about autism are diverse. Autism continues to be hard to define, continues to have no diagnosis based on blood tests or x-rays or other objective medical procedures, and continues to evoke emotion.

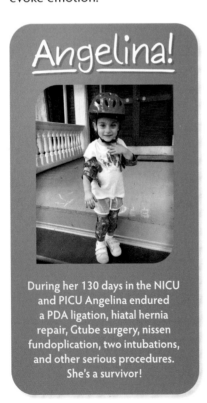

Angelina!

During her 130 days in the NICU and PICU Angelina endured a PDA ligation, hiatal hernia repair, Gtube surgery, nissen fundoplication, two intubations, and other serious procedures. She's a survivor!

Following is my list of only a few of the many autism controversies. (And I am very aware that it can be controversial to use only one paragraph to summarize any autism controversy.)

VACCINATIONS – How do you argue with a parent whose child was "perfectly normal" until she was vaccinated, after which followed regression and autism? How do you argue with lots of families who have had the same experience? Or with noted celebrities who say the same thing? This is of course the autism controversy that is most visible among the general public – that vaccinations cause autism. And even though exhaustive scientific research has discovered no link between vaccinations and autism, the anti-vaccination contingency persists. And if it were Angelina who had gone from pre-vaccination normal to post-vaccination autism I'd probably feel the same way.

DENIAL – It's common for families to be in denial after receiving a diagnosis of autism, and it's common for denial to persist even in the face of an exhaustive diagnosis by experienced specialists. Denial can persist for many years.

CAUSES – It's common for families to blame someone or some-

GRANDPARENT CONFIDENTIAL

"My grandson is autistic and doesn't speak. His parents haven't looked for any therapies or support; I wonder if they're in denial."

thing for autism: poor parenting, stress, poor nutrition, television, cell phones, family dynamics, spankings, and on and on. But it has been proven that none of the above causes autism. The most recent research indicates that genetics is the most significant factor. And "genetics" means that autism is inherited based on the genome of a person or persons somewhere in the child's family tree that spans many, many generations. Blaming a person or an event or an activity or a lifestyle isn't helpful.

DIET – There are widespread opinions about the relationship of diet/nutrition to autism – including the belief that diet can cause or cure autism. But scientific research is clear: diet doesn't cause or cure autism, and there is no evidence that diet in itself can be therapeutic. What science does indicate is that autistic children/adults are more susceptible to gastrointestinal issues and eating disorders – issues that can cause pain and discomfort and malnutrition, etc. that in turn can be counterproductive to the autistic person's development and emotional well-being – just as with all of us.

ABA THERAPY – ABA therapy (Applied Behavior Analysis) has long been the most widely used and respected therapy for children with autism. It's organized around a child's individual needs and uses a continual series of steps and rewards. But there is a growing contingency of persons – especially autistic adults who had ABA therapy as children – who are adamantly opposed to it. They contend that its routines are cruel and/or that it tries to force children to conform to "normality" rather than accepting their neurodiversity.

EDUCATION – "Inclusion" or not? Should Angelina's formal education be in a "normal" school, or should it be in a "special" setting? Is it better for Angelina's education to focus on academics or on social skills? Is it better for her to be among neurotypical schoolmates, or among schoolmates who are developmentally delayed? The answers are never easy and are always dependent on the dynamics of the individual child and family. This can be a contentious issue for autism families and can include strong opinions on every side.

DIFFERENCE OR DISORDER? – Words such as "disorder," "disease," "cure," and "prevent," when referring to autism can be considered hurtful. There are highly contentious opinions on whether autism should be considered a disorder or simply a "difference." Is autism a negative condition that needs to be repaired, or is autism a difference that should be celebrated? Should autism and its neurodiversity be respected as naturally different, or considered an abnormal condition in need of therapy and repair? The Autistic Self Advocacy Network (ASAN – autisticadvocacy.org) is a major national organization that is run totally by autistic persons. (Note: they adamantly use the term "autistic persons" rather than "persons with autism.") ASAN professes the strong opinion that autism

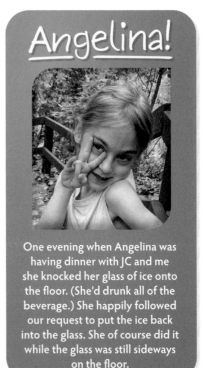

is unfairly and unproductively portrayed and researched and treated in ways that produce negative views about autistic persons. But the widespread and majority opinion outside of ASAN is that autistic persons can benefit most, and can lead the most productive lives, by receiving help and support grounded in proven practices. It's important to be aware of ASAN's thoughts on this. Their website provides their "Position Statements."

RESEARCH – As with most other types of research, autism research is terribly underfunded. The controversies surrounding autism research center on what specific research should be funded and who should do it. For example, should there be research to detect autism in-vitro? Would this lead, as it has already done with Down syndrome, to termination of pregnancies? Should there be research to determine a "cure" for autism? (Research shows that autism can't be "cured.") Should there be research regarding vaccinations causing autism? (Lots of significant research – all with the same definitive and conclusive result – has already been done.) And on and on.

Angelina!

One evening when Angelina was having dinner with JC and me she knocked her glass of ice onto the floor. (She'd drunk all of the beverage.) She happily followed our request to put the ice back into the glass. She of course did it while the glass was still sideways on the floor.

AUTISM SPEAKS – America's biggest nonprofit autism organization has been a target of controversy since soon after its 2005 start – by originally trying to stay neutral in the very heated debate about vaccinations, by originally promoting research to "cure" or prevent autism (amid an ever growing sentiment that autism is a difference and not a disease), by being a champion of ABA therapy (now condemned by many), by using the puzzle piece as its logo (see below), and on and on. Today the organization, always well-meaning and with a wealth of excellent resources on its website, continues to have a full lineup of all-star champions and supporters, but it also has a number of detractors. Localized nonprofit autism service organizations contend that Autism Speaks uses its national marketing budget to engage donor participation in lots of localized Autism Speaks events throughout the nation, thereby diminishing donor funds that could be going to the local organizations that provide actual in-person services for their communities. Autism Speaks might counter that it uses those funds to pay for significant research and political advocacy that local autism organizations don't have the abilities to fund, and that it also uses the funds to provide a robust website that provides free information and education.

AUTISM ORGANIZATIONS – There are lots of local, regional, and national nonprofit organizations and they have differences in the way they see and relate to autism. The bottom line for autism families is to understand that no matter which nonprofit autism organizations we decide to help or be involved with, we may expose ourselves to criticism: "How can you support an autism organization

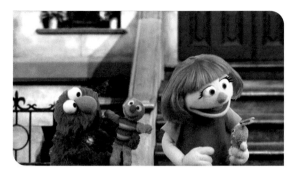

that . . ." My vote is to focus on the good things about each organization.

SESAME STREET – The controversy connected with this beloved and wonderfully educational television show is Julia, the autistic puppet character who made her debut in 2015. The general public views Julia as a wonderful addition to "Sesame Street" – an example of the show's trademark celebration of diversity and inclusion. The Autistic Self Advocacy Network provided consultation and involvement with the introduction of Julia, but when the show began a partnership with Autism Speaks in 2019, ASAN broke its ties and discontinued its approval and believes that the Autism Speaks partnership has introduced "regressive and dangerous narratives" about autism. I happen to like Julia and "Sesame Street," and although I do understand ASAN's complaints, I'm not ready to dismiss Julia or the show. (The main reason I list "Sesame Street" in this list of autism controversies is to demonstrate that just about anything connected with autism attracts controversy – even a longtime widely heralded public television show.)

THE PUZZLE PIECE LOGO – Many autistic persons strongly dislike the puzzle piece as a symbol for autism. The puzzle piece depicts autism as "puzzling" or a mystery, and autistic persons don't wish to be viewed as a puzzle that can't be understood.

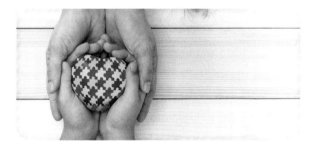

AUTISTIC ADULTS VS AUTISM PARENTS VS OTHER "EXPERTS" – Those of us who have a lot of knowledge about autism often think that OUR opinions are the correct opinions and that those of others are wrong. I applaud something that an autism parent recently told me: "I don't like being judged by the autistic adults who express contempt for parents or who feel that they know everything there is to know about autism across the very very wide spectrum based on how they personally experience autism. I acknowledge that my experience is limited and I try to show grace to folks who have had an experience or a kid who comes with struggles that I can't begin to fathom."

SUMMARY – There are three themes for us autism families. One is that we should be aware of the controversial nature of autism and should expect to be pulled into conversations about specific autism controversies. Second is that even though a little knowledge can often be dangerous, at least some knowledge can be helpful as we have discussions with friends and colleagues. And third is that both sides of every autism controversy are founded on the genuine feeling that that specific side is the most helpful side for autistic persons.

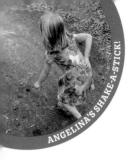
ANGELINA'S SHAKE-A-STICK!

Young and Stupid: The Author's Shame

I WAS YOUNG AND STUPID AND DIDN'T KNOW ANY BETTER." That's a line from the musical play that Dreamers Theater here in Richmond, Virginia presented about bullying – a play performed by autistic adults. During the talkback after the play, an audience member asked the cast, "What was one best moment in your life?" One cast member said it was when he encountered a former grade school classmate and asked him why he had bullied him so much. The classmate gave a heartfelt apology that included, "I was young and stupid and didn't know any better." Other cast members cited similar best moments: apologies from folks who had bullied them when they were younger.

I continue to feel guilty, ashamed, and embarrassed by the way I treated the Johnson family more than 50 years ago. (I've changed the names.)

Fresh out of graduate school in New York City, JC and I had moved to rural south Georgia to teach in a tiny junior college. After a couple of months, another new faculty member, Frank Johnson, invited us to dinner at his home where we met his wife Darla, his 4-year-old son Jack, and his daughter Connie who was perhaps a year old. The house wasn't tidy, the food was haphazardly cooked, 4-year-old Jack was loud and out of control, baby Connie just laid there on a blanket the whole time, eyes open, apparently unable to speak or do much of anything, and Darla tried way too hard to be our new best friend.

Although I liked Frank, the evening at his home turned me off. His son Jack was obviously severely undisciplined, his daughter Connie was way overdue at getting medical attention, and his wife Darla was way too needy. (JC, however, liked Darla and wanted to develop a friendship with her – but I didn't offer encouragement.)

One of the huge perks for the college's faculty members was 50-cent lunches in the college cafeteria for them and their families – which resulted in most faculty members bringing their families to lunch most days. The faculty members sat together in cliques, and JC and I were part of what I considered the IN-group clique – which didn't include the Johnson family.

Our lunch conversation sometimes targeted the Johnson family, especially the lack of discipline for little Jack. "Young hellion," is how one senior faculty member referred to Jack whenever he ran screaming around the cafeteria. And more than once I offered my negative opinions regarding the Johnsons.

"I was young and stupid and didn't know any better," of course isn't an adequate excuse. I wish I could now find that family and apologize. (I've tried unsuccessfully to locate them.) Jack obviously had developmental challenges, I'm sure they were doing all they could for baby Connie, and Darla,

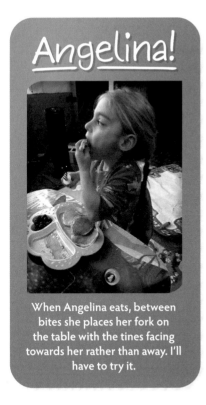

Angelina!

When Angelina eats, between bites she places her fork on the table with the tines facing towards her rather than away. I'll have to try it.

who of course had 24/7 challenges at home, desperately needed adult friends.

I'd like to similarly apologize to the odd-acting classmate in college whom many of us made fun of simply because he walked with a funny cadence and always greeted everyone with a broad-smiling "Hello" whether he knew us or not. And to the grammar-school classmate whom we relentlessly made fun of for putting peanut butter in his pockets and digging it out and eating it during classes. And to others throughout my youth – persons whom I blamed and ridiculed for their neuro-divergent behaviors.

Angelina was born in 2016 and it was only after her autism diagnosis, just before her second birthday, that I discovered the word "neurodivergent." I suspect (and hope) that most persons who have autistic family members have learned what I've begun to learn: often when children and adults behave in seemingly strange and/or unsettling ways, it's because of the way their brains are wired. The behaviors are, as Dr. Barry M. Prizant says in his landmark book, *Uniquely Human*, "strategies the person uses to feel better regulated emotionally and physiologically."

Angelina's Story:
Megan – the Killer Doll

ANGELINA WAS WITH US FOR A COUPLE OF HOURS. Kelly dropped her off on her way to work the night shift and Justen picked her up on his way home from working the day shift at the huge downtown hospital where he's a respiratory therapy and Kelly is a nurse.

Angelina and I were eating pizza at a card table in the living room when she asked, "Can we play school after dinner?" I made an O with my thumb and forefinger and then followed

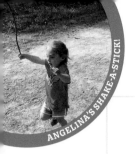

ANGELINA'S SHAKE-A-STICK!

it with a two-handed K. She repeated her question and I again finger-formed an O and a K and accompanied it with a verbal explanation – which pushed her creative button.

She lifted her hands, looked at her fingers and then looked into space as she contemplated. She returned to her fingers and contorted them into one configuration after another, none of which looked like a letter.

"What does that spell?" she asked me. I shook my head. "I spellded [sic] Megan," she smiled.

Megan? Who is Megan? She doesn't have any friends named Megan. I learned later, when Angelina's voice went haltingly monotone, that Megan must be a robot: "I am Megan, and I am here to protect you," she said with an expressionless face.

Days later I Googled "Megan Robot" and didn't like what I found: a movie in which Megan is an evil doll that does very bad things – definitely not suitable for children. I asked Justen and Kelly about it and they told me that there's a trailer for that movie imbedded in one of the children's educational programs on Angelina's tablet. Geez . . .

The "Cure" for Autism

THE INTERNET IS FILLED WITH CLAIMS THAT AUTISM CAN BE "CURED" and that various therapies, diets, food supplements, etc. can provide a cure. Here's the short answer: While there is lots of anecdotal evidence of cures, thus far there is no evidence-based science that demonstrates that an autistic brain can be transformed into a neurotypical brain. Reliable information can be found on websites of reputable autism research centers like the Kennedy Krieger Institute, reputable medical centers such as the Cleveland Clinic, and reputable nonprofit autism organizations such as the Autism Society of America. One thing that I find helpful when researching any therapy or medicine is to Google the name plus the word, "controversy." That's where you're likely to find a *Wall Street Journal* article about a specific medicine or therapy being outed as a sham. (For example, Google "GcMAF controversy" – a touted cure for cancer.)

There has been an increasing level of research regarding whether autism can disappear. What we do know is that some persons do "outgrow the autism diagnosis" – meaning that they no longer meet a specific group of standards. But research shows that these persons continue to have challenges that require various levels of support. And there is an increasing number of autistic adults who adamantly

Angelina!

I'm compelled to fish, and before she could walk I'd take Angelina in her stroller to some of my favorite fishing ponds, which, as I claim to be verified by these photos, interested her.

dismiss the notion that autism can disappear.

It has been proven that there are therapies that can improve language and motor skills and also lessen some types of challenging behaviors. But thus far there is no proof that anything can make autism disappear. It is a lifelong condition indicative of the way the brain is wired. One study of a few dozen children who no longer exhibited autism traits showed, via MRI scans, that they had "recruited" different areas of their brains for certain behaviors. So instead of "recovery," a better word is "compensation."

There are lots and lots of unproven medicines and therapies that are, essentially, selling hope. The Son-Rise Program got its start from a real-life story that was featured in a made-for-television movie in 1979 about a couple who developed their own therapy systems that "cured" their son's autism. Tens of thousands of families have now paid a lot of money for the Son-Rise Program's training sessions, and the website features praise from such luminaries as President Jimmy Carter, Deepak Chopra, and Coretta Scott King. But now, after more than 30 years and lots of anecdotal evidence, there is still no scientific evidence that Son-Rise cures autism.

Other non-proven "cures" for autism include the domain of integrative and functional medicine – nontraditional medicine. Proponents claim this to be the future "best practices" of the medical field, but its practices are currently absent of the scientific proofing rigor of traditional medicine. Hello, Health is one of the companies founded on integrative and functional medicine. On the website its founder tells how supplements were developed that cured her son of autism. The current products featured on the website contain non-FDA-regulated/inspected ingredients such as organic olive leaf extract, Indian frankincense, sunflower lecithin, fish oil, etc.

Wouldn't it be wonderful if autistic children didn't have violent meltdowns? If they were able to have friends and be invited to birthday parties? If they could all function wonderfully without the need for supports? And wouldn't it be great if there were a medicine or therapy that could make this happen? Beware of miracle "cures" that promise such.

ANGELINA'S SHAKE-A-STICK!

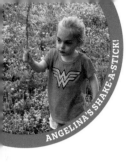

ANGELINA'S SHAKE-A-STICK!

ABA: Autism's Therapeutic Gold Standard – Or Not

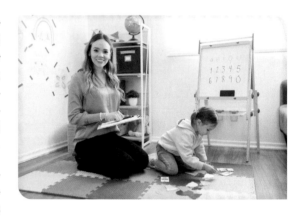

MY THOUGHT IS THAT EVERY CARE-TAKER OF AN AUTISTIC CHILD should be knowledgeable about ABA therapy – autism's most widely used and studied therapy. ABA therapy has the "best practice" recommendation of the U.S. Surgeon General and the American Psychological Association. Evidence-based research has confirmed the results of ABA therapy.

The number of newly-introduced "miracle therapies" for autism seems to continually increase as autism becomes more prevalent. Unproven therapies usually have three calling cards. First, they make use of amazing anecdotal stories: "My child experienced a miracle cure from autism." Second, their advertising and marketing materials are heavy on fantastic claims. And third, they site zero scientific evidence. (I just now Googled a few companies that provide ABA therapy, and none uses amazing anecdotal stories or fantastic claims.)

ABA therapy is probably unique in the amount of scientific study and scrutiny it has received. ABA's initial widely accepted "scientific proof" arrived in the much-lauded 1987 publication of a study of autistic children by Ivar Lovaas that proclaimed amazing results for 40 hours of ABA therapy per week. Even though Lovaas' study was later discredited, the "40 hours of ABA" recommendation continues to be recognized and enshrouded in "scientific proof." And that's exactly what I heard from local and national experts when Angelina was diagnosed.

More and more autistic adults are now speaking out forcefully against ABA therapy. They say that their childhood experiences with ABA were forceful indoctrination that tried to make them "normal" and tried to "fix" them rather than respecting their natural differences. An analogy is what used to take place in Catholic schools. (JC can confirm from her 12 years in a Catholic school in Nashville.) They would force left-handed children to write right-handed. This, they well-meaningly thought, would enable the children to function better in a right-handed world. And they used corporal punishment; JC's hands were smacked often by ruler-weilding nuns.

And a few current caregivers have told me about withdrawing their children from ABA because of the "Gestapo tactics" (one parent's unfortunate choice of words) used to mold their child's behaviors.

My first encounter with ABA therapy took place when Angelina was 2 and I visited her prospective

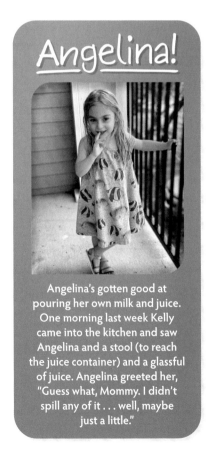

"Who can educate me about ABA? An ABA company evaluated my grandson for less than a half hour and want him to use a therapist who isn't certified."

"school" – an ABA therapy provider. They showed me a series of clipboards – one for each child – that had lots of blocks and lines and numbers and phrases and dates and times. The clipboards contained meticulous documentation of ongoing micro-strategies and results. If, for example, a micro-goal was for the child to orient towards the therapist when she calls his name, the clipboard would document every prompt and result and, when successful, the positive reinforcement. I learned that ABA therapy is one-on-one therapy that includes ongoing documentation of goals and results.

In this school each ABA program was customized for the specific child, and focused on what happens both before and after a specific behavior. A custom mixture of techniques is developed according to each child's abilities, challenges, and personality. They told me that ABA has been proven to be helpful for language and communication, attention and focus, social skills, self-control, self-help, motivation, etc. And it can be helpful in replacing problem behaviors (tantrums, aggression, self-injury etc.) with positive behaviors. They said that the overall strategy of ABA therapy is to use positive reinforcement techniques in a way that can be carefully measured and documented.

I learned that ABA therapists are of course human, and some are "better" than others. I also learned that there are "trained" ABA therapists and "Certified" ABA therapists. By law, "trained" ABA therapists must be supervised by Certified ABA therapists. (ABA therapists who are not Certified should be expected to be just as effective as those who are.)

I also learned that parents and caregivers are sometimes provided with enough ABA training to do various ABA techniques at home – techniques that produce positive results.

Of course we won't know until she becomes a reflective adult and can speak for herself, but I think we got lucky with Angelina's ABA therapy: 30+ hours per week beginning at age 2, tapering off beginning at age 4, and discontinuing at age 5. She was always happy both arriving and departing from therapy, we never had occasion to suspect any sort of emotional abuse, and she made remarkable strides in learning skills and behaviors that are helpful for her to enjoy and thrive in life.

Angelina!

Angelina's gotten good at pouring her own milk and juice. One morning last week Kelly came into the kitchen and saw Angelina and a stool (to reach the juice container) and a glassful of juice. Angelina greeted her, "Guess what, Mommy. I didn't spill any of it . . . well, maybe just a little."

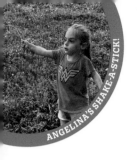
ANGELINA'S SHAKE-A-STICK!

"Autism Every Day" – The Widely-Condemned 13-Minute Film

THIS FILM, PRODUCED IN 2006 BY AUTISM SPEAKS, and that features a few mothers and their high-support autistic children, has been highly criticized and widely condemned for its presentation of autism as something that ruins the lives of the parents. Except for the film's final 45 seconds, there is nothing upbeat, nothing positive, nothing that celebrates anything good about autistic children. And the most criticized part of the film is when one mother, Alison Singer, says that she contemplated putting her autistic child in the car with her and driving off the George Washington Bridge.

Following are some of the things that we hear the film's mothers say. "I really had to give up my entire life." "Your heart is breaking all day long." " . . . expected to do things that no human being should be expected to do." "My life is completely insane." About broken marriages: "An angry time . . . we both felt so helpless and didn't know what to do and sort of turned on each other." About money: "We just keep taking out loans to pay the bills." About social life: " . . . trips and vacations and girlfriends – it's taken me a really long time to let those things go."

I discuss the film in this book to help educate persons who don't know much about autism. The film is startling and gripping and does provide a real-life depiction of a portion of the autism universe – a depiction that the general public needs to know about. BUT . . . But the general public needs to know that there is so much more, so very much more, than this film depicts. Sure, autism is usually accompanied by significant challenges, sometimes even by family-consuming challenges. But the film does not show the positive aspects of neurodiversity and the many ways that those of us who are in autism families benefit greatly in ways that we couldn't otherwise. Although the film implies that the featured children will continue into adulthood to be all-consuming negative drains on their families, the film doesn't show any autistic adults, including adults who contribute positively and productively to society.

GRANDPARENT CONFIDENTIAL

"*My 6-year-old grandson is nonverbal, always appears to be in pain, and squeals a lot. I'm also worried about his parents. I need support from other grandparents who are in similar circumstances.*"

The film's final seconds provide what I wish had been sprinkled throughout the film: hope and love and hugs and statements by the mothers such as, "He is my greatest teacher; he teaches me something every day," and, "He's very, very, loving."

Bottom line from my perspective: watch the film, because it's real and it's educational to see these children who represent a few individual places on a vast, vast spectrum. But know that there is much, much more to autism and to autistic persons than what this film depicts.

Wikipedia: "Both the film and Autism Speaks have received heavy condemnation from autistic people and groups advocating for autistics, with complaints about the film, including that it focuses more on the parents than the actual lives of autistic children themselves, as well as that it portrays autistic people as tragic burdens than as actual human beings who happen to be autistic – which most of them do not want to be 'cured' of or see it as a bad thing. It is also criticized for the fact that many of these interviews – most of which are about the things the parents can't do and how horrible it is to have a child with autism – are conducted with said child in the room, again without any regard for the fact that their children can hear and understand the parents talking about how horrible it is to have to take care of them. This is especially focused on with the aforementioned case of Alison Singer, who spoke about contemplating murder-suicide with her daughter Jodie in the room."

Alison Singer, the film's George Washington Bridge mother and a former executive with Autism Speaks, left Autism Speaks in 2009 because of its research regarding a discredited link between autism and vaccinations. She then founded (and heads) the Autism Science Foundation (autismscience-foundation.org). "At ASF, we believe the greatest gift we can offer our families is innovative autism research that will enable individuals with autism to lead fulfilling lives with dignity . . . Early diagnosis and early intervention are critical to helping people with autism reach their potential, but educational, vocational and support services must be applied across the lifespan. Science has a critical role to play in creating evidence-based, effective lifespan interventions." The website has a lot of good information. Start with the section, "Quick Facts About Autism."

What if You Don't Agree with Your Community's Autism Support Organization?

RECENTLY DISCOVERED A LOCAL NONPROFIT AUTISM SERVICE ORGANIZATION in another state that provides wonderful in-person services and activities and that obviously plays beneficial supportive roles in many families.

But its website has disturbing content: "Too many parents feel like there's no where [sic] to turn, you've been devastated by the news that you're [sic] child has autism, we don't know how they get it, and there's no cure or proven treatment for it. We are here to tell you that these things are just not true!" The website goes on to imply that autism can be cured: "There are thousands of children out there that . . . are recovering, getting into main-stream [sic] school, losing the diagnosis of autism all together [sic] !" And the website credits DAN! doctors for some of the organization's expertise.

DAN! stands for Defeat Autism Now! The DAN! protocol was introduced in 1995 and was embraced by autism parents and researchers who thought that autism could be cured by biomedical efforts such as nutrition, chelation (removal of heavy metals) and hyperbaric oxygen. DAN! methodology never passed scientific scrutiny and thus lost much of its following in the early 2000s, although thanks to continual purported success stories, it continues to have acolytes, including physicians who identify as "DAN! doctors." DAN! is one of perhaps hundreds of non-proven therapies and treatments that claim to be able to "cure" autism, and thus offers hope to many families.

I remember when I was a child and Laetrile got headlines as a purported cure for cancer in spite of scientific studies that showed otherwise and in spite of non-approval by the FDA. Folks with incurable cancer flocked to Mexico to be cured at Laetrile clinics that were legal there. They of course weren't cured and eventually Laetrile lost most of its allure. My father was a doctor and he shook his head at the fact that families were spending so much money on worthless treatments. But, as we all know, "Hope springs eternal."

It is often extremely difficult for science to dislodge strongly held beliefs – even beliefs by good, well-meaning people and organizations. What if your community's autism organization espouses information with which you disagree? My suggestion is to embrace and be grateful for all of the good things that the organization does.

Facilitated Communication and the Book, *Ido in Autismland*

IDO WAS MY PERSONAL INTRODUCTION TO FACILITATED COMMUNICATION (FC), and, as my review below confirms, the book made me a believer . . . UNTIL . . . until I became aware of other opinions about FC and of evidence-based information about FC. (RPM, or Rapid Prompting Method, is a sort of subset or side-set or even same-set of FC, and is basically the same, but with <u>rapid</u> prompting by the facilitator.) Although I've now talked with friends who say that they've personally seen it, and that it's impossible for what they've witnessed to be fake, and that they are absolutely certain that FC works, I still haven't been able to find scientific confirmation that it works. In fact, just the opposite. The scientific evaluations that I've reviewed have discredited FC. I've Googled "Proof of Facilitated Communication," and all I've found are conclusions such as, "Facilitated Communication is not an evidence-based intervention for

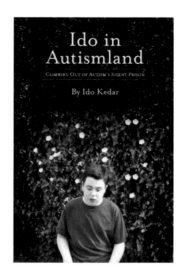

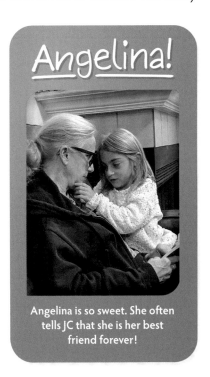

individuals with autism spectrum disorders and should be avoided." – Association for Science in Autism Treatment. Still, I want to believe. And I want to believe the heartfelt claims of my believing friends. And after you read my review of *Ido* (written before I researched FC) perhaps you will want to believe too.

Wikipedia: "Facilitated Communication is a scientifically discredited technique that claims to allow non-verbal people, such as those with autism, to communicate. There is widespread agreement within the scientific community and among disability advocacy organizations that FC is a pseudoscience."

The American Speech-Language-Hearing Association (ASHA): "Facilitated Communication (FC) is a discredited technique that should not be used. There is no scientific evidence of the validity of FC, and there is extensive scientific evidence—produced over several decades and across several countries—that messages are authored by the 'facilitator' rather than the person with a disability. Furthermore, there is extensive evidence of harms related to the use of FC. Information obtained through the use of FC should not be considered as the communication of the person with a disability." The ASHA similarly discredits RPM.

And, **worst case scenarios** for FC include an ever increasing number of charges of sexual abuse: autistic children, via facilitated communication, accusing parents of sexual assault, complete with "extensive, explicit, pornographic details." One highly publicized case in North Carolina was finally dismissed after a court-ordered, double-blind test proved that the autistic person who had made the sexual assault claims was illiterate. A Wikipedia listing says, "The number of cases continues to increase. In addition to accusations of sexual abuse, facilitators, reportedly, have developed sexual feelings for their communication partners and, relying on FC for consent, initiated sexual, physical contact with people in their care, raising serious ethical and legal problems for facilitators, protective service agencies, law enforcement, court officials, educators, and family members alike."

Angelina!

Angelina is so sweet. She often tells JC that she is her best friend forever!

My review (written prior to my investigation of Facilitated Communication):

The book, *Ido in Autismland*, by Ido Kedar, was published in 2012. Its fundamental message is something that everyone – especially autism families – should be aware of: a highly intelligent, deep-thinking mind is sometimes locked inside of a non-communicative, constantly-stimming, terribly-behaved, unresponsive person who is diagnosed with profound autism. Ido Kedar, who had made little progress during years of ABA therapy and was evaluated by all of the experts as having only minimal cognitive ability, found a teacher who used unconventional strategies and ignored the diagnoses of the experts and taught Ido to communicate. He credits her for saving his life.

Facilitated communication enabled Ido to reveal his high intelligence, and he went almost immediately from rudimentary "touch your nose" ABA drills to high-level performance in mainstream schools. His writings are professional level. His speeches are moving and profound. And if not for the unconventional teacher, he would still be locked inside of a physical body that he is unable to control and from which he is unable to communicate.

Ido has autistic friends who, as he was, are locked inside uncontrollable bodies with no way to communicate, and who are subjected to ABA therapies that don't work. (Over and over again Ido was given directives such as "touch your nose" which he understood but couldn't cause his body to do.) But Ido found an unconventional teacher who used the Rapid Prompting Method (RPM – which "experts" continue to say is inappropriate and ineffective for use in such cases) and spoke to him as she would to a neurotypical person – rather than with simplistic phrases used in early childhood ABA therapy.

Ido first learned to point to letters on a letterboard and immediately demonstrated that he could read and write and was highly intelligent. Today he uses an I-Pad that, as with Stephen Hawking, vocalizes whatever Ido types. He gives speeches, writes a blog, and has now published a novel.

Nevertheless, most experts continue to disregard Ido's plea that there are many other persons who, like him, can't communicate and have the "severe autism" label, but have a keen mind and intelligence locked inside. Most experts think Ido's "coming out" was a sham, a trick, some sort of manipulation by his unconventional teacher.

Ido has determined that his mission in life is to help autism experts embrace a new paradigm for dealing with persons with severe autism who can't communicate. He has friends who are this way and, via facilitated communication, he says he can often see that "spark" in their eyes.

A FINAL NOTE: *Ido in Autismland: Climbing out of Autism's Silent Prison* is included on proponent lists as evidence that Facilitated Communication (FC) works. The book focuses on traditional, touch-based FC and Rapid Prompting Method (RPM), where the facilitator holds a letter board in the air and/or cues from a distance. When facilitators are reliably blinded to test protocols, the resulting responses fall into three categories: 1) facilitator known responses, 2) unintelligible, and 3) correctly spelled words that are not relevant to the materials presented (e.g., facilitator generated messages). To date, there is no reliable evidence to prove that facilitated communication is produced independently.

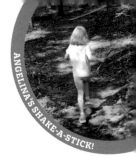

The Amazing Randi: Vaccinations and Facilitated Communication

'VE BEEN A LONGTIME ADMIRER OF JAMES RANDI (1928-2020) – first as a magician and later as a debunker of claims of paranormal phenomena and pseudoscience. You might be both educated and entertained by his 2010 TED talk that's available you YouTube: "Homeopathy, quackery and fraud."

Randi wasn't a disbeliever; he just yearned to see proof. For example, he placed a million dollars in escrow with a Florida Bank – money for the first person who could prove something paranormal. Proof was always first subjected to a very simple test.

One example was a man who arrived at Randi's office claiming to glow in the dark. Randi simply invited the man, along with a few persons who were standing at the nearby bus stop, to come into his office. Randi turned off the lights and nobody could see the man glow in the dark. For many years Randi was confronted with paranormal and pseudoscience claims – none of which ever evidenced proof.

Randi vehemently disapproved of persons who made money by using pseudoscience and fake paranormal stuff to prey on persons' emotions – such as claiming to talk with deceased persons and claiming to cure diseases.

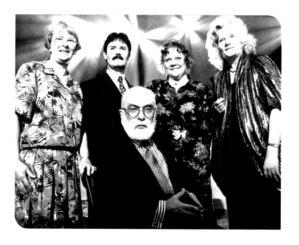

Randi knew two autism families that caused him to devote extensive study to two examples of what he recognized as pseudoscience: that vaccinations cause autism, and that facilitated communication can unlock reservoirs of intelligence that exist within persons who have never communicated and haven't shown signs of cognitive function.

His extensive findings, detailed with sophisticated chemistry and laboratory studies, and as published in the Vol 41, No. 2 issue of *Skeptical Inquirer* and scheduled to be included in his 11th book (he died before completion) are briefly summarized as follows:

Vaccinations (that they cause autism):

ANGELINA'S SHAKE-A-STICK!

"If there is one major concern that has taken my attention as a skeptic and served to inspire this book, it is the persistent and currently very popular delusion that tries to connect the process of childhood vaccination with . . . autism . . . The most erroneous and damaging misunderstanding about this condition started in 1998, when a British researcher, Dr. Andrew Wakefield, published in the prominent medical journal *The Lancet* a paper claiming that there was a connection between the use of MMR—a multi-purpose immunization vaccine used against measles, mumps, and rubella (German measles) – and the onset of autism in children. This is simply not true. MMR has been found to be a very effective prophylactic measure, and since the 1970s, well over 500 million doses have been successfully administered worldwide in some sixty countries . . . Then, in 2010, that *Lancet* paper by Wakefield was officially retracted upon the discovery of serious overlooked basic flaws in his protocol and the unethically close connection between the author of the paper and the industrial agencies that had financed his work. . . . But why do so many people continue to believe that there is a link, despite the overwhelming evidence? The answer is something that has more credibility than the best scientific study: personal experience. Here we encounter a basic error in logic that folks often make. Many parents . . . believe that vaccines caused their children's autism because the symptoms of autism appeared shortly after the child received a vaccination. On a psychological level, that assumption and connection seems to make sense, but on a logical level, it is a clear and common fallacy: *post hoc ergo propter hoc*— [It happened] after this, therefore because of this."

One of Angelina's favorite things about the Autism Society of Central Virginia is her friendship with Executive Director Ann Flippin's daughter, Kate, as per this photo at ASCV's annual Trunk or Treat event.

Facilitated Communication (that practitioners can unlock communication):

"I looked into the farce known as Facilitated Communication (FC). The resulting experience was most unpleasant, with little cooperation being offered me by those administering this blatant quackery . . . Consult the subject under Facilitated Communication on the Internet, and you will see this farce . . . As for the degrees of these behavior patterns they exhibit, I found that it varied from extreme – wild shouting and damaging bouts of flailing with arms and legs – to gentle, distant, and almost acceptable demeanors and attitudes . . . The staff at Syracuse had actually come to believe that these children might be using *telepathy*, and had called me in to find out if that might be the correct solution!"

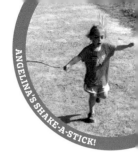
ANGELINA'S SHAKE-A-STICK!

A Note About Relentless, Loving, Autism Moms

GOOGLE "AUTISM MOMS" AND YOU'LL FIND LOTS OF OPINIONS, including this one: "I think that the self-proclaimed 'autism moms' whose entire personality is having an autistic child and form a superiority complex around it are obnoxious." It's of course unfair to paint everyone who self-identifies as an autism mom with such an unkind brush. But until I dove into the research and personal connections that have enabled this book, I had my own terribly unfair thoughts about a certain type of autism mom: the type who believes in "cures;" who, after traditional therapies fail, attach their hopes to scientifically dismissed methods such as chelation and parasitic worms and faith healers; who don't let miles or money get in the way of chasing every latest glimmer of, albeit unproven, hope – even when warned that a specific "cure" may be harmful. I used to think these type of moms aren't good moms.

But now I know a few of them personally and what I've seen is an intensity of motherly love that we should wish for every child. I've seen their non-complaining, full-speed-ahead, drive to enable their child to have the best life possible. Are many of their travels and expenditures worthless? Of course. But each provides hope. And each is testament to the mother's love.

Uninformed Novelist

KEEP THINKING ABOUT KAREN KINGSBURY. She's a best-selling author of "inspirational" novels – you know, filled with plotlines that feature the power of God and Jesus and prayer. A good friend recently told me that she reads Kingsbury's novels, so I decided to read one too and learned that there is one, *Unlocked*, written in 2010, that focuses on an autistic high school boy. After I read it I sent an e-mail to Kingsbury (she has about a half million followers on Facebook, so I didn't expect to get a reply) that included this: "I applaud your attempt to shine an understanding light on autism in your 2010 novel, *Unlocked*, but the novel presents information and themes that now, in 2024, we know are wrong, and also harmful – both to autism families and to the general public's understanding of, and relationships with, autistic persons. I have a three-part suggestion. First, remove the novel from the marketplace. Second, rewrite it using consultation from current autism experts. Third, re-release it as a new and improved edition."

The book has a variety of problems. One is that it continually implies that vaccinations cause autism.

(I understand why many folks believe that; there's a section elsewhere in this book that discusses vaccinations.) Another is that the book implies that autism can be cured (especially with God's help). It can't. And still another is that autistic persons are to be pitied, and so are their families. There are other problems with the book – as confirmed by the 25 pages I dogeared.

Two days later I received a reply to my e-mail. It was from Anne Kingsbury, "Karen Kingsbury's Mother and Assistant." The e-mail was long and it promoted Kingsbury's forthcoming movie, her newsletters, and her website that has info about "contests, movies, speaking events and new book releases!" The e-mail had only one sentence regarding the concerns that I expressed: "I think medical issues in a story will always need updating."

Bottom line: There are sincere, well-meaning, beloved writers who, in their attempts to shine a productive light on autism, are ill-informed and even harmful.

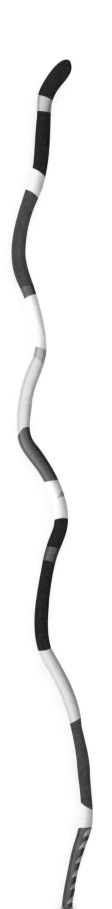

Online
Research and
Discovery

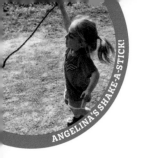

ANGELINA'S SHAKE-A-STICK!

Autism Society of America

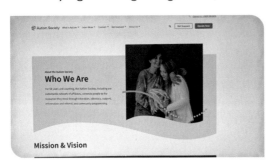

THE AUTISM SOCIETY'S WEBSITE (AUTISMSOCIETY.ORG) is a great place to start your online research and discovery. There is an explanation of autism, basic information about identifying and diagnosing autism, information about interventions and therapies, employment, housing, and on and on – a wealth of all sorts of information. One of my favorite things is the political advocacy information – not only about various pending legislation, but also a list of my personal elected officials, from national president down to my local representatives; all you have to do is enter your address. Go to the website and explore; you'll no doubt find resources that are helpful for your personal circumstances.

Autism Blogs are Great. Or Not.

GOOGLE "AUTISM BLOGS" AND YOU'LL SEE LOTS OF SITES including sites that list the top 10 autism blogs, top 40 autism blogs, and even top 100 autism blogs. I've found several productive things just by exploring autism blogs that can be helpful for Angelina, and I've let Kelly and Justen know about them. For example, a blog is where I got the idea for one of Angelina's favorite learning activities when she was 3 – an activity that involves containers of water and food coloring. I found a couple of her favorite books on blogs, and blogs have provided helpful insider advice for her IEP and 504 meetings.

Which blogs are best? Which blogs can we trust? Unfortunately, there is no guidebook. It has to be intuitive. Following are a few things that I've learned from continually browsing autism blogs.

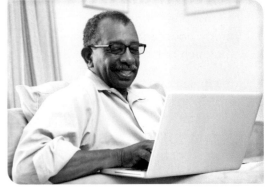

1: **Titles can be misleading.** I don't refer anyone to a specific blog until I first read it myself. For example, following are some seemingly obvious titles of blog articles that I've discovered but haven't yet read: "Using Video Technology

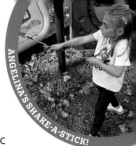

to Support Autistic Individuals," "Successful Adulthood Starts in Childhood," "The Do's and Don't's of Overcoming Sensory Issues at the Dentist," and "8 Ways Yoga Therapy Can Benefit Children With Autism." Hopefully each of these articles is helpful regarding the specific topic, but I've learned that it's not always the case.

2: **Be skeptical of miracle therapies.** The prevalence of autism is increasing, and so is the number of miracle therapies – and it seems that all of them find their way into autism blogs. Here's what I do when I read about a therapy that sounds miraculous: I simply Google the name of the therapy followed by the word "controversy" – for example, "Son-Rise Program Controversy." (That's a real therapy program that although now discredited, is still praised by lots of autism families.) If there are problems with the therapy, Google will find them.

3: **If a blog offers stuff for sale, be cautious.** I've found that there are a lot of autism blogs that provide opportunities to buy books and t-shirts, to donate to good causes, to participate in workshops, etc. Although commerce can be an indicator of negative things, that's not always the case. For example, one widely praised (including by me) blog site that offers commerce and philanthropy is "Finding Cooper's Voice."

You can explore autism blogs 24/7 and still not make a dent in what's out there; I try to devote a half hour or so every few days.

Angelina's Story:
The Dental Office

EVEN THOUGH SHE'S 8 NOW, and even though she's been brushing her own teeth for a couple of years, she still hasn't thoroughly mastered it. So sometimes when I'm with her during tooth-brushing occasions, she accepts my offer to help. And she's pretty good about letting me put the toothbrush in her mouth and demonstrating a thorough brushing routine.

But in her early years when her first teeth arrived Angelina hated to have things poked around in her mouth. And having a dental exam and cleaning was a major challenge. It would take two of us to hold her while she screamed as the dentist did the work. We always dreaded dental appointments.

But that suddenly changed after JC sat Angelina in her lap and read a little book to

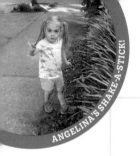

ANGELINA'S SHAKE-A-STICK!

her while showing her the pictures. It was about a little girl's visit to the dentist – a smiling, happy experience. (I can't remember the title, but there are lots of good children's books about going to the dentist.) Angelina's next visit to the dentist was a happy one: no screaming, no squirming, just smiles. We thought it was a miracle.

This introduces the topic of "social stories" and how they can often be helpful for autistic children.

Autism Parenting Magazine's website provides a good, basic description: "A social story is a narrative made to illustrate certain situations and problems and how people deal with them. They help children with autism understand social norms and learn how to communicate with others appropriately." Social stories can be helpful for autistic children in myriad ways: learning to share, riding in a car seat, taking a bath, riding an elevator, eating new foods, etc.

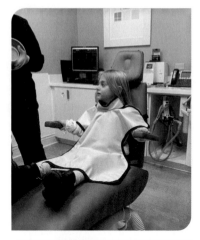

A social story is most effective when the protagonist has similar characteristics as the specific child. The social stories that I now make up for Angelina always start something like this: "Once upon a time there was a little girl who had blond hair, a big smile, and a dog named Max. Her name was Leena." And the story may continue with something like this: "Leena was so happy that she was going to go on a trip on an airplane!" And the story will continue with a happy, upbeat, step-by-step chronicle of Leena's flight. Almost always such social stories have been beneficial for Angelina.

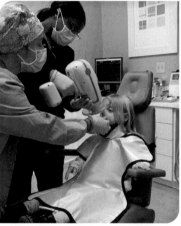

Autism Parenting Magazine

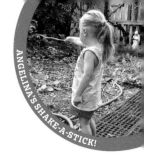

J UST LAST WEEK I READ SOMETHING written by a mother of a child with autism. She said that the moment her autism mother status became public, she started being bombarded continually by various stuff to buy: memberships, therapies, publications, trinkets, seminars, snake oil, and on and on . .

All of which I thought of today when receiving yet another unsolicited e-mail from "Mark from Autism Parenting Magazine": an invitation to join the "Autism Learning Network . . . a community for and by autism parents. All the support you need, when you need it." And much more: "Get over $1,400 worth of content for just $29/month." Following are a few of the sales pitches.

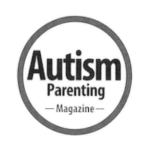

"Are you ready for your child to ditch diapers for good? Our course will show you how. Say goodbye to dirty diapers and say hello to a peaceful toilet routine . . ."

"Teach your child independence! You can learn to create and use visual schedules for meltdown-free transitions and clear communication."

" . . . symptoms like meltdowns, aggression and disrupted eating and sleeping habits. Get a spectrum of solutions . . ."

GRANDPARENT CONFIDENTIAL

"My 8-year-old granddaughter was only recently diagnosed. She masks her autism characteristics at school and has meltdowns in the evenings. I care for her 2 days each week. Her family has a lot of stress trying to address her challenges. How can I be more helpful and supportive?"

And there are quotes from satisfied customers like Lily Thompson: "Autism Learning Network has been a true lifesaver for us grandparents." Judith Del Valle: "Very useful information . . . can help these kids improve there [sic] method of communication." Becky Geis: "I am an occupational therapist . . . so many ideas that I can incorporate into my practice." Sunita Agarwal: " . . . extremely beneficial and top quality. I am a special needs educator . . . " (I wondered who these persons are, and later Googled and found a Sunita Agarwal whose profile relates to "special needs educator." She is the Learning Support Coordinator for Edubridge International School in Mumbai, India. I also found a Becky Geis who is listed as a non-Medicare-accepting occupational therapist in Bellingham, Washington, but I found no information about her practice.)

The site has a long-scrolling series of explanation-pointed su-

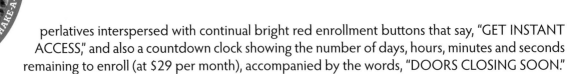
ANGELINA'S SHAKE-A-STICK!

perlatives interspersed with continual bright red enrollment buttons that say, "GET INSTANT ACCESS," and also a countdown clock showing the number of days, hours, minutes and seconds remaining to enroll (at $29 per month), accompanied by the words, "DOORS CLOSING SOON."

If you decide to enroll in the Autism Learning Network, please note that the giant nonprofit organization, Autism Speaks, has a <u>free</u> service called the Autism Care Network. (My guess is that there are other "Networks" out there, both free and fee-based, attached to the term "Autism.")

Behavioral Innovations: A Website With Great Blogs

THERE IS A TEXAS-BASED COMPANY whose website has some great blog articles – with new ones posted weekly. The company is Behavioral Innovations and its website is behavioral-innovations.com. Behavioral Innovations is an ABA company, but many of the blogs are not about ABA.

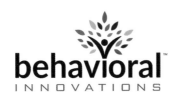

JC reads to Angelina when she is in our care, and one blog, posted on 2/18/2022, has been helpful: "Best Books by Age for Kids with Autism." The article begins by asking and explaining a few questions such as: What is your goal for your child? What are your child's special interests? And What skills do you want your child to develop? (You can find books about brushing teeth, getting along with siblings, etc.) The article tells about 14 different books. *All My Stripes: A Story For Children With Autism*, by Shaina Rudolph and Danielle Royer, is about a young zebra with autism and his feelings about being different from his classmates. Another recommended book is *Why Does Izzy Cover Her Ears?* by Jennifer Veenendall. Izzy experiences sensory overload and her behaviors are misunderstood.

Another helpful blog on the site, posted on 2/3/2022, is entitled "Aggression in Children With Autism – How to Manage Aggressive Behavior." A blog that JC and I relate to, posted on 1/31/2022, is entitled "7 Ways to Teach Independent Living Skills to Kids with Autism." For example, JC gets Angelina to help with various household chores, and when I cook I get her to do various steps by herself, like cracking eggs.

And the 1/26/21 blog features a 1-minute video entitled "Potty Training Tips." I wish I'd discovered it when Angelina was going through potty training. The major takeaway from the video is that successful potty training requires everyone (parents, grandparents, therapists) to be on the same page. It's not productive if different methods are used simultaneously by different persons.

At this writing the website's blog contains 145 articles, and I suspect that every autism family will find a few that are both helpful and relevant to their own situation.

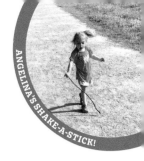

Child Mind Institute – A Great Go-To Source

'VE DISCOVERED A WEBSITE that not only provides all sorts of information and guidance regarding autism and its challenges, but does so in a well-organized and highly accessible manner. It's the website of the Child Mind Institute: www.childmind.org.

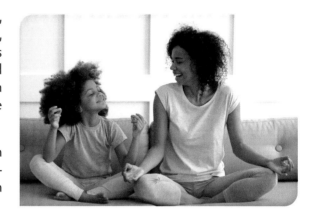

"The mission of the Child Mind Institute, founded in 2009 by Dr. Harold S. Koplewicz, Brooke Garber Neidich and Debra Perelman, is to: Offer best-in-class evidence-based clinical care. Engage the global scientific community in visionary research to discover more effective treatments."

When you go to the website, simply search "autism" and you'll find a wealth of information: more than 60 "guides" and more than 700 articles.

Click on "Complete Guide to Autism" and you'll find 13 topics including Sensory Issues, Rigid Eating Habits, Wandering, Medication, and others. And each topic is accompanied by lots of helpful information, guidance, and recommendations.

For example, the Sensory Issues section addresses such things as screaming when their faces get wet, and putting inedible things in their mouths.

The Rigid Eating Habits section talks about preferences for soft foods or crunchy foods, how to rule out GI problems, techniques for tackling various mealtime issues, and more.

The Wandering section includes things such as guidance on how to make homes safe and how to guard against wandering/eloping.

The Medication section begins with this: "There is no medication for the symptoms of autism." But it provides information about medicines that are often prescribed to lessen symptoms, and advises that all have concerning side effects. It states that Risperdal, for example, is widely used to treat children who are aggressive, but it comes with very significant side effects.

The website is searchable such that you can find most any topic of concern, and robust enough that you can explore and learn for hours.

I especially like that the Child Mind Institute is science-based, evidence-based. And I like this introductory information regarding autism: "Autism is a neurodevelopmental disability that starts in utero, isn't caused by vaccines or bad parenting, and, due to a broad spectrum of symptoms, manifests differently in everyone."

Angelina's Story:
JC's Art Studio

JC AND I KEPT ANGELINA ON SATURDAY from 6:30 am until 8:00 pm while Kelly and Justen were at work. I suspect that the highlight of the day for Angelina was going to JC's art studio that's located at Studio Two Three, an artists' collective – lots of artists making art using the facility's space and equipment. JC is one of more than a dozen artists who have personal studios there.

JC's studio has a purple and white checkerboard rug with 5-inch squares. She bought a set of 4-inch checkers to have available when Angelina is there, and the scenario was a big success on Saturday. It was Angelina's first experience with checkers; they played for almost an hour. Of course Angelina had her own thoughts about how the checkers should move.

Angelina also created a couple of artworks including one that she said was of me and

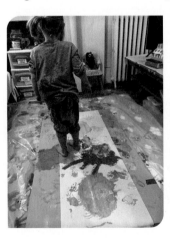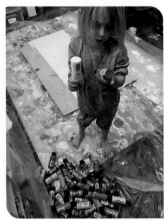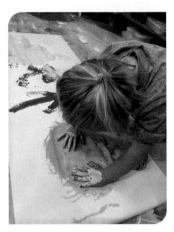

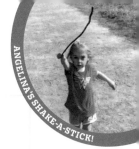

her dog, Max. JC is so good at igniting her interest in drawing and painting. Whenever I'm watching Angelina at our house I always suggest that we get out her art supplies (sketchpads, paints, color pencils, crayons, markers, etc.) and create art and Angelina almost always declines.

When she was younger she loved it when I would place a 6-foot piece of paper on the floor atop a plastic floor covering and give her little bottles of acrylic paint and some brushes. She would use not only the brushes but also her hands and bare feet. She would wear a little gray gym outfit each time – which we'd never wash. One year we put a photo of this on our Christmas card along with the message, "Wishing all of us a fresh season of joy as we embrace seemingly uncomfortable interactions between blues and reds, blacks and whites, browns and yellows, straights and curves, lights and darks, strongs and weaks, and on and on and on . . ." And we featured her again on our 2021 Christmas card with the message, "May a sweet angel paint your 2022 canvas with unbridled strokes of LOVE + KINDNESS"

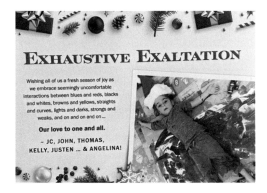

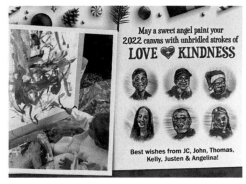

Almost Everything I Know About Autism, I Learned from Other Parents!

THAT'S THE TITLE OF AN HOUR-LONG PANEL DISCUSSION (link: https://autismakron. org/parent-panel) that is engaging, educational, and inspiring to anyone who takes the time to watch it. The panel was gathered by the Autism Society of Greater Akron (autismakron.org)

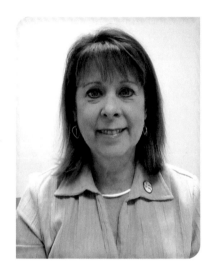

which is headed by Executive Director Laurie Cramer. I e-mailed Laurie and asked if she would be willing to provide an introductory essay about this wonderful panel discussion. She said yes, and here it is:

As the mother of a young man with "a lot of Autism" as we say in our house, and as the Executive Director of the Autism Society of Greater Akron, I have the unique opportunity to not only be the parent of a child with Autism, but also to walk beside many other parents on their Autism journey. I'm not sure where the phrase "Everything I know about Autism I've learned from other parents," came from, but I picked it up many years ago. I've also heard many other parents use it. It's the perfect phrase that describes both the journey of Autism as a parent and family and the mission of the Autism Society and its affiliates: We create connections, empowering everyone with the resources needed to live fully. Connecting, finding each other, learning together and providing support is what we do.

During the pandemic when everyone was struggling to provide services and we couldn't connect in person, ASGA found that our community had a strong desire and need to continue to be together, even when we couldn't. So when I decided to do a webinar with other parents of young adults with Autism, it was natural to name it after the familiar phrase. The parents on the webinar found that we had many similarities, including that the mothers blamed themselves for their children's Autism, that we were at a loss of how to help our children when they were newly diagnosed and underwent intensive and expensive treatments that didn't work, how the schools were not prepared for our involved children, and how we continue to worry about their health and safety in a broken disability system as they enter adulthood. We also found that we could laugh together and how much we all continue to lean on each other as we navigate the complex disability world.

I hope you enjoy this video and have your own "tribe" of parents to support your journey. It really does help to know that you are not alone.

YOU Can Participate in Autism Research.

AUTISM RESEARCH STUDIES ARE BEING CONDUCTED CONSTANTLY by reputable organizations, and they continually seek volunteers and they often pay the participants. And many of the studies are conducted remotely (questionnaires, communications, etc.) and do not require in-person involvement. Caregivers and guardians of persons with autism can often qual-

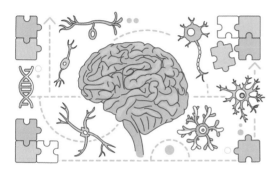

ify for research participation.

On its website the Autism Society of Central Virginia (ascv.org) lists a variety of current research studies that are taking place nationwide. Simply go to the website and search "research studies."

I looked at the list while preparing this book and it contained 28 research studies that were looking for participants. The ASCV groups the studies into six categories: infants, children, siblings, adolescents, adults, and gender diverse individuals.

Within the Infants category, for example, was Drexel University's study of communication tools used by infants with autism. They paid the participants.

The Children category included a study of significant sleep disorders in 3-to-7-year-old children with autism, a study of the impact of COVID-19, a study of auditory hypersensitivity, and others.

Examples in the Adolescents category included a study on sex education and one on transition planning (to adulthood).

The Adults category included studies on employment experiences, physical activity habits, experiencing pain, and others.

There are three fundamental ways that we can benefit from participating in research studies. First, we are likely to gain information and strategies that can be helpful to our own families. Second, we will form potentially beneficial relationships with autism experts. And third, we will help to elevate the overall understanding of autism.

Do You Know about Wanelda?

HAVEN'T BEEN VERY SUCCESSFUL IN GETTING MY FRIENDS INTERESTED in one of my favorite social media personalities, but if you want to see 100% authenticity regarding a mom and her autistic son, check out The Wanelda Diaries and Wanelda Hensley on Facebook. Most of Wanelda's Facebook posts in which she talks about Maverick (her autistic son) aren't as intense as the one posted on March 27, 2024, but that one confirms Wanelda's straight-ahead honesty. For a brief, upbeat post, look at the one from May 15, 2024. To be clear, most of her posts are not about autism, but from time to time they are.

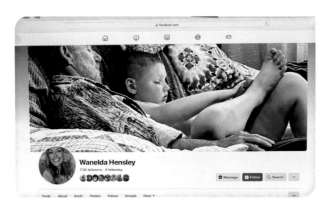

I became aware of The Wanelda Diaries a few years ago by accident and was immediately engaged by her West-Virginia-hollers accent and language, and especially by her authenticity. She backed into social media's viral universe unintentionally, and has been able to leverage things to make a seemingly good living. In 2022 she was even a guest on NBC's "Hoda and Jenna." (Google it; you'll find the video.)

A couple of years ago when I saw a Facebook post about Maverick, I contacted Wanelda about possible involvement with my first attempt at putting this book together. Her assistant responded that Wanelda was interested. But the communication discontinued after that. (I've learned over and over again that autism families almost always have more urgent priorities than providing content or information or interviews for a book.)

At any rate, although I'm not in touch with Wanelda and don't have any sort of endorsement from her, I herewith suggest her Facebook presence for your consideration.

9

Grandparents

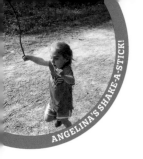

Grandparents' First 100 Days After Diagnosis

FOLLOWING IS MY SUGGESTION FOR A "FIRST-100-DAYS-AFTER-DIAGNOSIS LIST FOR GRANDPARENTS." The 6 items are listed in priority order – and, if schedule allows, in the order they might be accomplished. And it is reasonable to expect that all can be accomplished in 100 days.

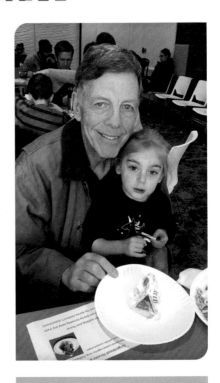

1: Resolve your issues regarding denial and blame. Denying an accurate diagnosis will be counterproductive for your grandchild because denial will result in delayed therapies and supports. Accepting an autism diagnosis that may later prove to be wrong won't do any harm at all. Even if therapies begin, they will be equally helpful to a child who is later found not to be autistic. And it's useless to assign blame for autism, because nobody yet knows what causes autism.

2: Have a talk with your grandchild's parents to discuss: how much time and energy you can provide; how much you can participate regarding money; and how much you're willing to be proactive in finding and taking your grandchild to participate in activities with others (faith organizations, sports teams, support groups, etc.).

3: Offer ways that you are willing to provide immediate support – such as providing money, providing caregiving, and doing online research (finding therapy providers, information to help with challenges such as meltdowns, investigating schools, etc.).

4: Join your local nonprofit autism support organization and get involved by volunteering for something. You'll meet good folks and learn good things.

GRANDPARENT CONFIDENTIAL

"I'm an early-70s single grandmother raising my 11-year-old granddaughter whose mother died. She's not toilet trained and has some challenging behaviors. I've moved to another city and have no family or friends here. I need others to talk to."

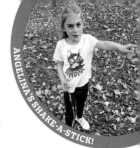

5: Join the following autism grandparents support group on Facebook: Grandparents of Children on the Autism Spectrum. It's well run, informative, and has frequent Zoom meetings that are helpful and supportive.

6: Order and read Nancy Mucklow's book, *Grandparent's Guide to Autism Spectrum Disorders*, and the short booklet, *Start Here – a guide for parents of autistic kids* (a 2021 publication of The Autistic Press).

The involvements of grandparents can provide significant benefits for our grandchildren – and the sooner the better!

The Club for Autism Grandparents

WHEN ANGELINA'S DIAGNOSIS WAS CONFIRMED, I immediately looked, without success, for support groups for grandparents. (Carol Vincent's grandparents Facebook group was yet to be formed, and our local Autism Society of Central Virginia had not yet formed its grandparent support group.) So I engaged an experienced autism professional, Dr. Kathy Matthews, to partner with me in establishing the online Autism Grandparents Club (www.autismgrandparentsclub.com) – a free organization with no fees and nothing to buy. The club offered consultation, chatting, and a blog that consisted of helpful essays, usually two or three each month. After a couple of years, Carol Vincent began administering the Club.

Following is one of the first blogs that I posted on the Club's website – information about Susan Moeller's 3/1/21 article published on AARP's website, "How to Grandparent a Child With Special Needs."

The article provides wonderful basic guidelines for us autism grandparents. The article's subtitle is, "Educate yourself, provide support, know your limits and find joy." And its first sentence begins, "When Jim Oricchio's grandson was diagnosed with autism at age 3 . . ."

It's a brief but poignant article and it's worthwhile for any of us, whether we're new grandparents or have been at it for a while. The article concludes with six suggestions:

Learn about your grandchild's diagnosis.

Use education as a defense against public comments about

> **GRANDPARENT CONFIDENTIAL**
>
> *"I can't find any information helpful to grandparents. My granddaughter is 4 and nonverbal. I want to be supportive to her and her family."*

your grandchild's bad behavior. That is, rather than getting angry, tell the person about your grandchild's challenges.

Know your grandchild's rights and advocate for them. Every state has various regulations and we can be advocates, for example, for our grandchild having an aide in school.

Understand your limits. It's wonderful for us to provide time and energy and money, but we need to be careful not to significantly jeopardize our own future.

Find support for yourself. The article says the best support is connecting with other grandparents who have grandchildren with similar challenges.

Discover joy. All of us autism grandparents know the wonderful joy in seeing progress, in receiving a smile.

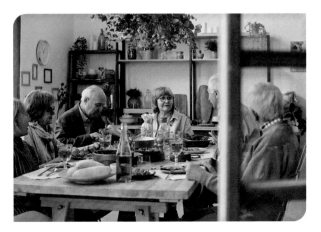

Importance of Grandparents

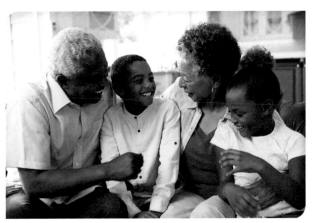

WE AUTISM GRANDPARENTS SOMETIMES FEEL like nobody else has the same challenges and family dynamics as us – that our situations are unique and nobody else can really understand. Of course our feelings are technically accurate in that each grandchild with autism is unique – and thus our own situation is unique. But there is knowledge and research about autism grandparents that can be helpful to all of us as we try to understand and make the best of our personal situations.

Dr. Jennifer Hillman has published several scholarly research articles about autism grandparents – all of which amplify the importance of autism grandparents. Following are 20 takeaways from her June 2007 article entitled, "Grandparents of Children With Autism: A Review with Recommendations for Education, Practice, and Policy."

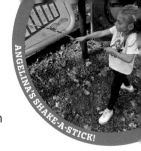

Even though the article was published nearly 20 years ago, it continues to be poignant and valuable. The article, which can be found via Google, sites dozens of research sources from which Dr. Hillman derives her information.

"One in 166 grandparents will become grandparent to a child with autism." (That number is much greater today.)

"Grandparents engage in a variety of activities that provide both emotional and instrumental, or practical, support to parents of children with autism. Emotionally supportive activities include listening and providing empathy and friendship."

"Maternal grandmothers receive highest ratings and reports of satisfaction [regarding their support] from both mothers and fathers."

"Close mother-daughter relationships have been associated with reduced parental stress."

"Specific areas of conflict [between parents and grandparents] may include disagreement over treatment or discipline for a child's behavioral problems."

"A lack of knowledge about a child's diagnosis and symptoms appears related to a state of role confusion among grandparents of children with autism."

"Research suggests that grandparents who maintain limited involvement with disabled grandchildren do so in response to poor relationships and previous conflict with their adult children, rather than their grandchild's disability per se."

"Although custodial grandparents in general appear to be a diverse group, they also share a common need for social support. Obtaining support through social service agencies and support groups can serve as a buffer for grandparental caregivers who must cope with a disabled child's health care or behavioral problems."

> ## GRANDPARENT CONFIDENTIAL
>
> *"My 29-year-old grandson lives with me. He has never received any therapies or supports, and I suspect he would be categorized as high functioning."*

"Because various studies suggest that nearly half of adolescents and young adults with autism suffer from anxiety and depression, positive interactions with grandparents can provide essential support."

"Educational needs [for autism grandparents] include the design of curriculums and programs that will help grandparents explore and define their role as grandparents of a child with autism."

"Limited knowledge about a child's disability can hamper grandparental involvement. . . . Open, guided communication between parents and grandparents to mutually define grandparental re-

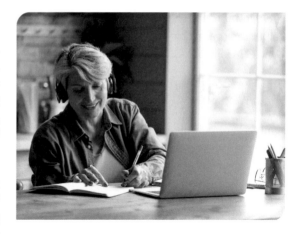

sponsibilities and roles is desirable."

"Life planning is another essential area . . . particularly for custodial grandparents . . . Talking openly between parents and grandparents about custodial arrangements in the event of a caregiver's untimely death can also be a challenging but critically important aspect of life planning."

" . . . few social workers engage grandparents in their work with autistic children, and nearly half expressed no interest in learning more about ways to incorporate grandparents into diagnosis or treatment. This apparent stigma or reluctance among professionals to learn about autism as it relates to grandparents must be challenged and rectified in order for all family members, including grandparents, to receive appropriate and effective help."

One thing we grandparents can continually do that will be helpful for our grandchildren and their families is to learn more and more about autism and about autism's relationship to grandparents. Dr. Jennifer Hillman has written several articles about this, and they can be helpful to us.

Angelina's Story: Hair and Fingernails

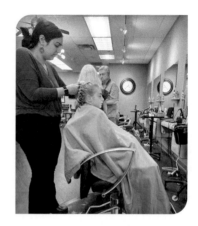

TODAY JUSTEN TOOK ANGELINA TO A REAL SALON TO GET HER HAIR CUT; she picked out a short-hair style. (Her hair was long.) Her sensory challenges regarding her hair have just about disappeared. She used to dislike getting it wet, getting it combed, getting it braided or pony-tailed, etc. All of this has gradually disappeared; no professional therapy was involved.

It's of course common for autistic children to have major sensibilities regarding their hair. Before I knew better I thought that one of Angelina's ABA therapy

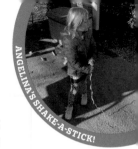

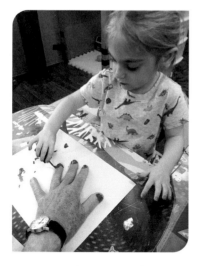

classmates had parents that didn't really care about her appearance; she would arrive at therapy each morning with her hair extremely messy and in tangles. Later, as I learned more about autism, I realized that the little girl was mega-sensitive about her hair.

Fingernail sensitivity is another common trait among autistic children. A couple of weeks ago Angelina's other grandmother took her to a nail salon for a manicure. Angelina loved it and proudly showed everyone her nails for a few days afterwards until she had picked off all of the polish. Angelina has never had a lot of sensory challenges regarding her nails. Even at a very early age she would let me put polish on her nails, and I'd let her polish mine. She is still resistant to me cutting her nails – fingers and toes. But if I attach the process to some sort of reward she'll let me, but will occasionally wince during the process.

As one would imagine, my fingernails were always blotchy messes whenever Angelina would polish them. Once after a nail-painting session, I was making a drive-through deposit at the bank and as I handed the check to the attendant she smiled and asked me if I have a granddaughter. I said yes and she replied that she liked my fingernails.

Challenges for Autism Grandparents

WHAT ARE YOUR CHALLENGES AS AN AUTISM GRANDPARENT? You of course have many in a wide variety of categories. Have you listed your challenges? Have you prioritized them? Do you know which ones are the most urgent? Which are the most important?

I wonder if my challenges as an autism grandparent are similar to those of other autism grandparents. I've been an autism grandparent for only a few years and it will be interesting to see how my list changes during the coming years.

Here are five of my challenges:

1. **A support group of other autism grandparents.** Right now my list of autism grandparents

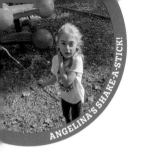

ANGELINA'S SHAKE-A-STICK!

who are my friends and live in my city is short. I hope it grows so I can have even more in-person camaraderie.

2. **Knowledge about autism.** There is a ton of information on the Internet, and my continual challenge is knowing what's good, what's current, and what's best.

3. **How to help Angelina's progress.** Should I select just one thing at a time – like teaching her to tie her shoes – and work on that one every time I'm with her? Or should I be open to a wide variety of things and work on them as opportunities arise?

4. **Relating to Angelina's parents.** JC and I have a great relationship with Kelly and Justen, but this is something we need to proactively work on. I assume that all grandparents believe that they know what's best for their grandchildren, and I assume that all parents resent THEIR parents giving them advice on how to raise their children correctly. We continue try to think of ever better ways for us to continue to have a best-case relationship with Kelly and Justen.

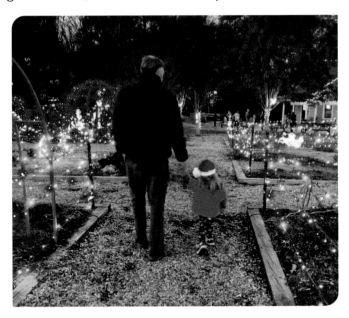

5. **Planning for Angelina's long-term future.** For many folks on the autism spectrum, odds are that they will need financial and other types of support throughout their lives. What's my role in this? And how do I make it happen?

What are YOUR challenges?

Financial Provisions for Our Grandchildren

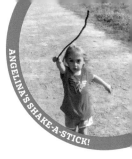

[A friend of mine who is a financial planner wrote the following about how we autism grandparents can provide long-term financial support for our grandchildren.]

IF YOU ARE A GRANDPARENT OF AN AUTISTIC CHILD, you may be wondering how you can help provide for your grandchild financially over the long term. There are many approaches you can take to address this need, each offering you a different level of control of the funds and varying tax implications for you and your beneficiaries. Keep in mind that some decisions may be irreversible, so it's important to seek legal advice, tax advice, and talk to a financial professional, preferably one who holds a Certified Financial Planner (CFP®) designation, to understand the pros and cons before you take action. Below are some broad ideas to get you started.

Assuming your grandchild is a minor, you can establish a joint bank or investment account with them or open a custodial account for their benefit and give up to $15,000 (in 2020) without triggering the gift tax. If you open a custodial account, make sure to set up a successor custodian in case something happens to you. As an alternative, you can give money to your grandchild's parents, but by doing so you will give up control of how the funds are spent. Even if you give money directly to a minor, his or her parent would control the

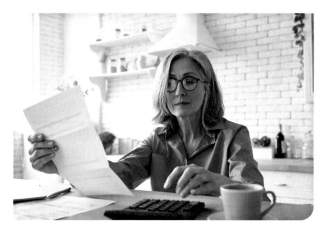

use of the child's money until they reach the age of majority (this varies by state). Since your grandchild has special needs, the parents may control these assets even beyond this age if the recipient is not capable of managing their own affairs and has a conservator.

Another simple way to gift assets to your grandchildren is through your will. This will be subject to estate tax rules, and most people will be able to make this gift tax-free. However there still remains a question regarding who is going to manage the money and how it is spent.

A trust is a different method that can give you control over how and when the money is used, even after you die. There are many types of trusts and a "special needs trust" is a popular route for many people. By using a trust, you can control the money as long as you are able and then assign a person or institution (like a bank or trust company) to manage the funds based on the directions you make when you set up the trust. This is a great way for you to control how your gift is spent over

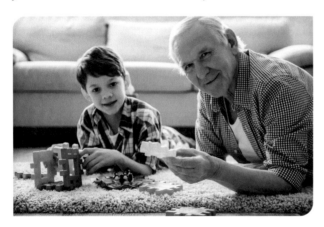

your grandchild's life, long after you are no longer here to oversee it yourself. Trusts can be funded gradually over time or as a lump sum, and the money in the trust can be invested in securities or used to purchase insurance (for example, to provide money when you or their parents die).

In addition to financial assets, you may wish to give your grandchild (directly or via a trust) a home to live in, furniture, and other things to make their life easier. As with financial assets, it will be important to think about how the property will be maintained, and by whom, and how the cost will be managed over your grandchild's lifetime. It's a lot to consider and every situation is as unique as your grandson or granddaughter.

Note from the author: The final sentence is key: ". . . every situation is as unique as your grandson or granddaughter." We autism grandparents want personal financial advisors who are trained to understand and evaluate our unique situations and then suggest appropriate financial planning options.

Permissive Grandparent Disorder

HAVE PERMISSIVE GRANDPARENT DISORDER – PGD. It's a term that I coined to describe something that I suspect is common among grandparents. We have a tendency to spoil our grandchildren, grant every wish, make things easy for them, and of course to never make them do anything they don't want to do. I realize that my PGD isn't helpful for Angelina. (JC loves Angelina just as much as I do, but fortunately she doesn't have PGD.)

Dr. Temple Grandin continually says how valuable it was for her that her mother pushed her to do things for herself – difficult things. Dr. Grandin recommends that this is generally good for persons on the autism spectrum.

I realize that my PGD does not contribute to Angelina's progress. For example, I'll help Angelina put her shoes on even though she can do it by herself. For example, I'll buckle Angelina into her car seat even though

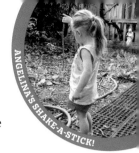

Kelly tells me that Angelina can do it by herself. For example, when I'm keeping Angelina I'll be attentive to her every second even though Kelly tells me that Angelina can spend a lot of time (an hour or more) playing by herself. There is a long list of similar even-thoughs.

I have now sought advice from a variety of sources, and the following is my new list of things I'm trying to put into practice.

1: I recognize that I have PGD and I commit to curing it.

2: I will "push" Angelina on things that are in her short- and long-term best interest.

3: I realize that successfully doing something difficult will give Angelina a feeling of accomplishment and confidence.

4: I will sometimes offer Angelina a time limit for doing a chore: "Let's pick up toys for five minutes and then you can stop."

5: I will sometimes use a play-based approach when encouraging Angelina to do something difficult: "Let's sing the happy song about the toys going to their homes."

> ### GRANDPARENT CONFIDENTIAL
>
> *"I need to brag about my 7-year-old grandson who has taught himself how to swim and even do the butterfly and flip turns. Life is so hard for him and his parents, and water is his happy place."*

6: I will recognize that even though it's easier and quicker for me to do things that are hard for Angelina, I'll try to remember that it's better to get Angelina to try to do those things for herself.

7: I will understand that Angelina is best motivated to do something difficult when she has lots of energy and has no stress or tension. And that the opposite is also true.

8: I will break difficult tasks into small steps that are attainable.

9: I will sometimes use things that Angelina enjoys as rewards for doing/trying difficult things.

10: I will shower Angelina with smiling praise when she accomplishes something difficult.

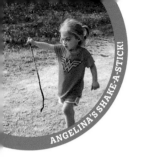

Support from Long-Distance Autism Grandparents

AS I'VE COME TO KNOW GRANDPARENTS WHO LIVE LONG DISTANCES from their autistic grandchildren, I've learned about ten ways that they provide their support.

1: Long-distance autism grandparents can be **loving and supportive** of the grandchild's parents. Parents are often confronted with an almost unimaginable group of physical, financial, and emotional challenges, and unconditional loving support from grandparents can be truly helpful. Grandparents can refrain from criticism, bury any unresolved hatchets, and confirm sincere approval of the parents' actions and decisions – and assure the parents that they are on their team.

2: Long-distance grandparents can continually **learn more and more about autism**. A primary source of knowledge is the Internet. Websites of Autism Speaks and the Autism Society of America are great places to start. Autistic children's parents are often so busy with daily challenges that they don't have time for such research. The world of autism contains continually new information about therapies, research, and life experiences – all of which grandparents can share with their grandchildren's parents.

> ## GRANDPARENT CONFIDENTIAL
>
> *"My 7-year-old grandson is nonverbal and has stomach problems. I live 3 hours away and have an up and down relationship with his parents because they don't like some of my suggestions. I need to know how to build a better relationship with them."*

3: Long-distance grandparents can **offer to do research** – but in a non-forceful manner and only when appropriate. For example, if the grandchildren's parents share that the grandchild is having problems with aggressive behavior, the grandparents can say, "If you like, I can do some research about that and let you know what I find." Or the parents might say something like, "All of the local developmental pediatricians have multi-month waiting lists." And grandparents can reply with, "If you want, I can do an Internet search of developmental pediatricians in your area and then start calling them. And I could let you know if I find one that doesn't have a long waiting list."

4: Long-distance grandparents can **become involved with an autism support group**. Just about every community has some sort of appropriate support group. It may be a local affiliate of the Autism Society of America, it may be an arm of the local government, it may be part of a college or university, or it may simply be a volunteer community group. An Internet search can usually

Angelina!

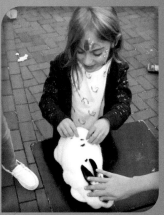

Angelina loves be helpful precisely as we request. For example, after supper recently we asked her to take her plate and put it in the kitchen. She did . . . in the middle of the kitchen floor. (We should have said " . . . on the kitchen counter.") Although the floor plate can't compare to the request from magician Jonathan Austin to pat the rabbit that had appeared from a flaming pan.

find such groups. And if not, a telephone call to the local school system can help locate such groups. Involvement with a support group will help grandparents learn more about autism, experience first-person examples of autism, and provide a support group of persons who can be sources of information and knowledge that can be helpful to their grandchildren.

5: Grandparents can send **snail mail** to their grandchildren. Everyone enjoys receiving personal snail mail, and snail mail can be a real source of joy and even education for grandchildren. Every grandchild is different, but here are three general tips that can result in enjoyment. First, make the envelope visually interesting. If the grandchild likes animals, perhaps glue photos of animals on the envelope. If the grandchild likes Halloween, give the envelope a Halloween theme. Or the envelope can feature a rainbow, etc. etc. Second, make the letter a one-pager (or even only one or two sentences) that includes at least one picture. And third, make the letter interactive – that is, the letter should provide an opportunity for a response. "Can you name this farm animal? What sound does it make?" Or, "Today's emotion is happiness. Do you know how to smile?" Or, "I am told that you can name all of the presidents. Can you name the three that are pictured here?" Grandparents may want to put their letters on notebook paper that can fit in a 3-ring binder, and that way the grandchild can collect them in a binder that he can continually enjoy.

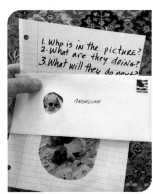

6: Grandparents can do **FaceTime** or Zoom or Skype or other types of electronic visual communication. Following is an excerpt from a blog written by Dr. Kathy Matthews: "First, let's identify what you are going to talk about as we want to avoid the uncomfortable interview that can happen. Again, keep in mind that random conversations are harder for children with autism. Instead, it is best to have an interaction that is familiar, easy, and with clear expectations. To do that, think of an activity-based call. Does the child like books? Like pictures? Like videos? Think about something the child really likes and center your call around that. It will help the child (and you) to have a targeted goal for the conversation and to work to meet that goal. Also, keep in mind

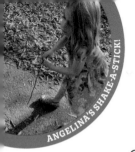

that this call is going to be short. The first few calls should focus on having a successful, meaningful interaction. I say QUALITY over QUANTITY when it comes to thinking about how long the call should be. I can share an example of a grandmother talking to her grandson. In this example, she made a FaceTime call to read a favorite story. She already knew that this story was his favorite and she took time at the beginning of the call to explain her plan to read it. He shared his excitement to hear the book. The call was short and sweet! They connected,

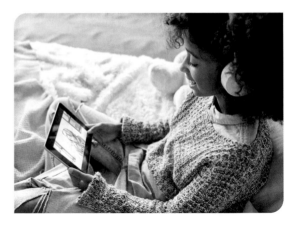

had a good interaction, and both left feeling positive about the experience. Next time she wants to call, she can think about expanding her interaction even more!"

7: Grandparents can, on a regular basis, **send care packages and gifts** to their grandchildren and their parents. This means directly from the grandparents – not from Amazon. Everyone likes receiving a home-wrapped package that contains personally selected contents. The key is to put some thought into it. A personally packaged gift sends a different message from an Amazon-delivered gift that resulted from pressing a few computer keys (although an Amazon gift can also be very positive). Grandparents can ask their grandchildren's parents what sorts of gifts are appropriate. Something as seemingly simple as a Mr. Rogers talking Bobblehead (inexpensive and it says wonderfully peaceful and calming things) might be appropriate. It's the thought that counts, not the amount of money spent.

8: Grandparents can provide **financial support** if they are able. Almost every autism family needs more money – if not for current expenses, then for establishing a fund for lifetime care. This can be a delicate area, and a good way to approach it is to be direct: "Tell us about your financial needs; we want to be as supportive as we can. We live too far away to provide in-person support, but one of the things we can do is help with money." (And of course if grandparents give financial support, there should be no strings attached.)

GRANDPARENT CONFIDENTIAL

"I'm 80 and live in another state from my 11-year-old autistic grandson. How can I learn more about him and autism and how can I form a relationship with him?"

9: Grandparents can **listen and commiserate**. Just about everyone who has challenges needs someone to unload on – to tell details about the challenges, to go on and on and on about the challenges. Grandparents can be wonderful listeners, and when there is a pause, we can say simply, "I understand." Grandparents can be an amazing relief valve for all sorts of mental and

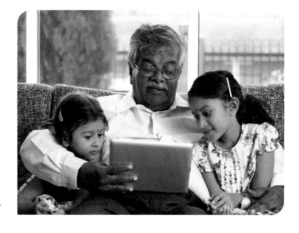

emotional stress that their grandchildren's parents are experiencing.

10: And finally, long-distance grandparents can be **understanding** when their grandchildren's parents forget the grandparent's birthday, when they are not appropriately concerned about the grandparent's life, when they don't thank the grandparent for something, when they forget to do something they said they'd do for the grandparent, and on and on. When grandparents become comfortable with this understandable phenomenon, it will make everyone's life even better.

THE WHOLE POINT – Grandchildren and their parents face a lifetime of challenges. And even grandparents who live too far away for in-person involvement can provide wonderfully meaningful assistance and support!

Zooming with Grandparents

JC AND I ENJOY MEETING OTHER AUTISM GRANDPARENTS, not only in our local community, but also nationally and internationally via FB groups and Zoom meetings. We encourage support groups specifically for grandparents. And we've learned that many autism grandparents who are heavily involved in their grandchildren's lives deal with challenging, complex, disruptive family dynamics. Grandparents are often tasked with trying to be the only stabilizing force in the family. And sometimes grandparents have assumed legal custody of their autistic grandchildren.

(JC and I are fortunate indeed that while our roles are important for Angelina, she has good, loving parents who take seriously their roles in her development.)

Last evening we were among the six grandparents who attended a national autism grandparents zoom meeting. (I was the lone grandfather in attendance. It's been our experience that autism grandmothers are much more involved than grandfathers.) One grandmother of two autistic grandchildren offered that the grandchildren's parents had separated after the mother had become pregnant by another man. Now the grandchildren spend designated weekends with their mother and her new baby and the baby's father – weekends that they dislike. Another grandmother is raising (has custody of) her teenage granddaughter who has all sorts of physical, mental, and emotional problems. Among the grandmother's children was a son who was autistic and deaf and who had recently died. Another grandmother at the meeting told about her 7-year-old autistic grandchild having eloped (unnoticed) from his public school; he ran across the street and wound up inside one of the homes in the neighborhood. He was found safely. And one other grandmother in the meeting is a relied-upon caretaker of one grandchild who is autistic and another who has Down syndrome. The parents of her grandchildren don't see eye-to-eye with her on how to raise the children.

JC and I have learned that while it takes a village, it's even better when the village includes grandparents who are able and willing to be involved.

Our favorite grandparents Facebook group is Carol Vincent's "Grandparents of Children on the Autism Spectrum," and she provides frequent Zoom meetings. There is never any planned agenda, we just talk about what comes up. Almost all of the Zoom participants have active caretaking roles. At a recent meeting one grandparent asked the rest of us how we handle meltdowns. She has tried talking in a soothing voice to her grandson, but it doesn't work.

GRANDPARENT CONFIDENTIAL

"My 6-year-old nonverbal grandson has random angry meltdowns. I don't know what causes them. He eventually calms down and wants to be hugged. I'm confused."

Another grandparent, who has custody of and has raised her 13-year-old granddaughter, said that therapists had helped by trying a variety of calming methods until they finally discovered one that usually works: running circles around a tree. And if the weather doesn't permit, around the kitchen table. This very physical activity relieves her anxiety. When she finally calms down, she stops running and says she's okay now.

In Rachel Pretlow's Autism 101 presentation she advises that unless a meltdown includes harmful activity, it's best not to intervene, but to simply stay away and let the meltdown run its course. Rachel also advises that decreasing all sensory stimulus can be helpful: turn out lights, turn off the radio/television, etc. She also advises that it often exacerbates the meltdown to touch or hug or speak, even in a calming voice. Better to just stay away.

That's one autistic trait that Angelina doesn't exhibit: meltdowns. She's almost always happy. Just about the only time she cries is if she falls down and skins her knee or has some other type of visible injury. And she rarely exhibits sadness – and when she does, it's usually for only a short while. Like when her puppy died. The memory of her puppy stayed, but the sadness went away quickly. (She got a new puppy a few weeks later.)

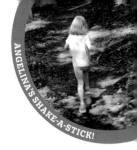

What to Ask Other Autism Grandparents

T'S WONDERFUL FOR US AUTISM GRAND-PARENTS TO BE ABLE TO TALK with other autism grandparents: to share stories, to compare situations, to ask for advice regarding our challenges, and to simply commiserate.

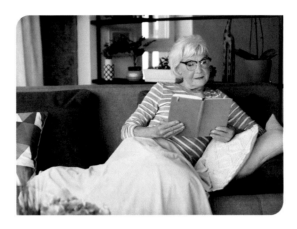

Sometimes it's hard to know where to start when we meet a new grandparent. "Tell me about your grandchild," seems like a good way to begin. But sooner or later – usually sooner – we tend to make the conversation about our own grandchild and we ask for ideas on how to deal with our grandchild's challenges.

All autistic persons are different, and thus other grandparents don't have grandchildren that are exactly like ours and thus any tips or advice they provide concerning our grandchild may or may not be appropriate. And while it can be emotionally beneficial to us to be able to tell another grandparent all about our own grandchild and his challenges, we of course don't learn anything simply by talking about our own situations.

Following are six questions that we can ask other autism grandparents – questions that may yield answers that can be beneficial to our personal situations.

1: **What are some of the things you do to foster and maintain a good relationship with your grandchild's parents?** *(This is a primary concern for all grandparents, and we can often benefit from knowing what works for others.)*

2: **In addition to in-person interactions with your grandchild, do you do any other types of communication that are helpful? Telephone, Skype, snail-mail?** *(If you're like me, you often feel lost on how to best to communicate with your grandchild other than in person.)*

3: **What is one of your grandchild's biggest challenges, and have you found ways to be helpful?** *(Each of us autism grandparents recognizes "biggest challenges" in our*

GRANDPARENT CONFIDENTIAL

"I have 4-year-old autistic twin grandchildren, and I live in another state. Their parents have more than they can handle; they both work. I'm going to start visiting for a few days each month to help with household things as well as babysitting. I need to learn a lot more about autism."

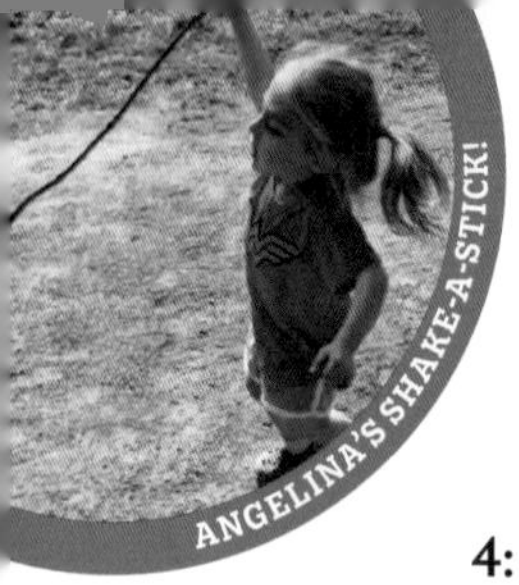

grandchildren; we can learn from how other grand-parents confront big challenges.)

4: **What are some of the helpful ways that you engage your grandchild's siblings?** *(If our autistic grandchild has siblings, there is always the challenge regarding how to treat them differently but appropriately.)*

5: **Do you have any tips on how to best relate to your grandchild's other grandparents?** *(This can be a sticky wicket, because grandparents have different views on things and different relationships with the grandchild's parents. But of course good grandparent-to-grandparent relationships can be wonderfully helpful.)*

6: **What are some of your methods for staying calm?** *(Even though we grandparents have more free time, get more sleep, see things in a broader perspective, etc., we are nevertheless subject to stress regarding our autistic grandchildren. All of us in the autism community can use as many calmness tips as we can get.)*

Those of us who are autism grandparents often get relatively few opportunities to talk with other autism grandparents. But when we do, we can learn a lot. A great place to interact with other grandparents is the Facebook group, Grandparents of Children on the Autism Spectrum.

> ## GRANDPARENT CONFIDENTIAL
>
> *"My 11-year-old granddaughter has only now been diagnosed. She has a lot of issues. I need to know how to handle her meltdowns."*

Angelina's Story: Time

"Are we there now?"

"Not yet."

"When will we be there?"

"In 20 minutes."

"When is 20 minutes?"

"In 20 minutes."

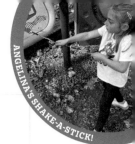

"When IS 20 minutes?"

"I'll let you know."

"But when IS 20 minutes?"

"It's hard to explain."

Angelina is now 8, and that was a portion of the conversation in the car as JC and I were taking her to an outdoor activities event presented by the Autism Society of Central Virginia. She was essentially asking, unlike a "normal" 8-year-old, about the very essence of "time."

So JC tried to explain: "What's that show that you watch on television where those tiny dolls talk and people's hands move them around as they talk?"

"LOL dolls!"

"Well, 20 minutes is how long one of those shows lasts, and that's how long it will be before we get there."

"Are we there now?"

Angelina wasn't trying to be annoying; she genuinely wanted to know. Just one of the indications that her brain isn't neurotypical. (Autism families learn that it's kinder to say "neurotypical" than "normal.")

Angelina doesn't exhibit or have any of the most severe manifestations of autism: persistent hand-flapping, aggression, uncontrollable meltdowns, lack of verbal communication, incontinence, lack of motor skills, and on and on and on. And our friends (who aren't themselves in autism families) sometimes say things like, "Are you sure she's on the autism spectrum?" and "I think you should have her re-diagnosed." And "She seems totally normal to me." We autism families appreciate such well-meaning questions, but at the same time we resent them. Do these folks think we haven't invested our energies into research and professional consultations? Do they think we haven't subjected Angelina to endless therapy sessions: physical therapy, speech therapy, etc.? Do they think we haven't had numerous conferences with Angelina's teachers and specialists and

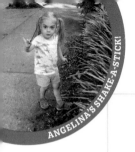
ANGELINA'S SHAKE-A-STICK!

developmental pediatricians?

All of us who are deeply involved with autism can spot an autistic creative brain. All you have to do is watch Angelina eat a banana: sideways and from the middle. Or use crayons to draw things on colored paper: pink crayons on pink paper, white crayons on white paper . . .

It's not surprising that autistic persons can often solve complicated puzzles that stump neurotypical persons: autistic persons try things that neurotypical brains don't/can't think of. I've seen Angelina stack blocks in seemingly impossible, never-before-imagined ways.

Another sign is toe-walking, walking on tiptoes. Not everyone who toe-walks is on the spectrum (Muhammad Ali toe-walked when he was a child), but it's often a sign of autism. Angelina does it. Sometimes this results in need for surgery for damaged tendons and muscles, but Angelina's doctors say that she's in good shape and they don't predict problems.

Angelina persisted in continually asking "Are we there now?" and "When will we be there?" and "When is 20 minutes?" JC and I were polite in our responses, although the repeated questions, without pause, soon began to irritate us. Later we asked Kelly what she does when this happens in her car and she had an answer that we'll try next time. Kelly says two things: "I'll let you know when we get close," and "Don't ask me again."

Books Written Specifically for Autism Grandparents

MY AGGRESSIVE SEARCH HAS FOUND ONLY SEVEN BOOKS written specifically for autism grandparents. I've now read all seven, and following are my brief comments. The seventh book is the best.

Autism & the Grandparent Connection, Practical Ways to Understand and Help Your Grandchild with Autism Spectrum Disorder, by Jennifer Krumins, Autism Aspirations, 2010, 235 pages

The author is knowledgeable, credentialed, and has first-person empathy, but the book reads like a long-day back-and-forth-between-topics discourse. Dip into the book anywhere and you'll find

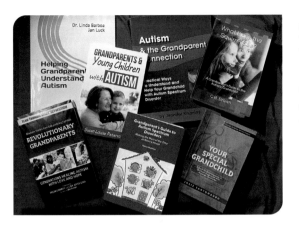

good stuff, but you may also find information on the same topic 50 pages distant. The book has helpful charts and lists and personal stories and guidance, etc., but – and this is a nice way to say it – everything is abundantly flavored with the author's heartfelt thoughts and feelings. The book is 8 ½ x 11 inches – the same size as standard paper. It looks like a manuscript fresh off the printer without benefit of a book designer, and thus is more cumbersome to read than if it were designed in a read-friendly manner. Also there are proofreading errors throughout.

Helping Grandparents Understand Autism, by Dr. Linda Barboa and Jan Luck, KIP Educational Materials, 2020, 23 pages

This slim book (with lots of white space) offers some very good basic tidbits about autism, all of which can be helpful for anyone who is just beginning to learn – but very little of which seems to be written specifically for grandparents. A full five pages are filled with a list of autism terms and acronyms and their meanings: "Auditory: The sense of hearing." "Calming Skills: Persons with autism may need to be taught skills to calm themselves," and so on.

Revolutionary Grandparents, Generations Healing Autism With Love and Hope, collected by Helen Conroy and Lisa Joyce Goes, Skyhorse Publishing, 2016, 166 pages

The book's Foreword states that vaccinations cause autism. The Introduction states that autism is a "disease" that can be cured. In the book's first chapter the authors state their mistrust of the medical/science community. The book features "Nineteen Stories from Extraordinary Families." The book is sincere and heartfelt but its challenge is in its dismissal of scientific research.

Your Special Grandchild, by Josie Santomauro, Jessica Kingsley Publishers, 2009, 48 pages

This little book is a poorly written hodgepodge of information, but it has its moments. For example, there is a good list of mannerisms that are common among autistic persons, some good information about the grief process that often follows an autism diagnosis, good comments from autistic persons, and a variety of good tips regarding autism.

Grandparents & Young Children with Autism, by Susan Louise Peterson, self-published, 2016, 35 pages

The value of this book is questionable. It briefly – very briefly – touches on some random aspects regarding autism, and does so with random organization. For example, the "section" on tantrums reads as follows (in total): "Tantrums: A tantrum can be a characteristic of autism as a grandchild resists a change of routine, but it can also be seen in a sick child. A grandchild who wants to go home may tantrum because he or she wants to rest or go to bed."

What Does the Squirrel See? A Grandparent's Guide to the Autistic Grandchild, by C.B. Brown, United Resource Books, 2018, 108 pages

My favorite thing about this book is the projects and activities that you can do with autistic children. They are sprinkled throughout and then there is a whole section at the end. The book contains lots of wonderful information – much of it directed specifically to grandparents – but it is not organized in a way that makes sense to me, and much of it, while appropriate for one autistic child, doesn't adequately address the wide variety of autism. For example, the "Making New Friends" section begins with this: "When you go someplace with people he doesn't know well, patiently reassure him. As you smile and say hello to a new friend or relative, encourage him to wave to the person." The book also presents some checklists and lists of bullet points that, when taken as a whole are a bit much, but when carefully considered item by item can be instructive. Again, the very valuable part of this book is the projects and activities that it presents.

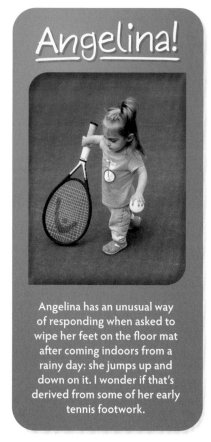

Angelina has an unusual way of responding when asked to wipe her feet on the floor mat after coming indoors from a rainy day: she jumps up and down on it. I wonder if that's derived from some of her early tennis footwork.

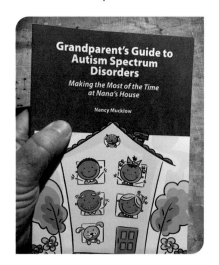

Grandparent's Guide to Autism Spectrum Disorders, Making the Most of the Time at Nana's House, by Nancy Mucklow, AAPC Publishing, 2012, 128 pages (This book is now out of print, but you can still find copies on Amazon and elsewhere, albeit at prices much higher than at the time of publication.)

This is the perfect book for autism grandparents. The author knows her stuff and she's walked the walk. It can be helpful for all varieties of autism – which means that there are portions of the book that will be especially relevant and helpful to each specific autism grandparent. My advice is to read the book with a yellow highlighter handy to highlight the portions that apply to your situation. Following is a review that I published earlier:

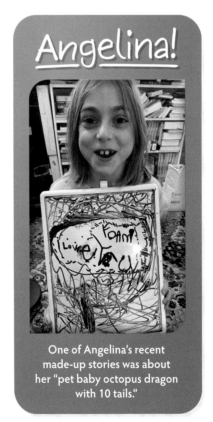

ANGELINA'S SHAKE-A-STICK!

GRANDPARENT CONFIDENTIAL

"Our grandson eats chicken nuggets and French fries. He makes noises but doesn't speak. He can take my hand and show me what he wants, but progress is very slow."

I've read a bunch of books on autism, and a clear favorite has now emerged: the 128-page *Grandparent's Guide to Autism Spectrum Disorders* by Nancy Mucklow. My thought is that everyone – autism families, autism friends, autism professionals, the general public – can benefit greatly from this easy-to-read, easy-to-apply-to-your-own-life guide.

I love the book's upbeat, encouraging, hope-filled tone – a tone that permeates even the book's attention to the most challenging and disheartening aspects of autism. And I love the book's theme of practicality – the constant message that problems and challenges can't always be solved right now: "Sometimes the right thing to do is to just let it go," and "Some issues can wait for another day."

Susan J. Moreno, CEO and founder, OASIS@MAAP says this: "This is a must-read for grandparents, their children, and all teachers, counselors and support staff who work with individuals on the autism spectrum. All levels of functioning and a cornucopia of circumstances are addressed."

A challenge for any book on autism is how to organize it. Nancy Mucklow has organized this book in a wonderfully engaging and readable manner. There are nine chapters, but the book's organizational brilliance is in its four categories of materials that are sprinkled throughout.

One category is short autism stories that illustrate certain topics. For example, the book's first page tells how three-year-old Leisa's grandparents reacted to Leisa's diagnosis and began their interaction with her.

Another category is called "Quick Tips," such as "Quick Tips for Dealing with a Meltdown." I've found every Quick Tip in the book not only helpful, but also revealing of the author's deep understanding and personal experience. (She's an autism grandparent herself.)

A third category isn't named, but I'll call it "Boxed Information." Sprinkled in appropriate places throughout the book are boxes containing special information with titles such as, "How to Respond to Friends who say 'What's Wrong with Him?'" or "What If You Don't Agree With What the Parents Are Doing." I

Angelina!

One of Angelina's recent made-up stories was about her "pet baby octopus dragon with 10 tails."

love some of the guidance in this specific box, such as, "Remember that the parents are doing this for the first time too, so your support will be much appreciated," and "Your job is to support their decisions and make the child's life as calm and happy as possible."

And the fourth category is one that I simply call "Charts." For example, there is an annotated chart that lists all of the senses (taste, touch, vision, etc.) and lists the various ways that a child with ASD may either seek or avoid each sense. Another example is a chart that's titled, "Common Communication Challenges In Children With ASD," that lists and describes the causes and emanations of those challenges.

I've found a great way to enhance the book's benefit to me. I've highlighted everything that relates to my situation. For example, Angelina doesn't have depression or pessimism, so the part of the book that deals with that isn't highlighted. But the book's box entitled, "The Ten-Minute Tidy-Up," is highlighted.

And finally, the book offers an analogy that can possibly be beneficial for everyone's overall understanding of autism: autism is a cat living in a dog's world. (At least for everyone who is familiar with the ways that dogs and cats see and relate to the world.)

Closing
Thoughts

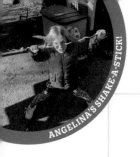

Angelina's Story:
"The Worst Day of My Whole Life!"

WHEN ANGELINA CAME HOME FROM SCHOOL ONE DAY LAST WEEK, she wasn't her normal happy self. She even got into an unwarranted, uncharacteristic argument with Justen – an argument that escalated into Angelina yelling and screaming and telling Justen that he is a bad father.

Angelina was crying uncontrollably, even shivering, when Kelly came downstairs to see what was wrong. Kelly calmly told Angelina to get all of her crying out and then they would discuss things. Angelina finally stopped crying and Kelly asked her what was the matter. No answer. She then asked if something happened at school today. Angelina nodded her head. Angelina eventually told her that several of the other first-graders had confronted her on the playground and told her that since she is 8 years old and still in first grade she must not be smart. They also told her that she's a scaredy-cat. Angelina said that only one kid came to her defense – an African American first-grader who is a friend of Angelina's. He told the other kids to stop, and that Angelina hadn't done anything to them. Angelina, crying again, told Kelly that it was the worst day of her whole life. And Angelina continued by saying that maybe she isn't smart and maybe she is a scaredy-cat.

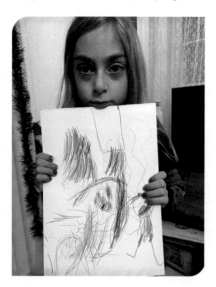

Kelly assured her that she she's smart and not a scaredy-cat. And then Angelina followed with this, "And I'm kind." Which of course made Kelly cry (and me too when I was told about it). And Angelina told Justen that she was sorry for saying he's a bad father.

[More to the story after the following info regarding bullying.]

Autistics, as you would suspect, are frequent targets of bullying – starting as early as kindergarten and first grade and reaching its most devastating impact during teenage years. Bullying usually occurs most often when there is some sort of difference between people – which of course positions autistics as prime targets.

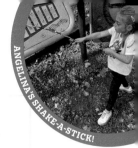

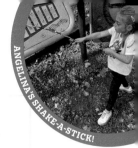

ANGELINA'S SHAKE-A-STICK!

Often autistic children are unwilling or unable to report bullying, even to their parents. Thus it is important to recognize signs of bullying, signs that can include the following: bruises or physical injuries, anxiety, depression, anger, sullenness, faking sickness, increased aggression, increased elopement, increased self-injury, change in eating habits, difficulty sleeping, loss of interest in school, frequent visits to the school nurse or office to avoid classes, avoidance of formerly-enjoyed social situations, etc.

Just as Kelly did with Angelina's sullenness and anger, parents should be proactive in trying to determine the cause of the unusual behavior. And parents should also regularly do the following:

Talk with your child about bullying, why it's wrong, and why kids do it.

Describe examples of bullying and tell social stories about the examples.

Role-play bullying situations. Tell your child how, and to whom, to report bullying. If your child is being bullied, arrange for your child to be near school personnel during lunch and recess. And enlist a "buddy" to accompany your child during lunch, recess, and transitions. (Angelina now has two buddies who say they'll stick up for her!) And of course always – whether bullying is taking place or not – look for continual ways for your child to build self-confidence and friendships.

Kelly immediately sent a descriptive e-mail to Angelina's teacher, including the name of the girl who was the lead bully, and including that Angelina said that this was the second time the girl had done it. The teacher responded immediately, saying that she would talk with the girl's parents as well as with the school administration. The following day Angelina came home from school happier. Her teacher had talked with Angelina and with the bully, and the bully had apologized to Angelina.

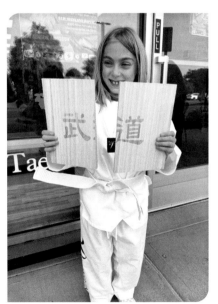

And that evening Angelina went to her Tai Quan Dao class where she happily and enthusiastically regained some confidence by breaking the board and earning her White Belt while the rest of the class applauded.

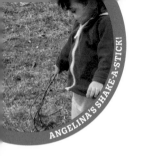

Thomas – The Author's, Late-Breaking, Embarrassing Realization

A COUPLE OF DAYS AGO WHEN I WAS JUST ABOUT FINISHED WITH THIS BOOK, my 39-year-old son Thomas came into my office while I was unsuccessfully trying to repair a palm-size electronic gizmo. I of course handed it to him and he of course had it working in about a minute. He showed me the two switches that he adjusted.

He's always been like that, able to quickly diagnose and repair things: automobile stuff, electronic stuff, even our refrigerator's ice machine after two different authorized technicians had said it couldn't be repaired.

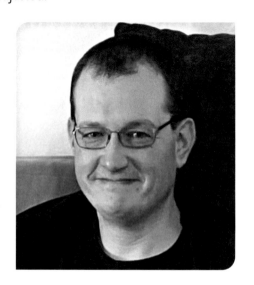

While talking with Thomas I saw a copy of John Elder Robison's book, *Look Me in the Eye*, on my desk and I pointed to it and told Thomas that he reminds me of Robison – able to diagnose and repair things. I told him about Robison having been the person who enhanced all the amplifiers for KISS and who had also rigged their guitars to emit smoke and shoot rockets and flames. And I said, "Of course Robison is on the autism spectrum and you're not." To which Thomas replied, "Uhhh . . ." which I interpreted as "Don't be so sure."

I told him that he has a few traits that are common with autism, such as being highly sensitive to noise and being awkward in certain social situations. He followed with saying that he avoids eye contact except with close family and friends. (I guess I'd never noticed; I'd always just figured that he didn't WANT to look at most persons.)

One thing led to another and I asked him if he would be willing to take an online self-test for autism. He nodded and sat down. Google took us to a UK company, Clinical Partners, that offers a free 30-question online evaluation. Thomas' result stated: **"There is a strong probability that you are autistic."** (Later JC and I also took the test – almost zero chance that either of us is autistic.)

Thomas responded to the evaluation with a matter-of-fact shoulder shrug; he's brilliant and has probably known for a long time. The website stated that the test result isn't a formal evaluation, and that only an evaluation by qualified professionals can produce an accurate diagnosis. Thomas, with a brief smile, said he didn't need a diagnosis.

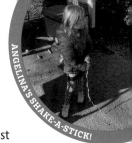

Here I am, an educated guy who has been all in regarding autism research and involvement since Angelina was diagnosed over 6 years ago, and who is engaged with a few prominent autism persons and organizations, and I haven't, until now, realized that my son is almost certainly autistic.

Now I understand the fundamental reason for Thomas' many childhood challenges. Now I feel huge guilt for blaming him for things that weren't his "fault." Now I know why he covered his ears at the circus, why he has always been able to notice and memorize every small detail in every room he enters, why his sessions with the psychologist weren't productive, and maybe even why, during the first several weeks after his birth, he cried and cried and cried in the crib at bedtime and well into the night. Now I know why, even though he made perfect scores on all the national standardized tests, he didn't finish high school. Now I know why for lots of things . . .

While writing this book I've communicated with a few autistic persons who didn't know they were autistic until they were adults. All of them told me that learning that they are autistic has greatly alleviated their feelings of failure, inadequacy, and low self-esteem. It has lessened their guilt about their difficulty at making and keeping friends, inability to keep a job, unknowingly saying rude or hurtful things, and on and on.

JC and I wonder how many parents these days are just now realizing that their adult children are (and of course have always been) autistic. I wonder how many parents, like us, took their children to psychologists and psychiatrists without ever hearing the word, "autism."

Now JC and I can understand many of the challenges that Thomas has experienced from childhood through adulthood. And we also have a greater appreciation for some of his amazingly wonderful characteristics – such as with Tony and Angelina. (Tony was JC's Down syndrome brother.)

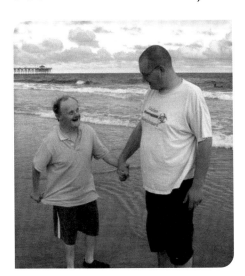

It's common for autistic persons to relate better to other autistics than to neurotypicals. Throughout most of his life, Tony would travel from his home in Nashville to spend a few weeks each summer with our family here in Richmond. Thomas always loved Tony's company, and even though all of us greatly enjoyed Tony and related well to him, Thomas was the best.

Angelina lived with us the first four years of her life and now continues to be with us often. Thomas, from the beginning, has always loved being with her: playing with her, laughing with her, teasing with her, letting her ride on his back and shoulders, etc. I don't know if anyone in the family could be judged "best" at relating to Angelina, but Thomas would certainly be in the running.

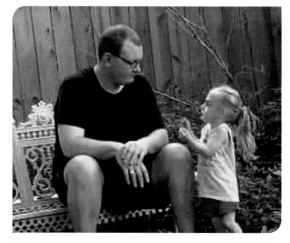

Ditto with cats (JC and I are cat people). We've always had cats. Thomas would definitely win first prize in his love of, and relationships with, our cats. I bring up cats because I have a copy of Kelly Hoopman's book, *All Cats Are on the Autism Spectrum*.

I don't know if the realization that Thomas is on the spectrum will change the way he relates to us, but I do know that it has already changed the way I relate to him. For example, since he is often a person of few words, I've always assumed that he isn't really interested in carrying on an extended conversation with me. So when he engages me about anything, I sort of respond in a perfunctory manner and then get back to whatever I was doing. (But he and JC always have long conversations – which I had assumed were HER doing rather than his.) Now I realize that he probably wants and welcomes long interactions – just like a lot of neurotypicals think that, since autistic persons are often alone, they WANT to be alone. The opposite is usually the case.

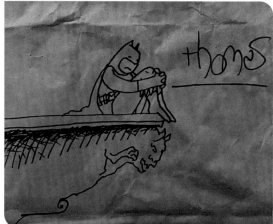

As I write this, my realization that Thomas is autistic is only a couple of days old. Over the coming days and weeks I will no doubt continue to think about it, to hopefully "improve" the way I relate to Thomas, and to be an ever better father and friend.

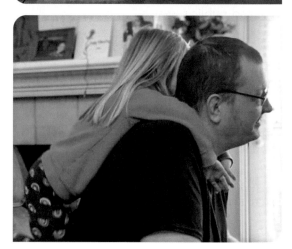

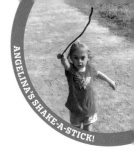

Afterword – Science Leads the Way

By Andy Shih, Chief Science Officer, Autism Speaks

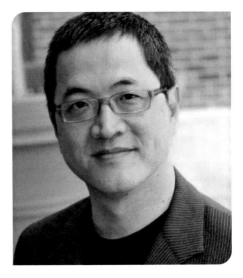

WHEN I JOINED THE AUTISM COMMUNITY OVER TWO DECADES AGO to facilitate and support research, I found a community with more questions than answers: What is autism? What caused it? Is there a treatment? What does the future hold?

Many parents, caregivers and families I met were confused and scared, struggling with stigma and basic childhood routines like going to school or seeing a pediatrician. They desperately wanted to help their children but didn't know how. Researchers were similarly stymied. Most thought of autism as a rare disease, some believed it was caused by environmental toxins, and all worked hard to collect evidence to shed more light on a medical mystery.

That knowledge gap was fertile grounds for ideas and conjectures about autism, some based on rigorous albeit at the time limited research, while others were not at all supported by evidence. Many of these ideas, like the "refrigerator mother" hypothesis, only further traumatized autistic people and their families.

Today, thanks to those parent and self-advocate pioneers, and investments in science made by private and public research funding agencies like Autism Speaks, SFARI and NIH, we have more answers. We know, for instance, that autism is not caused by "bad" parenting. We also know vaccines do not cause autism. We recognize with timely access to evidence-based support and services, autistic people could thrive and reach their full potential like the rest of us. We learned autism is not a disease but a disability.

While we have made much progress as a community, there are still many important questions to be answered. This is especially true as we begin to explore with increasing urgency transition to adulthood, aging and other lifespan issues. It is essential to understand the needs and challenges of autistic adults, especially as they grow older and age. We must make sure that they are not left behind by accelerating progress in science and medicine, and are able to access effective, quality care like the rest of us.

In these days of polarization and misinformation, it is ever more important for the autism community to be extra vigilant and demand most rigorous research to deliver the answers that will change our collective future. Together, we must redouble our efforts to support the best science and insist on the most robust evidence to help enhance the quality of life and wellbeing of autistic people and their families. Our community deserves nothing less.

We need to close the knowledge gap so we can begin to answer the question that I have heard from families since my first days in the community over 20 years ago: What is going to happen to my child when I'm gone?

Today there are divergent views regarding what should be considered socially accepted behavior. Negative subjective pathology language is widely used, and there is a need for an overall shift to positive language. (Example: the D in ASD stands for Disorder: a highly pejorative term.)

Andy Shih, Chief Science Officer for Autism Speaks, joined the organization in 2006, after its merger with the National Alliance for Autism Research where he served as chief science officer. Under Dr. Shih's leadership, Autism Speaks supports ministries, government agencies and leading nongovernmental organizations in more than 70 countries to deliver better outcomes and quality of life for tens of millions of individuals and families. With emphasis on human rights, science-driven advocacy and policymaking, and the development and implementation of innovative tools and programs, the team aims to help address knowledge and health disparities for individuals and families affected by autism and developmental disabilities worldwide, including underserved communities in the U.S. and other high-income countries. Dr. Shih holds a Ph.D. in molecular cell biology from New York University School of Medicine.

ANGELINA'S SHAKE-A-STICK!

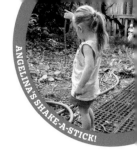

Epilogue

By Ann Flippin, Executive Director, Autism Society of Central Virginia

EVEN WITH A LIFELONG IMMERSION IN AUTISM, this book has unveiled new perspectives for me. It has given a special look into John and his wife JC's wonderful relationship with, and support for, their granddaughter, Angelina, whom I've had the pleasure of getting to know through her participation in many of our Autism Society of Central Virginia programs.

In this Epilogue, I'd like to offer three suggestions for both novices and experts in the field of autism. Firstly, seize every opportunity to deepen your understanding of autism's evolving role in our society. Secondly, spend time with individuals on the autism spectrum, forging relationships with them – their insights and experiences will teach you invaluable lessons and enrich your life. Lastly, emulate the spirit I've observed in Angelina at ASCV's events: embody acceptance, inclusivity, friendliness, and kindness.

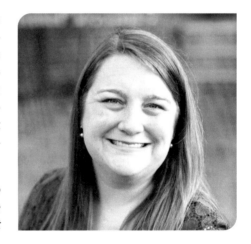

PS – Even if you reside far from Virginia, we welcome you to join the Autism Society of Central Virginia. We have ample online and virtual opportunities for education and support at ascv.org.

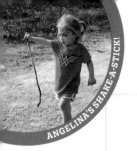

ANGELINA'S SHAKE-A-STICK!

Postscript

By Angelina

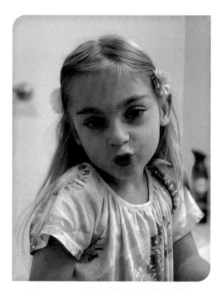

A S I WAS PROOFREADING THIS BOOK, my phone beeped with an incoming text. It was from Angelina. She was at JC's art studio and JC had handed her the phone and asked if she'd like to send a message to Papa John (me). I later learned it was the first text message she'd ever sent. I couldn't resist using it as the Postscript for this book, sans a bunch of emojis. The wording is of course a bit disjointed, but the message is clearly heartfelt.

I love me like you are my favorite person in my heart and soul forever my dear isn't. Papa John I am proud to say you have been my best person and my biggest supporter and friend ever since my heart and I will forever be proud to have been a fan and a fan of you and I will always be proud of that I am a huge part and a part and proud that you're my best friends forever.

Angelina later told us that "you're my best friends forever" refers to both me and JC.

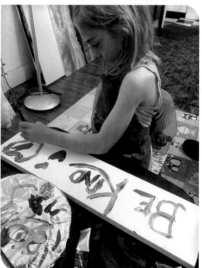

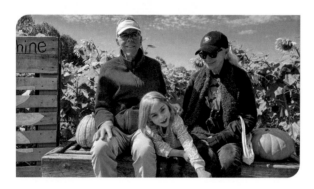

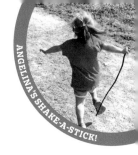

About the Author

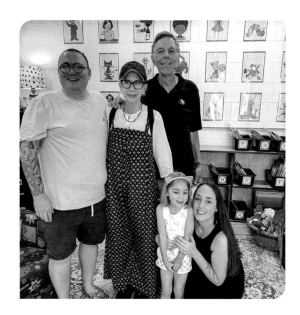

JOHN BRYAN'S WRITINGS HAVE AP-PEARED IN SUCH PUBLICATIONS as *Sports Illustrated, Delta SKY*, and *Parade.com*. His books have addressed topics ranging from art to religion to fly-fishing to Down syndrome, and have had Introductions and Forewords written by notables such as Virginia Senator Tim Kaine, *The New York Times* Executive Editor Howell Raines, The Conference Board CEO Jonathan Spector, and President Jimmy Carter. John and his wife, artist JC Gilmore-Bryan, live in Richmond, Virginia where they enjoy spending time with their 8-year-old granddaughter, Angelina, and her parents, Kelly (nurse) and Justen (respiratory therapist). John can be contacted by e-mail at jbryanfish@aol.com.

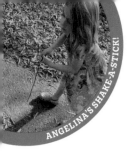

ANGELINA'S SHAKE-A-STICK!

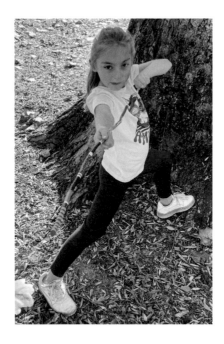

One Last Thing

For information on how to get your own, authentic, Angelina's Shake-A-Stick! (personally shaken by Angelina), and/or an original signed print by James Prosek (see page 217) go to www.AngelinasShakeAStick.com.

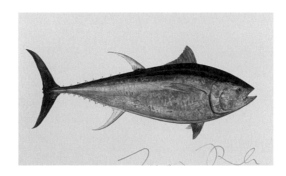

Appendix:

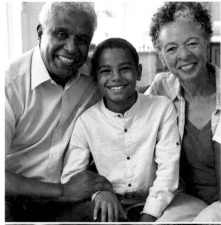

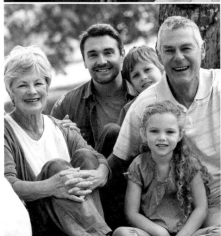

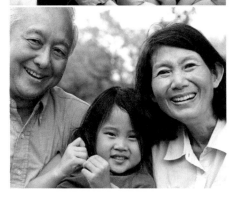

2021

National Autism Grandparents Survey Executive Summary

BY KATHY MATTHEWS AND JOHN BRYAN

Dr. Kathy Matthews, an autism parent, has nearly 30 years of professional experience supporting individuals and families impacted by autism and related developmental disabilities through nonprofit organizations, university teaching, research, and special needs planning. John Bryan, an autism grandparent, is a volunteer layperson who has local and national involvements with autism.

Overview

There are roughly 4 million autism grandparents in the United States. Prior to 2021, the only national study of autism grandparents was a survey conducted in 2009 by the Kennedy Krieger Institute of Johns Hopkins University. Since then there have been significant changes in the autism community, including a 100% increase in the percentage of children who are diagnosed with autism (1 in 88 in 2009, 1 in 44 in 2021).

The Survey's overall findings were consistent with the desires of most grandparents, with or without special needs grandchildren: they care immensely for their grandchildren, want to spend time with them, and want to support them into the future.

It should be noted that simply completing the Survey is an indicator of the participants' willingness to have productive involvements with autism; the Survey's length requires a minimum of 30 minutes, and several open-ended questions provide opportunities for much more time. Plus, nearly half of the participants spent even more time providing "Additional thoughts or comments" at the end of the Survey.

Survey Findings and Recommendations for Autism Professionals

1. Survey results indicate that it will be beneficial for autism professionals to take a more direct approach in involving grandparents.

The Survey finds that even though the majority of autism grandparents are involved in decision-making regarding therapies, education, etc. for their grandchildren, only 30% of grandparents receive information from the professionals who provide those therapies, education, and other services. The majority of grandparents receive their information about autism from the Internet and from their grandchildren's parents. Although 80% autism grandparents say they have at least a moderate amount of knowledge about autism and about their own grandchildren's specific cases of autism, they desire to know even more about how to address their grandchildren's specific needs.

The very nature of autism treatment is intensive. It is customized to meet the needs of the individual with autism, which includes considering what the treatment is, how it is delivered, and the associated treatment schedule. As such, there are often multiple professionals involved, including special educators, behavior analysts, learning aides, speech pathologists, occupational therapists, physical therapists, psychiatrists, case managers, feeding or nutritional experts, counselors and a host of other providers working in support of the child and family. Although grandparents are learning about autism from a variety of sources, the lack of contact with their grandchildren's professional providers could be the reason why they want to learn more about how to be helpful with the specific challenges of their own grandchildren. This is where the professional providers can help.

There appears to be a gap between autism grandparents, who are ready and willing to help, and a clear pathway inviting them and guiding them to a closer connection with the professional service providers.

Autism is a spectrum disorder in which the severity of the condition ranges broadly from impacting communication, causing social interactions to be challenging, and full dependence on others to the complete opposite spectrum where the individual is fairly independent in the areas of social, educational, and daily living skills. As such, a mere diagnosis of autism can shed little light on the specific needs of the person afflicted. Rather, those in the individual's life gain an understanding of the specific needs and then create a system of support and lasting care to meet those needs.

One barrier to including grandparents is the required process for professionals to obtain consent for treatment. The primary caregiver or guardian, typically mom or dad, consents and provides a list of other individuals to whom the professional may speak on their child's behalf. Usually, those persons are pediatricians and therapists. Rarely does the onboarding process actually list grandparents as possibilities for contact and involvement. And once services begin, it can be hard to engage or communicate with anyone outside of the prescribed treatment team.

Furthermore many professionals are prohibited from asking persons who are receiving services to render their opinions or feedback regarding their experiences. Someone receiving services may feel compelled to respond to surveys or requests for information favorably, as any other response might jeopardize service delivery. Therefore, it may be challenging for a therapist to reach out to gauge the family experience, which would include finding out if a grandparent or other family member has concerns or wants more information. A work-around in this situation would be to include grandparents from the very beginning.

It may be helpful for service providers to state that grandparents are welcome at the initial meetings, and also to actually list grandparents on the application/contractual forms as eligible to be "team" members. In initial meetings service providers may want to offer simple questions, such as, "Are grandparents involved in your child's life, and if so, how? Can we include them in planning sessions? How can we help them attend our meetings?" This is a far different approach than simply asking, "Is anyone else involved in caring for your child?"

Also, professionals can make meetings accessible via phone, zoom or in person. One result of Covid is flexibility. Service providers can consider the many avenues now available to getting grandparents involved.

And finally, service providers can include grandparents in regular communications by copying them on emails, mailings, and reports.

The day-to-day goings-on of autism parents can be overwhelming, Caring for a child with autism takes considerable time and effort, particularly when multiple therapies and activities are in place. It can feel impossible for a parent to feel like they can carve out time to strategize and ask for help. Encouraging grandparents to offer their help can be productive in rising above the day-to-day struggles.

Again, professional service providers can discuss all of this with mom and/or dad at the beginning. It would even help to share this survey to moms and/or dads and say, "We are learning that grandparents would really like to know more so that they can better connect with, and be helpful for, their grandchildren with autism. How can I support you to include grandparents in our work together?"

2. Autism service providers can be even more helpful by taking an approach that is family-centered rather than person-centered.

There is evidence of the unique value of a "family-centered approach" (Margetts, Couteur, & Croom, 2006). Most autism service plans are focused on services for one individual, and insurance and other funders assess the benefits and progress of those services. Although a person-centered approach is designed to protect the individual receiving services from getting a "canned" treatment, it does not consider the needs of other members of the family. What if financial problems result in a lack of transportation to therapy treatments? What if the attention requirements of siblings result in a lack of parental monitoring of the child's IEP progress? The goal of a family-centered approach is for all family members to be doing well and able to support the child with autism, thus helping treatments to be effective and lasting. Autism grandparents can fit in nicely as part of a family-centered type of support.

Survey Findings and Recommendations for Autism Grandparents

1. Autism grandparents can ask for a seat at the table.

The Survey shows that the majority of autism grandparents live near their grandchildren and spend in-person time providing caretaking, transportation, etc. for them. And the majority of autism grandparents report that autism has made their grandparent-parent relationships stronger rather than weaker. Parents are drowning in the day-to-day, and they may not realize that they have an opportunity to have grandparents more directly involved in treatment. Grandparents may want to offer simple questions, such as, "I'd love to join you at the next meeting," and even better, to follow with, "Do you have a few minutes to talk about how I can play a more supportive role?"

2. Autism grandparents can help assure the long-term future for their grandchildren.

In the Survey grandparents expressed a concern for the future of their grandchildren. Research shows that grandparents can plan for the long-term on behalf of their children and make sure the support is there (Prendeville & Kinsella, 2019). Special needs planning services can help identify a funding stream to support the child for life, establish legal protections such as special needs trusts and microboards to ensure a safe transfer of funding and overall well-being, and identify the services that may be needed now or in the future.

3. There is opportunity for more autism grandparents to proactively seek involvement with, and support from, nonprofit autism organizations and social media groups.

Only a minor percentage of grandparents are currently having such involvement and support.

Conclusion

Perhaps the most important of the Survey's findings is that a significant majority of autism grandparents care about their grandchildren, have important involvements with them, and want to learn how to be even more helpful and knowledgeable. Research shows that grandparents are a source of unconditional love and advocacy for their grandchildren (Hillman, Wentzel, & Anderson, 2017). It is hoped that this Survey will result in two things: the autism professional community's increased understanding of the roles that grandparents can and do play in enhancing their grandchildren's progress and quality of life, and their eagerness to proactively engage grandparents; AND autism grandparents being even more proactive in engaging direct involvement and communication with their grandchildren's professional service providers.

In summary, the Survey captured the experience of grandparenting a child with autism. Although autism poses unique challenges for many, grandparents have the patience, drive, and love to partner in the planning and support.

Data Summary

DEMOGRAPHICS OF GRANDPARENTS

The majority of Survey participants are healthy, white, married, females over 50 years old – half of whom have completed at least 4 years of college. Most do not work full-time, and half have annual incomes over $75,000.

Ethnicity
85% - White
10% - Black
5% - All Others

Sex
2/3 - Female

Age
1/3 - 65+
1/3 - 50-64
1/3 - Under 50

Health
87% - Good or even better

Education
50% - At least 4 years of college

Marital Status
2/3 - Married (not including widowed)

Work Status
36% - Working full-time
34% - Fully retired
30% - Other

Income
50% - $75,000+

DIRECT, IN-PERSON, INVOLVEMENT WITH GRANDCHILDREN

The majority of participants provide important in-person involvement with their grandchildren at least a few times per month.

Provide Transportation
61% - A few days or more per week

Provide In-Person Care
70% - A few times or more per month (including 50% a few times or more per week)

Distance from your grandchild?
70% - Live less than 25 miles away.

FINANCIAL AND MATERIAL SUPPORT

Most grandparents provide at least some financial involvement (gifts), and half provide/ spend $500 or more annually.

Grandchild lives with you
15%

Provide Cash
40%

Established Long-Term Trust
15%

Used Personal Savings
31%

Spend Money On
41% - Food
52% - Clothing
62% - Gifts
34% - Daily expenses
15% - School

Yearly dollar amount provided/spent
50% - $500 or more
(Including 36% who provide $1,000 or more)

Relocated to be near grandchild (or vice versa)
19% - Relocated
23% - Grandchild's family relocated

ABOUT THEIR GRANDCHILDREN

- ¾ are Male.
- 90% are younger than 18.
- Nearly ¾ are 12 or younger.

- 85% are the only autistic grandchild.
- 60% diagnosed at age 4 or younger.
- 71% first suspected at age 4 or younger.

KNOWLEDGE OF AUTISM

Most autism grandparents have only 1 autistic grandchild, and know at least a moderate amount about autism and about their grandchild's specific case of autism.

Sources of Information *(top 3 responses)*

57% - Internet research

52% - Grandchild's parents

30% - Autism therapy providers and professionals

Topics for desired additional information (top 2 responses from list of 24 topics)

42% - Fun Activities

37% - Treatment for Challenging Behaviors

What Causes or Contributes to Autism? (top 2 responses)

58% - Genetics

23% - Difficulties with pregnancy/birth

(14% said Vaccinations)

Member of Autism Organization(s)?

Majority said no.

Your knowledge of autism?

33% - Lots of under-standing and research

47% - Moderate, want more

20% - Little or none

Your knowledge of your grandchild's specific case of autism?

81% - Moderate or greater (including 34% who say great amount).

33% - First person to suspect autism

How many autistic grandchildren?

85% - 1

Your level of stress and/or sadness?

50% - Feel fine, rare stress or sadness.

40% - Feel fine half of the time.

Your personal support system?

83% - Spouse provides positive support.

85% - Family/relatives provide positive support.

69% - At least half of friends provide positive support.

49% - Community members provide positive support.

56% - Requested/received support for stress/anxiety from medical profession.

37% - Receive support from online support groups.

22% - Receive support from faith community.

12% - Receive support from nonprofit organizations.

How often do you meet with family members?

2/3 meet at least once or twice a week.

How often do you feel that you lack companionship?

2/3 feel this way rarely or never.

Has autism impacted your relationship with your grandchild's parents?

52% - Closer than before autism

38% - No change

10% - Autism has created conflicts.

Relationship with grandchild's other grandparents?

30% - Closer than before autism

59% - No change

11% - Autism has created conflicts.

Disagreements with parents regarding therapies?

84% - No

Disagreements with parents regarding reactions to behaviors?

77% - No

Your involvement with decisions regarding treatment/therapy.

42% - All of the time or a lot.

26% - Some

32% - None

What activities/involvements have had positive effects on your grandchild?

(Top 2 responses from a 7-item list including history activities, library activities, science activities, sports activities, and other.)

60% - Nature activities (outdoor trails, gardening, lakes and streams, etc.)

54% - Arts activities (painting, drawing, music, dance, theatre, etc.)

All others (history, literary, science, sports, other) were 35% or less.

Which, if any, have doubted the autism diagnosis? (Top 3 of 11 choices)

12% - Relatives

11% - My grandchild's parent who is not my child

10% - My spouse or significant other

What is the relationship status of your grandchild's parents?

87% are together.

Open-Ended Questions

(Rather than assuming that participants would know the accurate meanings of a list of terms that they could select from, the Survey used this open-ended question to elicit an "in-your-own-words" description of the grandchild's autism.) The responses were spread evenly throughout the spectrum, from severe to high functioning and including Asperger. One indicator of the grandparents' knowledge of, and interest in, their grandchildren is that a great many of them provided paragraph-long answers. Others provided short answers such as "High Functioning" and "Level Three." A great majority of the paragraph-long answers, even the ones that described challenging symptoms of severe autism, are flavored with love and positivity.

WHAT TYPE OF ACTIVITIES RELATED TO AUTISM WOULD YOU LIKE TO PARTICIPATE IN?

One commonly cited activity that respondents referenced were support groups or meetings, both in-person and online. For example:

"Support groups that have new ideas to help make life for my grandchild easier. [I'd] like to know what I can do to help make things easier for him to deal with."

"Anything that brings together parents of children with autism to talk about their experiences."

Another common activity mentioned was awareness of educational events or classes. Many respondents said that they would like activities to spread awareness about autism to the community and also to learn more about autism themselves. Some examples include:

"Anything to help and support my grandkid and gain a better understanding and knowledge of autism and what to expect[.]"

"Classes teaching strategies for dealing with behaviors[.]"

"Helping others become aware of support that families and people with autism need and finding ways to get this support[.]"

"I would like to be trained in ways to help my grandson. I want to be able to interact with him and help with his education. It's not enough to be asked to help fundraise. Fundraise for what?"

"More advocacy campaigns to make the public aware [of] the issue."

"Raising awareness of how hard it is to have an autistic child and expensive it is. That states have different resources and how little resources there are and that it takes so much work and research to find out what resources you are eligible to receive."

Grandparents also frequently mentioned that they would like to participate in donation-related activities such as walks or marathons. For example:

"Walks to raise awareness and money"

"Raising money that would go directly to find a cause and cure for autism."

"I would do walks for autism fundraisers."

"Fundraising for research and spreading awareness are probably the two most important topics. Removing the stigma surrounding autism and bringing awareness of just how many people that autism personally affects."

AS AN AUTISM GRANDPARENT, WHAT ARE YOUR GREATEST JOYS?

One very common theme within the responses was to just be with their grandchild. For example:

"Having my grandson in my life and being a part of his."

"Just spending time with my grandson[.]"

"Just having my granddaughter in my life brings joy to me. It is usually simple things that I enjoy with her. Sometimes it is just sharing a craft project or swimming in the pool. Often [it] is just her hugs that brings me happiness."

Some responses mentioned getting to see the progress that their grandchild has made in various aspects of their life. Examples include:

"I appreciate being able to see my grandson's growth in social skills and behavior gains."

"I have seen him grow in reading, math and social activities. Shows improvement in judgement."

"Loving my grandchild and hearing about the new things they have learned."

"Personal rapport and relationship with my grandson. Watching his progress. Being a facilitator of his progress when/however possible[.]"

AS AN AUTISM GRANDPARENT, WHAT ARE YOUR GREATEST CHALLENGES?

One commonly mentioned challenge was a lack of knowledge about autism in general or specific aspects of autism such as how to effectively respond to some of their grandchild's behaviors. Some examples include:

"Just not understanding autism completely[.]"

"Knowing what to do when he has a meltdown or starts yelling[.]"

"One of my greatest challenges fully understanding autism and how to be a better grandparent[.]"

"Sometimes not knowing how to react when he does something he should not be doing."

"I think one of the greatest challenges is not fully understanding all the specifics of how autism actually presents itself. I often find myself questioning why all the time, as in what the cause is. I think that level of unknowing disturbs me."

Communication difficulties were also frequently mentioned—grandparents experienced problems communicating with or connecting with their grandchildren.

"Trying to connect to my granddaughter. She's socially awkward and it's difficult for her to communicate"

"Trying to understand and communicate verbally (we're getting there) and dealing with people who don't[.]"

"Communication is difficult and I do not get visit enough to be able to figure out the words or to understand the emotions. It breaks my heart when he cries. Grandkiddos parents are wonderful but I worry about their stress."

Another frequently cited challenge was seeing their grandchild struggle or knowing that their grandchild will struggle in the future. For example:

"I cry to think that my severely autistic grandson will never be able to live independently. I worry about my other grandson "fitting in." I so want him to have friends."

"I ache for my children having to go through this[.]"

"Worry for her future and the stress on her parents[.]"

"[W]orrying about their future and the impact this has on their parents and siblings, also grieving some about the loss of "normal" for them and how much harder things are for them[.]"

Grandparents also mention difficulties with handling disruptive behaviors due to their grandchild's autism, such as:

"Watching him have a meltdown, with high pitched screaming."

"When she has a [meltdown] (sometimes daily although less now) or she can['] t go somewhere because of her anxiety. Changed her meds yet again and she is able to go out [occasionally] again."

"The main challenge is it difficult and embarrassing when she demonstrates unusual behaviors in the house/public and extreme displays of affection or the opposite[.]"

"He runs off. When he's upset he doesn't know how to deal with it. He lashes out. He has meltdowns."

AS AN AUTISM GRANDPARENT, WHAT ARE YOUR GREATEST CONCERNS?

Grandparents commonly mentioned concerns about their grandchild's future in general and continuing or growing difficulties as their grandchild ages, particularly in adulthood. Within this, future independence was a common concern.

"I wonder how far he will go in life and how he will be cared for when he's 18."

"I am fearful for my [granddaughter's] future and how she will make her way in the world when the day comes and she is alone."

"How she'll be able to take care of herself as an adult, jobs, basically any thought of independent living[.]"

"What he will be when he grows up, can he work, live independently."

Grandparents also worried about the treatment of their grandchild from the rest of society—for instance, some grandparents worry that their grandchild will be bullied for their autism or be taken advantage of. Some examples include:

"The future. Bullying from other kids and ignorance of others, having a negative impact on him."

"That my grandchildren will be judged and made fun of for being unique."

"That my grandchild will be a social outcast[.]"

"People taking advantage of his trust and hurting his soul[.]"

"My grandchildren being marginalized by society and not appreciated for sweet, funny, smart, creative children they are."

WHAT ARE YOUR GREATEST JOYS WHEN PROVIDING DIRECT CARE?

One commonly mentioned joy cited by grandparents while providing direct care was interacting or spending time with their grandchild.

"Spending time with grandchild and watching them learn and grow[.]"

"Just being a part of his life. I [love] all of my grandchildren equally[.]"

"I thoroughly enjoy the time that I get to spend with my grandchildren. I also enjoy being able to witness their growth in person[.]"

Similarly, grandparents also mention receiving physical affection or witnessing signs of joy from their grandchild as their greatest joy when providing direct care.

"The smiles, the hugs, the laughter."

"Seeing the smiles on my grandson's face, and hearing his laughter, and seeing that he has progressed."

"My greatest joy is spending time with them and getting their hugs[.]"

"Hearing him laughing and enjoying himself. And knowing that he feels safe and comfortable[.]"

Another joy cited in the responses is getting to help or experience their grandchild growing or learning. For example:

"I love spending time with my grandchildren. I enjoy teaching the new things and watching them learn."

"Watching his excitement when we read together or be successful when we try something new."

"I get to watch my grandchild grow up and flourish[.]"

When asked what their greatest challenges were when providing direct care, many grandparents mentioned having patience or handling frustration as a challenge. Some examples include:

"Patience with them making a mess in the house, [yelling] at me for making direct eye contact[.]"

"Being patient enough to handle any unexpected behaviors."

"One of my greatest challenges is dealing with frustration when dealing with my grandchild. I am not fully qualified to deal with autism and I am still learning and educating myself[.]"

"One of my greatest challenges is dealing with frustration when dealing with my grandchild. I am not fully qualified to deal with autism and I am still learning and educating myself[.]"

Grandparents also mentioned challenges with handling disruptive behavior such as meltdowns or temper tantrums from their grandchild.

"How to redirect his tantrums. How to redirect when he does something that's no right, but continues no matter what it is."

"Getting used to screaming outbursts."

"My greatest challenges are dealing with the emotional meltdowns especially when I'm exhausted and dealing with the youngest at bedtime[.]"

"Navigating the behavioral challenges[.]"

PARTICIPANTS' THOUGHTS ABOUT THE SURVEY

The Survey's "Additional thoughts or comments" section prompted a great many participants to praise the Survey. For example, "I very much appreciate this survey. I have written down the names of several of the organizations you listed to reach out to get more information regarding Autism and how I can be more of a help to my grandchild. THANK YOU – THANK YOU!!" and, "This was one of the most relevant and important surveys I have ever taken. It has inspired me to seek out platforms to be more supportive of my grandson." Only 2 of the 594 participants expressed negative, albeit brief, comments about the Survey: "Too many clicks," and "Too many personal questions – would have rather not answered a lot of questions."

NOTE: *Although this Executive Summary often uses the words "most" and "majority," the grandparents who completed this Survey included outliers on almost every topic. Following are some examples. Two participants expressed strong pushback on the term "non-binary" as a gender description: "There are only TWO genders." A small minority of grandparents have close family members who doubt the autism diagnosis: "My husband still thinks he will come out of it." One grandparent reports that she continues to be blamed for her grandson's autism because she was the first to suspect it. Another shared that her grandson has gender-transitioned to become her granddaughter. Also of note is that among "challenges" the participants cumulatively listed almost everything imaginable: violent attacks, destroying property, head banging, elopement, eating disorders, sleeping disorders, stimming, cursing, potty-training, etc.*

Hillman, J.L., Wentzel, M.C. & Anderson, C.M. Grandparents' Experience of Autism Spectrum Disorder: Identifying Primary Themes and Needs. J Autism Dev Disord 47, 2957–2968 (2017). https://doi.org/10.1007/s10803-017-3211-4

Margetts JK, Le Couteur A, Croom S. Families in a state of flux: the experience of grandparents in autism spectrum disorder. Child Care Health Dev. 2006 Sep;32(5):565-74. doi: 10.1111/j.1365-2214.2006.00671.x. PMID: 16919136.

Prendeville P, Kinsella W. The Role of Grandparents in Supporting Families of Children with Autism Spectrum Disorders: A Family Systems Approach. J Autism Dev Disord. 2019 Feb;49(2):738-749. doi: 10.1007/s10803-018-3753-0. PMID: 30229360.

Index: